Practical Angioplasty

Practical Angioplasty

Editor

David P. Faxon, M.D.
Section of Cardiology
The University Hospital
Boston University Medical Center
Boston, Massachusetts 02118

Raven Press ⚓ New York

Raven Press, Ltd., 1185 Avenue of the Americas, New York, New York 10036

Made in the United States of America

Library of Congress Cataloging-in-Publication Data

Practical angioplasty/edited by David P. Faxon.
     p. cm.
    Includes bibliographical references and index.
    ISBN 0-7817-0084-1
    1. Angioplasty. I. Faxon, D. (David)
    [DNLM: 1. Angioplasty. 2. Coronary Disease—surgery. WG 300
P8945 1993]
    RD598.5P68   1993
    617.4'13—dc20
    DNLM/DLC
    for Library of Congress   93-18672
                                             CIP

9 8 7 6 5 4 3 2 1

To my wife, Monica, and
children, Kimberly and Nathaniel

Contents

Contributing Authors

Donald S. Baim, M.D. *Harvard-Thorndike Laboratory, Cardiovascular Division, Beth Israel Hospital, 330 Brookline Avenue, Boston, Massachusetts 02115*

Peter B. Berger, M.D. *Division of Cardiovascular Diseases, Mayo Clinic, 200 First Street Southwest, Rochester, Minnesota 55905*

Seth D. Bilazarian, M.D. *Section of Cardiology, The University Hospital, Boston University Medical Center, 88 East Newton Street, Boston, Massachusetts 02118*

John E. Brush, Jr., M.D. *Evans Memorial Department of Clinical Research and Section of Cardiology, The University Hospital, Boston University Medical Center, 88 East Newton Street, Boston, Massachusetts 02118*

Andrew P. Chodos, M.D. *Evans Memorial Department of Clinical Research, and Section of Cardiology, The University Hospital, Boston University Medical Center, 88 East Newton Street, Boston, Massachusetts 02118*

Jesse W. Currier, M.D. *Division of Cardiology, Medical College of Wisconsin, 8700 West Wisconsin Avenue, Milwaukee, Wisconsin 53226*

John S. Douglas, Jr., M.D. *Emory University School of Medicine, and Cardiovascular Laboratory, Emory University Hospital, 1364 Clifton Road Northeast, Atlanta, Georgia 30322*

Neal Eigler, M.D. *Cedars-Sinai Medical Center, 8700 Beverly Boulevard, Los Angeles, California 90048*

Bradley H. Evans, M.D. *The Thoracic Clinic, 507 Northeast 47th Avenue, Portland, Oregon 97213*

David P. Faxon, M.D. *Section of Cardiology, The University Hospital, Boston University Medical Center, 88 East Newton Street, Boston, Massachusetts 02118*

Robert F. Fishman, M.D. *Harvard-Thorndike Laboratory, Cardiovascular Division, Beth Israel Hospital, 330 Brookline Avenue, Boston, Massachusetts 02115*

David P. Foley, M.B., ChB *Thoraxcenter, Dijkzigt Academic Hospital, Erasmus University, 3000 DR Rotterdam, The Netherlands*

Gary R. Garber, M.D. *Section of Cardiology, The University Hospital, Boston University Medical Center, 88 East Newton Street, Boston, Massachusetts 02118*

Geoffrey O. Hartzler, M.D. *University of Missouri at Kansas City, and Mid-America Heart Institute, 4320 Wornall Road, Kansas City, Missouri 64111*

Walter R. M. Hermans, M.D. *Thoraxcenter, Dijkzigt Academic Hospital, Erasmus University, 3000 DR Rotterdam, The Netherlands*

David R. Holmes, Jr., M.D. *Division of Cardiovascular Diseases, Mayo Clinic, 200 First Street Southwest, Rochester, Minnesota 55905*

Alice K. Jacobs, M.D. *Section of Cardiology, The University Hospital, Boston University Medical Center, 88 East Newton Street, Boston, Massachusetts 02118*

Mark L. Leitschuh, M.D. *Division of Cardiology, Medical College of Wisconsin, 8700 West Wisconsin Avenue, Milwaukee, Wisconsin 53226*

Frank Litvack, M.D. *Cedars-Sinai Medical Center, 8700 Beverly Boulevard, Los Angeles, California 90048*

Carlo di Mario, M.D. *Thoraxcenter, Dijkzigt Academic Hospital, Erasmus University, 3000 DR Rotterdam, The Netherlands*

Bernhard Meier, M.D. *Cardiology Center, University Hospital, 1211 Geneva 4, Switzerland*

Benno J. Rensing, M.D. *Thoraxcenter, Dijkzigt Academic Hospital, Erasmus University, 3000 DR Rotterdam, The Netherlands*

Nicholas A. Ruocco, M.D. *Section of Cardiology, The University Hospital, Boston University Medical Center, 88 East Newton Street, Boston, Massachusetts 02118*

Thomas J. Ryan, M.D. *Section of Cardiology, The University Hospital, Boston University Medical Center, 88 East Newton Street, Boston, Massachusetts 02118*

Patrick W. Serruys, M.D. *Thoraxcenter, Dijkzigt Academic Hospital, Erasmus University, 3000 DR Rotterdam, The Netherlands*

Richard J. Shemin, M.D. *Department of Cardiothoracic Surgery, The University Hospital, Boston University Medical Center, and Department of Thoracic Surgery, Boston City Hospital, 88 East Newton Street, Boston, Massachusetts 02118*

Joseph M. Sutton, M.D. *Department of Cardiology, The Cleveland Clinic Foundation, 9500 Euclid Avenue, Cleveland, Ohio 44915*

Eric J. Topol, M.D. *Department of Cardiology, The Cleveland Clinic Foundation, 9500 Euclid Avenue, Cleveland, Ohio 44915*

Preface

Interventional cardiology has developed from a concept nearly 30 years ago to a major subspecialty field within cardiology. Its growth would not have been possible without the inspiration and guidance of Andreas R. Greuntzig, who performed the first coronary balloon angioplasty in 1977. The concept of angioplasty, however, predated the birth of coronary angioplasty by nearly 15 years, and was the idea of another pioneer in interventional radiology, Charles Dotter. We are indebted to them for what they have done for the practice of cardiology and the care of patients.

The growth of angioplasty and the explosion of literature and textbooks on this subject attest to its importance at the present time. The concept for this book stems from numerous discussions with interventional cardiology fellows over the past years, who have felt a strong need for a more practical text on angioplasty. In the early years of the procedure, patient selection criteria were more restrictive and the equipment simpler. Dr. Greuntzig initially indicated that the learning curve for angioplasty was no more than 20 cases. However, today, the remarkable advances in balloon catheters, guidewires, guiding catheters, and the development of new interventional techniques including laser, atherectomy, and stents have greatly expanded the knowledge base and skills necessary to optimally perform the procedure, so that now at least 150 cases are usually recommended to develop expertise. It is generally accepted that at least one full year dedicated to learning angioplasty is essential. Many also feel that the knowledge base is unique enough to support the formation of a subspecialty certification.

While there are numerous textbooks on the topic of interventional cardiology, few directly address the knowledge and techniques necessary to perform interventional cardiology procedures. The purpose of this book is to address this need. The book is intended to assist interventional cardiology fellows during their training experience. Additionally, it provides a comprehensive textbook for the practitioner who is currently performing angioplasty. It will provide interventional cardiologists with a general knowledge base of clinical and technical factors important in daily practice. Periodic updates and expansion into new and available techniques are planned to continue to make this reference up-to-date and useful. I am indebted to all those contributors who have so generously provided their time and efforts to put this book together.

David P. Faxon, M.D.

Practical Angioplasty

Practical Angioplasty,
edited by David P. Faxon.
Raven Press, Ltd., New York © 1993.

CHAPTER 1

Introduction and Historical Background

David P. Faxon

The evolution of angioplasty from concept to an established treatment for coronary artery disease is one of the most remarkable developments to occur in medicine in the last century. Like many important advances in medicine the concept of angioplasty began by accident. In 1964, Charles Dotter, a vascular radiologist from Portland, Oregon, noted that when a diagnostic catheter accidentally passed through a high-grade iliac lesion the stenosis became less severe. Encouraged by this observation he used a tapered teflon dilating catheter to successfully dilate an 82-year-old diabetic's severely occluded superficial femoral artery. Subsequently he developed a series of graduated catheters to further enlarge the lumen. After the passage of a guidewire the smallest catheter would be passed through the stenosis followed by the next larger catheter and so on, gradually enlarging the vessel lumen. The technique, similar to that used to dilate esophageal strictures, is often referred to as the Dotter technique. Doctors Dotter and Judkins published a report on the first series of 11 cases in 1964 (1) and then subsequently reviewed a collection of 155 cases performed by their group up until 1967 (2). It is of interest that the coauthor was Melvin Judkins, M.D., who subsequently distinguished himself in the development of coronary angiography. Doctor Dotter envisioned that the technique worked by compressing or redistributing the atherosclerotic plaque as walking in fresh snow or driving a nail through wood compresses the snow or wood into a smaller space (3).

The genius of these observations was not initially realized in the United States, and little further work was accomplished until investigators began to use the technique in Europe to treat peripheral vascular disease. The

impetus for using the technique was that in the 1970s there was a considerable delay in scheduling patients for vascular surgery and alternative therapies were actively sought. The Dotter technique gained widespread popularity and was used extensively by a number of active centers including that of Doctor E. Zeitler (4). A number of investigators attempted to modify the catheter system (Fig. 1) by developing a balloon, and most notable in this regard was an elastic balloon developed by Doctor Werner Postmann. Doctor Andreas Gruentzig (Fig. 2) spent time as a guest in the radiology department of the Aggertalclinic in Engelskirchen near Cologne in West Germany, under the direction of Professor Doctor E. Zeitler, in order to become acquainted with the technique of percutaneous transluminal angioplasty. During his tenure with Doctor Zeitler, he also began to experiment with modifications of the Dotter technique by use of a double-balloon catheter. Doctor Gruentzig returned to Zurich, and in 1974 developed the first double-balloon catheter for the dilation of vascular stenosis in peripheral vascular occlusion. This was also the topic of his habilitation granting him the degree of "privatdozen" (PD) at the University of Zurich. The double-balloon catheter was made of a rigid balloon material that assumed a fixed diameter at balloon pressures up to six atmospheres. A distal lumen allowed pressure to be measured and contrast agents to be injected (Fig. 1). A soft distal guidewire allowed atraumatic passage of the balloon catheter. After preliminary animal studies, Doctor Gruentzig reported 75 cases of peripheral vascular disease successfully treated with this balloon catheter. The initial success rate was 75% (5). The small shaft, flexibility, and rigid balloon catheter allowed a safer, more effective procedure. Encouraged by the results, he developed a smaller version of the catheter for coronary use. It should be noted, however, that the concept of treating coronary stenoses with angioplasty, as well as with intracoronary stents, was in fact first suggested by

D. P. Faxon: Section of Cardiology, The University Hospital, Boston University Medical Center, Boston, Massachusetts 02118

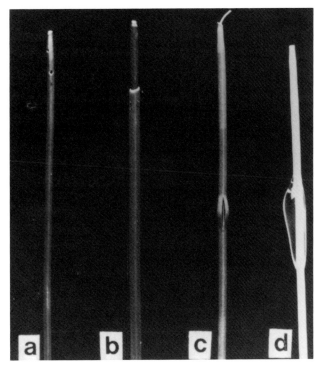

FIG. 1. The development of angioplasty catheters. **a:** An angiographic catheter. **b:** A coaxial dilation catheter used in the Dotter procedure. **c:** The corset balloon developed by Porstmann. **d:** an early example of the double-balloon catheter developed by Gruntzig. From Mathias (18), with permission.

Doctor Charles Dotter, although he never performed these techniques.

The initial studies in the coronary arteries were performed in dogs, where ligatures were placed surgically around the coronary artery (6). Following healing, balloon dilatation was successfully accomplished (Fig. 3). However, the dogs were susceptible to ventricular tachycardia and fibrillation and initial studies therefore required active perfusion of blood through the balloon catheter. An additional early concern was the possibility of embolization of atherosclerotic material. In collaboration with Doctor Richard Myler, the first patient underwent angioplasty in San Francisco during an operative procedure where dilatation of a saphenous vein graft was accomplished. Collection of the effluence showed no evidence of embolization.

The first patient to undergo angioplasty was a 37-year-old insurance salesman with a proximal left anterior descending stenosis (7). The procedure was performed on September 17, 1977. While distal blood perfusion was planned, it proved unnecessary and the procedure was successful. It is of note that the patient has done well and has undergone repeat cardiac catheterization at both 5 and 10 years after the initial procedure, with no evidence of progression of disease or restenosis. Four more cases were performed over the next year, and the first publica-

tion of the first five cases was reported in *Lancet* in February of 1978 (8).

By the following year, considerable interest in the procedure was in evidence, and several other groups had begun angioplasty. A workshop was organized by the National Heart, Lung, and Blood Institute (NHLBI), and a registry of all centers currently performing the procedure was instituted. Over 110 centers worldwide participated, and over 3,000 cases had been collected by 1981 (9).

Over-the-wire systems were first developed by Doctors John Simpson and Edward Roberts, who devised a coaxial balloon and shaft that permitted a large enough central lumen to permit independent passage of a guidewire through the center of the catheter while balloon inflation occurred through the outer lumen. The catheter was introduced in 1980 and soon became the standard, as the independent wire motion allowed access to more tortuous vessels and to distal stenoses. Further catheter refinements, using thinner and stronger balloon materials, more torqueable and flexible guiding catheters, and more flexible and steerable guidewires, developed over the ensuing years.

Initially, angioplasty was restricted to patients who had single vessel disease with proximal, single, discrete and nonocclusive stenosis. These restrictions were primarily related to limitations of both the guiding catheters and the balloon dilation systems. One study done during this period indicated that the number of patients

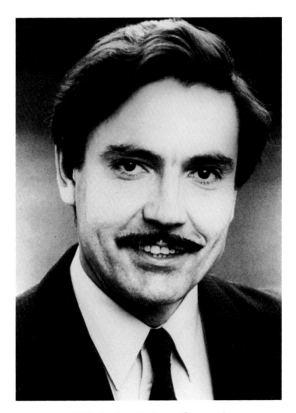

FIG. 2. Dr. Andreas Gruentzig

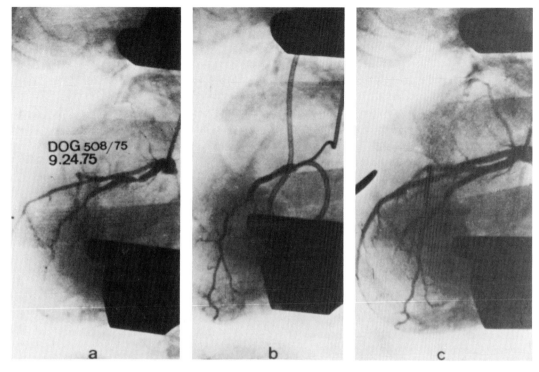

FIG. 3. a: A subtotal stenosis in the intermediate branch of the circumflex of a dog created by a 6.0 silk ligature. **b:** Using continuous distal perfusion, the lesion was dilated. **c:** Good angiographic result. From Gruentzig (19), with permission.

qualifying for percutaneous transluminal coronary angioplasty (PTCA) was small, comprising less than 5% of the coronary disease population needing revascularization (10). However, as technology improved, and as physician and patient enthusiasm and experience increased, use of the procedure rose dramatically (Fig. 4). By 1985, it was estimated that 100,000 patients were undergoing the procedure in the United States (11). Due to the changes in the practice of angioplasty, 16 centers who were originally part of the initial NHLBI PTCA registry

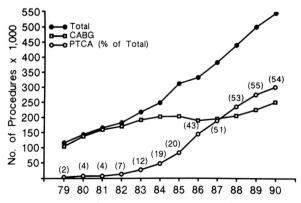

FIG. 4. The growth of coronary angioplasty in the United States since its inception 15 years ago. Currently more than 300,000 procedures are performed, exceeding the number of coronary bypass operations.

reopened the registry, and collected data on an additional 3,000 patients between 1985 and 1986. This data has proved invaluable in documenting the changes in angioplasty and helping to explain its growth and popularity (12–16).

In comparison with the early registry experience between 1977 and 1981, the latter registry (1985–1986) patients were significantly older, had worse left ventricular function and more prior myocardial infarctions (37% versus 21%) (12). A greater number also had prior bypass surgery (13% versus 9%) and, more importantly, the majority had multivessel coronary disease (57% versus 25%). In addition, multilesion angioplasty increased from 8.5% to 40%. Not unexpectedly, as multivessel disease increased, lesion complexity also increased, with more tubular, diffusely diseased, calcified, and totally occluded stenoses.

Despite significant increases in clinical and angiographic complexity, the success of the procedure, defined as a greater than a 20% change in stenosis with a residual stenosis of less than 50%, increased from 67.5% to 91%. Successful dilation of all lesions rose from 64.7% to 82.2%. As success increased, complications fell, with an overall mortality of 1.0%, need for emergency bypass surgery in 3.4% and elective bypass surgery in 2.2%.

A more recent experience would suggest that these changes have continued to move in a favorable direction. At Boston University, of 968 patients undergoing the procedure in 1990, 45% had multivessel disease, and more than 50% of patients had multilesion angioplasty. The success of the procedure, defined as angiographic success without the occurrence of in-hospital myocardial infarction, emergency bypass operation, or death, was 94%. Acute complications were likewise low, with a death rate of 0.4%, myocardial infarction rate of 3.2%, and the need for emergency bypass surgery occurring in only 1.2%.

In the United States, it is estimated that more than 300,000 angioplasties will be performed in 1993. Bypass surgery has also grown, but angioplasty appears to be more commonly performed today than bypass surgery. In one large multicenter trial in patients needing revascularation, angioplasty was done 53% of the time (17). In patients with single vessel disease angioplasty was the preferred treatment in 75%, in double-vessel disease, 50% of the time, and in triple vessel disease, only 25% of the time. The major reason for not performing angioplasty was the presence of a chronic total occlusion. At our medical center, a chronic total occlusion accounts for 50% of the exclusions of patients from angioplasty. The other reasons for exclusion are diffuse disease in 20%, left main disease in 12%, and other unfavorable anatomical characteristics such as extreme tortuosity, ostial lesion, or severe calcification in a smaller number of cases.

The current practice of angioplasty is also faced with a new and equally challenging problem. Data from the currently conducted randomized trials, indicate that 30% to 35% of all patients undergoing revascularization have had a prior revascularization procedure, either surgery or angioplasty (17). In fact, nearly 20% have had both procedures. Given the known failure rate of saphenous vein grafts after 10 years, it is not surprising that the incidence of prior revascularization is growing exponentially and will likely become a major issue in care of the cardiac patient in the future.

The challenge of angioplasty and new interventional techniques will be to further expand indications, establish the proper role of angioplasty in relationship to bypass surgery, and to deal with the emerging patient population who require repeat procedures. The subsequent chapters in this book are aimed at describing the current state of the art of angioplasty with a major focus on the practical approach to the conduct of angioplasty. With rapid changes in technology, it is likely that specific catheters mentioned in this book will change and that new technology will replace those discussed. However, the basic principles of angioplasty are not likely to change. It is hoped that the subsequent discussion will provide an understanding this basic foundation to those learning, as well as to those actively involved in the procedure.

REFERENCES

1. Dotter CT, Judkins MP. Transluminal treatment of atherosclerotic obstruction: description of a new technique and a preliminary report of its application. *Circulation* 1964;30:654–670.
2. Dotter CT, Rosch J, Judkins MP. Transluminal dilation of atherosclerotic stenosis. *Surg Gynecol Obstet* 1968;127:794–804.
3. Dotter CT. Transluminal angioplasty—pathologic basis. In: Zeitler F, Gruntzig A, Scheuer W (eds). *Percutaneous vascular recanalization.* New York: Springer Verlag, 3–12.
4. Zietler F, Gruntzig A, Schever W (eds). *Percutaneous vascular recanalization.* New York: Springer Verlag.
5. Gruntzig A. Die perkutan rekanalisation chronischer arterieller verschlusse (Dotter-Prinzid) mit doppellumigen dilatationskatheter. *Fortschr Rontgenstr* 1976;124:80–86.
6. Gruntzig AR, Turiner MI, Schneider JA. Experimental percutaneous dilating of coronary artery stenosis. *Circulation* 1976;54:81.
7. Hurst JW. The first coronary angioplasty as described by Andrew Gruentig. *Am J Cardiol,* 1986;57:185–186.
8. Gruntzig A. Transluminal dilation of coronary artery stenosis. *Lancet* 1978;1:263.
9. National Heart Lung and Blood Institute. Percutaneous Transluminal Coronary Angioplasty Registry. *Am J Cardiol* 1989;53:1–150.
10. Gosselin AJ, Fisher L, Judkins MD, et al. An estimate of the number of possible candidates from the CASS registry: proceedings of the workshop on percutaneous transluminal coronary angiography June 15–16, 1979. *NIH* 1980;80:2030:89–100.
11. National Center for Health Statistics 1986 summary: National Hospital Discharge Survey, Hyatsville, MD. National Center for Health Statistics 1987.
12. Detre K, Hollubkov R, Kelsey S, Cowley M, Kent K, Williams D, Myer R, Faxon DP, et al. Percutaneous transluminal coronary angioplasty in 1985–1986 and 1977–1981. The National Heart Lung and Blood Institute Registry. *N Engl J Med* 1988;318:265–270.
13. Holmes DR, Holubkov R, Vlietstra RE, Kelsey S, Reeder GS, Dorros G, Williams D, Cowley M, Faxon D, Kent K, Bentivoglio L, Detre K. Comparison of complications during percutaneous transluminal coronary angioplasty from 1977 to 1981 and from 1985 to 1986: The National Heart, Lung and Blood Institute Percutaneous Transluminal Coronary Angioplasty Registry. *J Am Coll Cardiol* 1988;12:1149–1155.
14. Detre K, Holubkov R, Kelsey S, Bourrassa M, Williams D, Holmes D, Dorros G, Faxon D, Myler R, Kent K, Cowley M, Cannon R, Robertson T. One-year follow-up results of the 1985–1986 National Heart, Lung and Blood Institutes percutaneous transluminal coronary angioplasty registry. New Eng J Med: 1989:80(3):421–428.
15. Detre KM, Holmes DA, Holtivo R, Cowley MJ, Bourassa M, Faxon DP, Dorros GR, Bentiogilo LG, Kent KM, Myler RK. Incidence and consequences of periprocedural occlusion: The 1985–86 National Heart, Lung and Blood Institute's Percutaneous Transluminal Coronary Angioplasty Registry. *Circulation* 1990;82:739–750.
16. Kelsey SF, Miller DP, Holtivo R, Cowley MJ, Faxon DP, Detre KM. Results of percutaneous transluminal coronary angioplasty in patients ≥65 years of age. From the 1985–1986 National Heart Lung and Blood Institute Percutaneous Transluminal Coronary Angioplasty Registry. *Am J Cardiol* 1990;66:1033–1039.
17. The BARI investigations. BARI survey of revascularization practice. *Circulation* 1991;84:II:250.
18. Mathias E. Percutaneous transluminal dilation (PTD) of carotid artery stenosis. In: Zeiter E, Gruntzig A, Shoop W, eds. *Percutaneous vascular recanalization.* Berlin: Springer-Verlag; 1978:62.
19. Gruntzig A. Transluminal dilation of coronary artery stenosis—experimental report. In: Zeitler E, Gruntzig A, Shook W, eds. *Percutaneous vascular recanalization.* Berlin: Springer-Verlag; 1978:59.

Practical Angioplasty,
edited by David P. Faxon.
Raven Press, Ltd., New York © 1993.

CHAPTER 2

Mechanisms of Angioplasty and Pathophysiology of Restenosis

David P. Faxon

ACUTE EFFECTS

It is remarkable that our understanding of the pathophysiology of angioplasty occurred well after the widespread acceptance of the technique clinically. Initially, angioplasty was conceptualized as enlarging the lumen by compression or redistribution of the atherosclerotic plaque, a concept initially suggested by Doctor Charles Dotter and supported by Doctor Andreas Gruentzig (1). However, studies of angioplasty in postmortem atherosclerotic vessels suggested that angioplasty resulted in severe damage to the blood vessel wall, with disruption of the atherosclerotic plaque often leading to neointimal tears or dissection (2). Evidence that this process may occur in man was first suggested by Block and colleagues who reported on three patients who died after angioplasty (3). The common occurrence of neointimal tears after angioplasty was further confirmed by experimental studies. Our group, utilizing a rabbit model of atherosclerosis, demonstrated that intimal tears and dissections were common following transluminal angioplasty of stenotic iliac vessels (4) (Figs. 1 and 2). Sanborn, using quantitative histology techniques showed that compression of the atheroma did not occur, but stretching was the primary mechanism of angioplasty with tearing of the neointimal plaque (5) (Fig. 3). When the stenosis was concentric, tearing uniformly occurred but was less frequent in eccentric lesions, where stretching of the least diseased portion of the vessel occurred (6). More recently, intravascular ultrasound studies have confirmed that stretching routinely occurs (7).

In the process of balloon dilatation, not only is the vessel dilated, but the endothelial lining is removed, and the subendothelium is exposed to circulating blood. There is little question that these acute events—namely stretching, deendotheliazation, and tearing of the neointima, with exposure of the subendothelial plaque—set into motion the subsequent healing events that result in the development of restenosis or renarrowing of the vessel lumen (8).

RESTENOSIS

Human pathological studies and histopathological examination of atherectomy specimens have demonstrated that neointimal hyperplasia is the most common pathological pattern associated with restenosis (9–11). This process appears to be histologically distinct from the underlying atherosclerotic process and is composed of proliferating smooth muscle cells that fill in the vascular lumen and bring about renarrowing the vessel (10) (Fig. 4). A large component of this process is extracellular matrix composed of glycosaminoglycans, collagen, and elastin. In fact, experimentally, approximately 50% to 80% of the volume of the intimal hyperplasia region is composed of extracellular matrix (12). The process that results in renarrowing of the artery is analogous to generalized wound healing and is a fundamental repair process of a blood vessel to any form of injury (13). As such, restenosis is not an abnormal process, but a normal one that occurs in response to vascular damage and, as shown by quantitative coronary angiographic studies, develops in nearly all patients to some degree or other (14). The phases of this process can be described as an initial injury phase, a granulation phase, and a remodeling phase (Fig. 5).

The initial injury to the blood vessel wall by the balloon results in removal of the endothelium. In experimental studies removal of the endothelium is sufficient

D. P. Faxon: Section of Cardiology, The University Hospital, Boston University Medical Center, Boston, Massachusetts 02118

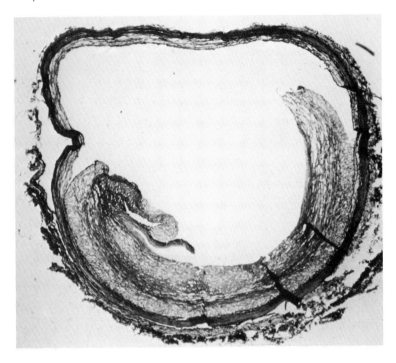

FIG. 1. An example of the acute effect of angioplasty in a rabbit model of atherosclerosis. The neointima has been torn away from the underlying media, with flaps folded into the vessel.

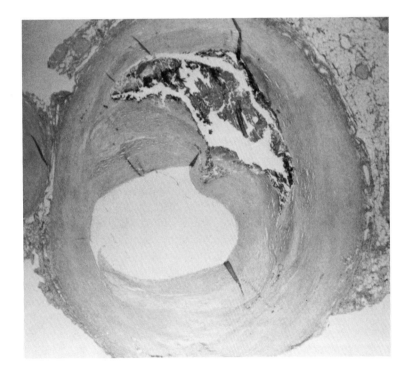

FIG. 2. An example of acute effective angioplasty in a patient who died early after angioplasty documenting dissection with flaps folder into the lumen. (By permission of Dr. Christian Haudenschild.)

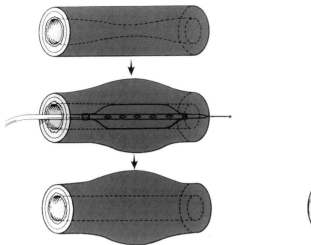

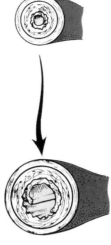

FIG. 3. Mechanism of angioplasty is illustrated rather than compression or redistribution of the plaque. Angioplasty results in stretching the entire vessel with creation of a localized fusiform aneurysm. From Sanborn (5), with permission.

to induce neointimal proliferation, although it is often very self-limited (15). Greater degrees of vascular damage induced by balloon angioplasty, particularly in the setting of atherosclerotic disease, result in splitting or tearing of the neointimal plaque with extensive exposure of the collagen, lipid, and extracellular matrix to circulating blood. Since the artery has considerable elastic components it immediately recoils from this stretching process to assume a diameter that is significantly smaller than the dilating balloon catheter. Studies done by Serruys, Rensing, and others have clearly demonstrated

that in nearly all patients significant recoil of the vessel is evident by quantitative angiography immediately following balloon angioplasty (16,17). Immediately following balloon dilation of the artery, platelets begin to deposit and form a carpet along the denuded surface. Significant accumulation of platelets occurs, particularly within the crevices crated in the neointima, and often leads to the development of macroscopic thrombi. In experimental studies, our group has shown that platelet deposition occurs rapidly, peaking within 4 hr in a rabbit atherosclerotic model (18), and within 24 hr, in a swine model of

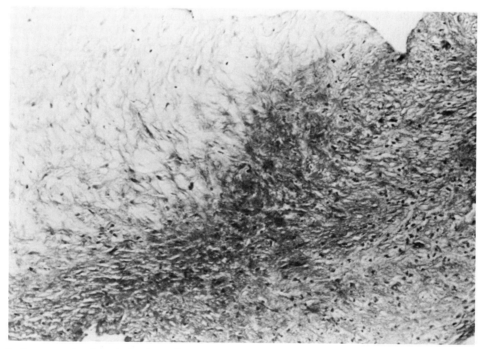

FIG. 4. An example of neointimal proliferation from an atherectomy specimen in a patient with restenosis. A loose and dense fibrocellular process is evident throughout. This is histologically distinct from the underlying atherosclerotic plaque and may occur in de novo lesions as well. (By permission of Dr. Christian Haudenschild).

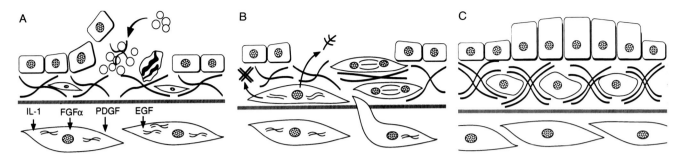

FIG. 5. A: The initial phase of restenosis. The endothelium is removed and platelets adhere and form small thrombi within the neointimal tears. An inflammatory response with infiltration of macrophages occurs within a few days following the initial injury. **B:** The granulation phase. The smooth muscle cells (SMC) within the neointima and media are activated by growth factors from platelets, macrophages, and damaged SMC. These mobile synthetic SMC migrate into the damaged area, proliferate, and produce extracellular matrix. **C:** The remodeling phase. The endothelium regrows over the damaged area, although the function of this endothelium may remain abnormal. The SMC convert back into their quiescent phenotype following organization of the connective tissue and collagen matrix. From Currier (8), with permission.

vascular injury (19) (Fig. 6). The degree of platelet accumulation is nearly tenfold higher than might be expected from removal of the endothelium alone. Following this initial thrombotic phase, platelet accumulation rapidly falls and seems not to play a major role during longer term follow-up. Thrombus, however, does continue for several weeks to months following initial injury. There is a correlation between the degree of vascular damage and the degree of platelet accumulation and thrombus formation (18,19) (Fig. 7).

The importance of thrombus in restenosis in man is emphasized by the necropsy study of Nobyoshi and colleagues (11) (Fig. 8). In 36 patients who died following angioplasty, the authors found histologic evidence of mural thrombus in up to 60% of patients within the first month, with a significant decline in its incidence thereafter. Thrombus formation and platelet accumulation are potent stimulators of smooth muscle cell growth and mi-

gration (20). Platelets release platelet derived growth factor, platelet factor IV, serotonin, epinephrine, and endothelial growth factor (EGF), all of which have been shown to result in proliferation and migration of smooth muscle cells in culture (21). In addition, thrombin has been shown to induce proliferation of smooth muscle cells, as well as to attract monocytes and macrophages. These inflammatory cells can release cytokines, which also contribute to the proliferative process (22).

GRANULATION

Injury to the vascular wall results not only in stimulation of thrombosis but in damage to the underlying intimal smooth muscle cells themselves. One of the central processes in the development of intimal hyperplasia is activation of the smooth muscle cell. A growing number of growth factors and cytokines appear to be important in this process (23). A list of the important growth factors is shown in Table 1 and Fig. 5. It has been shown by Reidy and others that damage to the smooth muscle cell releases growth factors, including fibroblast growth factor and platelet derived growth factor (PDGF) from within the cell, which can serve as a mitogen to adjacent undamaged smooth muscle cells (24). In addition, platelet derived growth factor and thrombin are also mitogenic for smooth muscle cells. Current evidence would suggest that platelet derived growth factor is more important in the migratory action of smooth muscle cells than in their proliferation (25). In addition, endothelial cells and macrophages produce interleukin 1 (IL-1) and fibroblast growth factor, as well as TGF beta that also contribute to the process (22). Angiotensin II is also felt to play an important role, both directly, and via its stimulatory effect on fibroblast growth factor and TGF beta (26). Other factors of potential importance include insu-

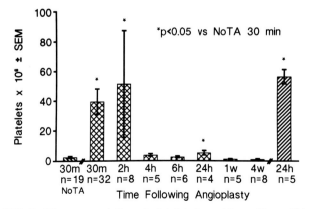

FIG. 6. The accumulation of platelets is rapid, peaking within 2 hr in the rabbit model. After 24 hr the surface does not attract further platelet deposition (so-called passivization), despite lack of an endothelium lying. From Wilentz (18), with permission.

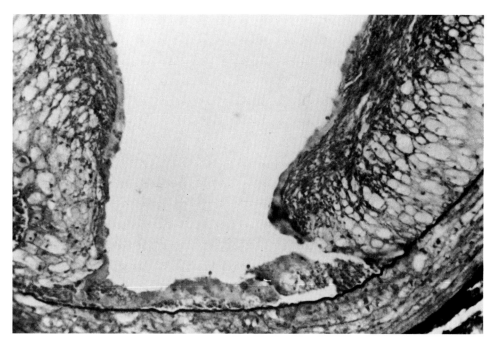

FIG. 7. The degree of platelet deposition depends on the severity of the vascular damage, but far exceeds that seen with only removal of the endothelium. As shown in this experimental study, platelet thrombi are usually located within the neointimal tears.

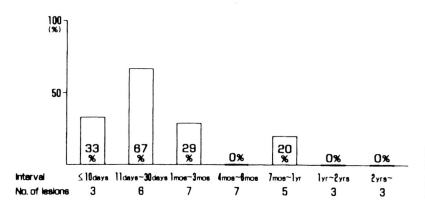

FIG. 8. The incidence of thrombosis in 20 patients with restenosis studied at necropsy. The peak incidence is within the first month. From Nobyoshi (11), with permission.

TABLE 1. *Growth factors*

Stimulators	Inhibitors
Platelet derived growth factor (PDGF)	Transforming growth factor beta (TGF$_B$)
Endothelial cell growth factor (ECGF)	Heparin-like factors
Fibroblast growth factor (FGF)	Vasorelaxant substances (EDRF)
Smooth muscle cell dervived growth factor (SDGF)	Prostaglandins (PGE, PGE$_2$, PGI$_1$)
Interleukin 1 (IL-1)	Interferon-y (glFM)
Interleukin 6 (IL-6)	
Transforming growth factor beta (TBF$_B$)	
Low density lipoproteins (LDL)	
Vasoactive substance—Angiotensin II	
Thrombin	
Leukotrienes (LTB$_4$, LTC$_4$, LTD$_4$)	
Prostaglandins (PGE$_2$, PGI$_2$)	

EDRF, endothelial derived relaxing factor.

TABLE 2. *Smooth muscle cell phenotype*

Characteristic	Contractile	Synthetic
Cell division	Quiescent	Proliferative
Location	Unaffected media	Within placque
Shape	Ribbon or fusiform	Broad or flat
Myofilament	High	Low
Synthetic organelles	Few	Numerous
Lipid accumulation	Resistant	Susceptible

lin growth factor, endothelin, thrombosporin, and IL-6 (23). While some growth factors are stimulatory, others have an inhibitory effect on this process, and such agents include heparan sulfate, (tumor necrosis factor) TNF, TGF beta, and gamma interferon. TGF beta may in fact have a dual action, showing both stimulatory and inhibitory actions, but it is recognized to be an important factor in the stimulation of extracellular formation from the smooth muscle cell (27).

Prior to balloon injury the smooth muscle cell is largely (>50%) in a quiescent stage or contractile state (Table 2). This is characterized by a fusiform shape, high microfilament density, and few organelles (28). Once injury occurs and the smooth muscle cells are stimulated by both growth factors and cytokines, a phenotypic change occurs in the smooth muscle cell. These phenotypically changed synthetic smooth muscle cells are characterized by a flat shape, low number of microfilaments, and numerous synthetic organelles. Of importance is that these cells are capable of migration and proliferation as well as secretion of extracellular matrix. Experimental studies in a rat artery injury model suggested that migration of these cells into the neointima occurs rapidly within the first few days of injury, and that nearly 50% of these migrating cells subsequently proliferate (29). Nobyoshi, in a necropsy study, showed that after 11 days there was a dramatic increase in intimal hyperplasia, with 83% of histologic specimens showing evidence of intimal hyperplasia (11) (Fig. 9). This figure rose to 100% by 1 to 3 months. Phenotypically, these smooth muscle cells were predominantly of the synthetic type, however, after 6 months, the predominant cell type was the quiescent, contractile smooth muscle cell.

REMODELING

The final phase of restenosis involves reconversion of the smooth muscle cell back to the quiescent phenotype, re-endothelialization of the damaged area, and organization of the extracellular matrix. Regrowth of the endothelium in the rabbit iliac model occurs within 2 weeks. The data from other experimental studies indicate that regrowth is dependent upon the extent of de-endothelialtion (30). In addition, the regenerated endothelium does not appear to be normally functional and the relationship of this dysfunction to restenosis has not been well studied (31). Similarly organization of the extracellular matrix is poorly understood. Studies in the rat injury model indicate that 50% to 80% of the neointimal thickening is due to matrix formation. The contribution of collagen and elastic fibers and contraction of collagen into an organized scar are important final events that contribute to the healing process.

The potential to reduce the complications of angioplasty, namely abrupt closure and late restenosis, depends on our better understanding of the pathophysiological events involved in restenosis. Great progress has been made in this area; however, further understanding is clearly necessary. Our previous lack of success in preventing restenosis most likely reflects our lack of complete understanding of vascular healing. It is possible that animal models do not accurately reflect the process in man. Certainly each animal model has some aspects that are similar but also others that differ from the human experience. For example the rat model is primarily a smooth muscle cell proliferative model and has few macrophages or lymphocytes present. In addition, it is a primary injury model that occurs on a normal artery rather than an atherosclerotic vessel. In the rabbit model, the plaque is comprised largely of lipid-laden macrophages, while the swine stent model appears to have a large component of thrombosis (32). In addition, the pig is known to have a much more potent fibrolytic system than man, while the rabbit metabolizes lipids poorly. Despite these limitations, experimental studies continue to provide useful information about the physiologic pro-

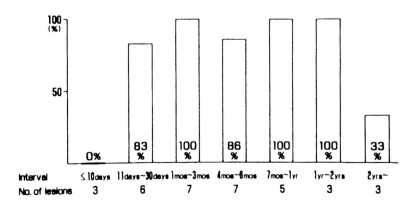

FIG. 9. The incidence of intimal hyperplasia in 20 patients with restenosis was nearly 100% and peaked between the first and third month following the procedure. The degree of intimal hyperplasia was correlated with a degree of vascular injury. From Nobyoshi (11), with permission.

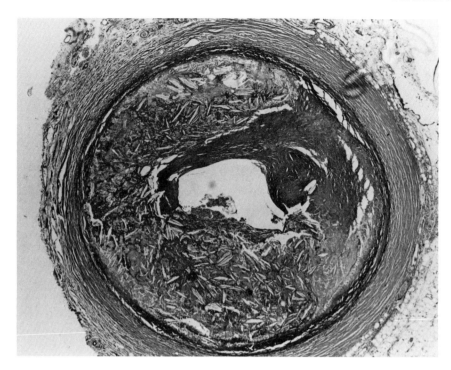

FIG. 10. An example of restenosis in a patient who died following angioplasty. The older atherosclerotic plaque is seen with a new fibrocellular neointima, which further narrows the lumen. (By permission of Dr. Christian Haudenschild.)

cess involved and can provide a useful testing ground for potential new drug and device interventions (Fig. 11). Another limitation of animal models is that they are histologically homogenous. Studies of atherectomy specimens suggest that the process of restenosis is quite heterogeneous (9). In some patients thrombosis may be a more important component, while in others, smooth muscle cell proliferation, or late recoil and healing events may be more important. The true frequency of these components in any individual patient is currently unknown.

As documented later in this book, no pharmacological therapy has been shown to reduce restenosis. However, our knowledge of restenosis has grown considerably and

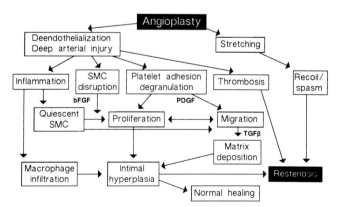

FIG. 11. A potential mechanism that leads to restenosis. Angioplasty results in deendothelialization, deep arterial injury, and stretching of the vessel. Vascular injury leads to platelet aggregation, thrombosis, and inflammatory response, all of which result in activation of the smooth muscle cell and neointimal hyperplasia.

the methods to inhibit the various contributing factors has also greatly expanded. It seems highly likely that effective treatment will be developed as a result of these advances.

REFERENCES

1. Dotter ST, Rosch J, Judkins MP. Transluminal dilation of atherosclerotic stenoses. *Surg Gynecol Obstet* 1968;127:794–804.
2. Baughman KL, Pasternak RC, Fallon JT, Block PC. Transluminal coronary angioplasty of post mortem human hearts. *Am J Cardiol* 1981;48:1044–1047.
3. Block PC, Myler RK, Stertzer S, Fallon JT. *N Engl J Med* 1981;305:382–385.
4. Faxon DP, Weber VJ, Haudenschild C, Gottsman SB, McGovern W, Ryan TJ. Acute affects of transluminal angioplasty in three experimental models of atherosclerosis. *Arteriosclerosis* 1982;2:125–133.
5. Sanborn TA, Faxon DP, Haudenschild C, Gottsman SB, Ryan TJ. The mechanism of angioplasty: evidence for aneurysm formation in an experimental atherosclerosis. *Circulation* 1983;68:1136–1140.
6. Faxon DP, Sanborn TA, Haudenschild C. The mechanism of angioplasty and its relationship to restenosis. *Am J Cardiol* 1987;60:513–519.
7. Honye J, Mahon DJ, Jain A, White CJ, Ramee SR, Wallis JB, Al-Zarka A, Tobis JM. Morphological affects of coronary balloon angioplasty *in vivo* assessed by intervascular ultrasound imaging. *Circulation* 1992;85:1012–1025.
8. Currier JW, Haudenschild C, Faxon DP. Pathophysiology of restenosis: clinical implications. In: Ischinger T, Gohlke H, eds. *Strategies in Primary and Secondary Prevention of Coronary Artery Disease.* W. Zuckschwerdt Verlag 1992: 181–192.
9. Garratt KN, Holmes DR, Bell MR, Bresnahan JF, Caufmann UP, Vlietstra RE, Edwards WD. Restenosis after directional coronary atherectomy: differences between primary atherometous and restenosis lesions and influence of subintimal tissue resection. *J Am Coll Cardiol* 1990;16:1665–1671.
10. Waller DF, Pinkerton CA, Orr CM, Slack JD, van Tassel JW, Peters T. Restenosis 1–24 months after clinically successful coro-

nary balloon angioplasty: a necropsy study of 20 patients. *J Am Coll Cardiol* 1991;17:58b–70b.

11. Nobuyoshi M, Kimura T, Ohishi H, Oriushi H, Nosaka H, Hamasaki N, Yokoi H, Kim K. Restenosis after percutaneous transluminal coronary angioplasty: pathologic observations in 20 patients. *J Am Coll Cardiol* 1991;17:433–439.

12. Wight LN. Cell biology of arterial proteoglycans. *Arteriosclerosis* 1989;9:1–20.

13. Forrester JS, Fishbein M, Helfant R, Fagin J. A paradigm for restenosis based on cell biology: clues for the development of new preventive therapies. *J Am Coll Cardiol* 1991;17:752–757.

14. Rensing BJ, Hermans WR, Deckers JW, deFeyter PJ, Tijssen JGP, Serruys PW. Luminal narrowing after percutaneous transluminal coronary angioplasty following Gaussian distribution. A quantitative angiographic study in 1,445 successfully dilated lesions. *J Am Coll Cardiol* 1992.

15. Fingerle J, Johnson R, Clowes AW, Majesky MW, Reidy MA. Role of platelets in smooth muscle cell proliferation and migration after vascular injury in rat carotid artery. *Proc Natl Acad Sci* USA 1989;86:8412–8416.

16. Rensing B, Hermans WR, Beatt K, Laarman GJ, Suryapranata H, VandenBrand M, deFeyter PJ, Serruys PW. Quantitative angiographic assessment of a last degree coil after percutaneous transluminal coronary angioplasty. *Am J Cardiol* 1990;66:1039–1044.

17. Serruys PW, Foley DP, deFeyter PJ. Angiographic assessment of restenosis after coronary angioplasty and other devices: is it time to compare approaches based on quantitative angiography? *J Am Coll Cardiol* 1993; (in press).

18. Wilentz JR, Sanborn TA, Haudenschild C, Valari CR, Ryan TJ, Faxon DP. Platelet accumulation in experimental angioplasty: time course in relation to vascular injury. *Circulation* 1987;75:636–642.

19. Ip JH, Fuster V, Israel D, Badimon L, Badimon J, Chesebro JH. The role of platelets, thrombin and hyperplasia in restenosis after coronary angioplaty. *J Am Coll Cardiol* 1991;17:77b–88b.

20. Berk C, Taubam MB, Grendling KK, Cragoe EJ, Fenton JW, Brock TA. Thombin-stimulated events in cultured vascular smooth muscle cells. *Biochem J* 1991;274:799–805.

21. Fuster V, Badimon L, Badimon J, Chesebro JH. The pathogenesis of coronary artery disease and acute coronary syndromes. *N Engl J Med* 1992;326:242–250.

22. Libby P, Hansson GK. Involvement of the immune system in human atherogenesis: current knowledge and unanswered questions. *Lab Invest* 1991;64:5–15.

23. Marmur J, Taubman MB, Fuster V. Pathophysiology of restenosis: the role of platelets and thrombi. *J Vasc Med Biol* 1993; (in press).

24. Lindner V, Reidy MA. Proliferation of smooth muscle cells after vascular injury is inhibited by an antibody against basic fibroblast growth factor. *Proc Natl Acad Sci* USA 1991;88:3739–3743.

25. Ferns JA, Raines EW, Sprugle K, Hspruge L, Motani AS, Reidy MA, Ross R. Inhibition of smooth muscle cell accumulation after angioplasty by an antibody to FGF. *Science* 1991;253:1129–1132.

26. Dzau VJ, Gibbons GH, Pratt RE. Molecular mechanisms of vascular renin-angiotensin system in myointimal hyperplasia. *Hypertension* 1991;18:II-100–II-105.

27. Sporn D, Roberts AB. Transforming growth factor-beta: multiple actions and potential clinical applications. *JAMA* 1989;262:938–941.

28. Gown A, Tsukada T, Ross R. Human atherosclerosis-II immunocytochemical analysis of the cellular components of human atherosclerotic lesions. *Am J Pathol* 1986;125:191.

29. Clowes AW, Reidy MA, Clowes MM. Kinetics of cellular proliferation after arterial injury, I. Smooth muscle cell growth in the absence of endothelium. *Lab Invest* 1983;49:327–333.

30. Reidy MA. Reassessment of endothelial injury and arterial lesion formation. *Lab Invest* 1985;53:513–520.

31. Weidinger F, McLenachan JM, Cybulsky et al. Persistant dysfunction of regenerated endothelium after balloon angioplasty of rabbit iliac artery. *Circulation* 1990;81:1667–1679.

32. Muller DW, Ellis SG, Topol EJ. Experimental models of coronary artery restenosis. *J Am Coll Cardiol* 1992;19:418–432.

Practical Angioplasty,
edited by David P. Faxon.
Raven Press, Ltd., New York © 1993.

CHAPTER 3

Patient Selection: Current Status

Thomas J. Ryan

The proper selection of patients for coronary angioplasty demands careful review of the clinical and anatomic features of each case. Patients with single vessel disease who have significant symptoms undoubtedly constitute the largest, and probably the most suitable, group of patients undergoing coronary angioplasty. At the same time, the generally excellent prognosis for patients with single vessel disease should be a paramount consideration before undertaking an interventional procedure in such patients. It is imperative that there be some assurance that the symptoms are indeed due to the coronary lesion proposed for dilation. It is also important to recall that coronary angioplasty was first introduced as an alternative form of revascularization of the ischemic myocardium. This implies that patients selected for revascularization by coronary angioplasty will have failed medical therapy or, at least, have found its side effects and curtailment of lifestyle unacceptable. It is only in recent years that coronary angioplasty has been viewed as a preferred alternative to successful medical therapy. While there are certain data to support this point of view (1), it is incumbent on the clinician making this selection to be thoroughly familiar with the natural history of coronary artery disease in a wide variety of patient groups. The clinician must also be thoroughly familiar with pharmacotherapy of coronary artery disease and have a working knowledge of a wide array of therapeutic agents available for medical therapy.

During the early years of its application, coronary angiography was used predominantly to treat patients with discrete, proximal, noncalcified subtotal occlusive lesions in a single coronary artery. In subsequent years, the technique has been applied successfully to patients with multivessel disease, multiple subtotal stenoses in the same vessel, accessible complete occlusions of recent vintage, partial occlusion of saphenous vein or internal mammary artery grafts, and recent total thrombotic occlusions in acute myocardial infarction, as well as to isolated high-risk patients with congestive heart failure and cardiogenic shock. Clearly, the procedure has gained wide clinical acceptance and there is currently an extraordinary expansion of its use, with an estimated 300,000 procedures performed in the United States in 1992 (2). Such growth is attributed not only to demonstrated clinical benefit but also to recent technical advances that have lead to improved techniques and higher success rates.

SUCCESSFUL ANGIOPLASTY AND ITS DETERMINANTS

A successful angioplasty procedure is defined as one in which a greater than 20% change in luminal diameter is achieved, with the final diameter of the stenosis being less than 50%, without the occurence of death, acute myocardial infarction, or the need for emergency bypass operation. Atherosclerotic coronary stenoses are considered significant if they have the potential of impairing coronary blood flow under physiologic circumstances. Experimental data indicate that coronary flow reserve declines as coronary diameter is reduced beyond 50%. It is acknowledged that the visual assessment of coronary narrowing on cine angiograms is associated with substantial interobserver and intraobserver variability. Determination of coronary narrowing by caliper techniques is a readily available methodology that correlates closely with sophisticated computer quantitative methods. It is, thus, no longer acceptable to estimate the severity of a coronary stenosis by visual assessment and a significant stenosis is now defined as one that results in the 50% reduction in coronary diameter as determined by caliper method.

After more than a decade of experience it is now reasonable to expect an overall success rate of greater than

T. J. Ryan: Section of Cardiology, The University Hospital, Boston University Medical Center, Boston, Massachusetts 02118

or equal to 90% for single lesion dilations, within any angioplasty program. This same experience indicates that, in addition to operator experience, procedural success relates to certain patient characteristics and, very importantly, to angiographic characteristics of the lesion or lesions to be dilated.

Patient-related factors influencing a successful dilation (see Table 1) are primarily age (<65 years) and sex (male), but clinical variables, such as the history of hypertension, diabetes, prior myocardial infarction, prior bypass surgery, and impairment of left ventricular function, are known to be associated with procedural mortality.

Angiographic patterns outlining the morphologic characteristics of vessels and defining lesion-specific characteristics have also been shown to influence the likelihood of a successful dilation. It is, thus, possible to stratify patients into low-risk and high-risk categories based on clinical and angiographic variables. These variables may serve as a guide for estimating the likelihood of a successful procedure, but, more importantly, the likelihood for abrupt coronary occlusion and/or cardiovascular collapse should angioplasty fail.

Based on an American College of Cardiology/American Heart Association Task Force report that promulgated Guidelines for Percutaneous Transluminal Coronary Angioplasty (PTCA) (3), it is now common practice to designate a coronary artery lesion as Type A, B, or C based on its angiographic appearance. These angiographic characteristics are summarized in Table 2.

Type A lesions have those characteristics that allow a high anticipated success rate (≥85–90%) and have a low risk of abrupt vessel closure (<4%).

Type B lesions have those characteristics that result in a lower than optimal success rate, ranging from 60% to 85%, or have a moderate risk of abrupt vessel closure (<8%), or both. It is recognized that lesions with these characteristics, although associated with some increase in abrupt vessel closure, may in certain instances be associated with a comparatively low likelihood of a major complication. This is often the case, for example, in unsuccessful attempts to dilate total occlusions that are less than 3 months old, or in the dilation of some Type B lesions in which the distal vessel is supplied by abundant collaterals.

TABLE 1. *Patient-related factors influencing successful PTCA*

Age (<65 years)
Sex (male)
Hypertension
Diabetes
Prior myocardial infarction
Prior bypass surgery
Impaired left ventricular function

TABLE 2. *Characteristics of type A, B, and C lesions*

Lesion-specific characteristics
Type A lesions (high success, >85%; low risk)
Discrete (<10 mm in length)
Concentric
Readily accessible
Nonangulated segment, <45°
Smooth contour
Little or no calcification
Less than totally occlusive
Not ostial in location
No major branch involvement
Absence of thrombus
Type B lesions (moderate success, 60–85%; moderate risk)[a]
Tubular (10–20 mm in length)
Eccentric
Moderate tortuosity of proximal segment
Moderately angulated segment, >45°, <90°
Irregular contour
Moderate to heavy calcification
Total occlusions < 3 months old
Ostial in location
Bifurcation lesions requiring guide wires
Some thrombus present
Type C lesions (low success, <60%; high risk)
Diffuse (>2 cm in length)
Excessive tortuosity of proximal segment
Extremely angulated segments, >90°
Total occlusion > 3 months old
Inability to protect major side branches
Degenerated vein grafts with friable lesions

[a] Although the risk of abrupt vessel closure is moderate, in certain instances the likelihood of a major complication may be low, as in dilation of total occlusions less than 3 months old or when abundant collateral channels supply the distal vessel.

Type C lesions have those characteristics that result in an unacceptably low success rate (<60%) or have a high risk of abrupt vessel closure (>8%), or both. Attempts to dilate such lesions should not be undertaken when they are present in vessels supplying large or moderate areas of viable myocardium.

RISK STRATIFICATION

Low Risk

Patients generally considered to be at low risk for an angioplasty procedure are those who are below 70 years of age; are of the male sex; have single vessel and single lesion coronary artery disease, with no history of congestive heart failure and a left ventricular ejection fraction greater than 40%; who present with stable angina; and have less than 90% stenosis of a Type A coronary lesion.

High Risk

Patients with the following characteristics, as enumerated in Table 2, are generally considered to be at high risk for an angioplasty procedure: age greater than or equal to 70 years, female gender, multivessel and multilesion PTCA, diabetes mellitus, history of congestive heart failure, left ventricular ejection fraction less than or equal to 40%, left main equivalent coronary disease, inadequate platelet therapy, and unstable angina pectoris; additionally, patients with lesions exceeding 90% narrowing, stenosis bend angulation greater than 45 degrees, excessive proximal vessel tortuosity, interluminal thrombosis, and Type B or C characteristics, as enumerated in Table 2.

Although these correlates of procedural complications may serve to stratify groups of patients according to anticipated risk, they generally have a low positive and negative predictive value and it must be remembered that abrupt vessel closure remains largely unforeseeable. Highly experienced angioplasty operators seek to identify patients at risk for cardiovascular collapse if abrupt coronary occlusion complicates the angioplasty procedure. The four most important variables that prospectively identify patients at risk for cardiovascular collapse are (i) the percentage of myocardium at risk, (ii) the percent diameter of coronary stenosis, (iii) multivessel coronary artery disease, and (iv) diffuse disease in the coronary segment to be dilated.

In-Hospital Complications

Because coronary angioplasty requires visualization of the coronary anatomy as well as systemic arterial and venous access, patients undergoing the procedure are at risk for the same potential complications that are known to be associated with diagnostic cardiac catheterization. Included are arterial or venous obstructions, vessel perforations, bleeding, hypersensitivity reactions, and infection. Myocardial infarction, stroke, and death can also occur as a result of cardiac catheterization, but are infrequent.

Specific complications can occur that are directly related to the coronary angioplasty procedure. Balloon inflation results in localized trauma to the coronary artery

TABLE 3. *Untoward events related to elective percutaneous transluminal coronary angioplasty[a]*

Event	Frequency (%)
Death	1
Nonfatal myocardial infarction	4.3
Emergency coronary artery bypass surgery	3.5

[a] From the NHLBI Registry (4).

TABLE 4. *Factors associated with in-hospital mortality[a]*

Factor	Risk ratio
History of congestive heart failure	8.5
Age > 65 years	8.0
Triple vessel disease	4.5
Sex (female)	3.1
Diabetes	2.9

[a] From the NHLBI PTCA Registry (4).

wall; the net result is usually atheroma fracture and arterial expansion that produce an increase in the luminal area available for blood transport. At times, balloon inflation or guidewire or catheter manipulation can cause more extensive arterial wall damage, with medial dissection and the creation of an occlusive intimal flap. Thrombus formation also may occur at the dilation site. Either of these two latter consequences can exacerbate coronary narrowing and result in progression to abrupt, total coronary artery occlusion. In the absence of a well-developed collateral circulation, acute coronary occlusion usually results in severe myocardial ischemia and myocardial infarction.

Data from the National Heart, Lung, and Blood Institute (NHLBI) Registry (derived from very experienced centers) indicate that the procedure is associated with a 1% in-hospital mortality rate and an incidence rate of nonfatal myocardial infarction of approximately 4%, although the need for emergency bypass surgery is 2% to 3% (4) (Table 3). A number of single centers report large series of patients undergoing angioplasty to have death rates ranging from 0.2% to 0.5% for patients undergoing elective angioplasty (5).

Fortunately, when coronary occlusion occurs during a procedure, recrossing the occluded segment and repeating balloon inflation, inserting a perfusion catheter, or using thrombolytic or vasodilator agents can frequently reestablish coronary artery patency and relieve ischemia. The use of intraaortic balloon counterpulsation in the setting of acute coronary occlusion may reduce the magnitude of ischemia and augment systemic perfusion. Percutaneous cardiopulmonary bypass has also proven to be effective in this setting. However, prolonged maneuvers to reestablish coronary patency are discouraged because emergency surgical revascularization may be delayed. The probability of myocardial infarction is high and mortality is increased when coronary artery surgery is undertaken on an emergency basis: reports (6,7,8) indicate a 25% to 40% incidence rate of nonfatal new Q wave infarctions among patients undergoing emergency surgery after a failed angioplasty.

Other infrequent complications unique to coronary angioplasty include intracoronary embolization of atherosclerotic or thrombotic material, coronary perforation, and laceration or rupture of a coronary artery with subsequent hemopericardium and tamponade.

RESTENOSIS

Angioplasty outcome is also limited by restenosis, the phenomenon of renarrowing of the dilated arterial segment, usually within 3 to 6 months of the procedure. Symptomatic restenosis occurs in 20% to 25% of the patients, whereas angiographic studies suggest that the rate of restenosis is as high as 30% to 40% (9,10). The restenosis rate following angioplasty has remained quite constant over the past decade, in spite of the advances made in the initial success rates of the procedure over the same time frame. The rate of restenosis in native coronary arteries depends partly on its definition; in the National Heart, Lung, and Blood Institute Registry, restenosis was defined as a loss of 50% of the gain achieved in luminal diameter at the time of the successful angioplasty, or a 30% increase in narrowing at the site of stenosis (9). The most frequently applied definition in clinical practice is the finding of a greater than 50% diameter stenosis at follow-up angiography at the site of initial dilation. Quantitative angiographic analyses have proposed that a change greater than or equal to 0.72 mm in minimal lumen diameter represents restenosis. The present trend is to relate the extent of restenosis to the size of the vessel by using the change in minimal lumen diameter at follow-up normalized for the reference vessel diameter (relative loss).

The pathogenesis of the restenotic response to mechanical injury is incompletely understood but appears to be multifactorial. It includes growth factor stimulation of smooth muscle proliferation, elastic recoil, and organization of thrombus adherent to the site of arterial injury. Fortunately, restenosis can be managed very successfully by repeat angioplasty (11), even though the procedure exposes the patient to additional morbidity, mortality, and cost. Nevertheless, angioplasty is viewed as less expensive and inherently less invasive than is bypass surgery and is a more attractive alternative to many patients because a rapid return to normal functional status is possible.

The factors associated with restenosis are currently thought to be: recent onset of angina (<3 months), unstable angina, variant angina, diabetes, elevated blood insulin levels, multivessel disease, stenoses at the origin of vessels, lesions in the proximal anastomosis or body of a

TABLE 5. *Factors associated with abrupt closure^a (multivariate analysis)*

Percentage of post-PTCA stenosis
Initial tear or dissection
Post-PTCA heparin infusion
Branch point stenosis
Fixed bend point
Other stenosis > 50% in the same vessel

[a] From ref. 5 Ellis et al.

TABLE 6. *Factors associated with restenosis*

Recent onset angina
Unstable angina
Variant angina
Diabetes mellitus
Elevated blood insulin levels
Multivessel disease
Stenosis at the origin of vessel
Stenois in proximal or mid portion of saphenous vein graft
Chronic total occlusion
Presence of thrombus
Severity of residual lesion

vein graft, chronic total occlusions, presence of thrombus, and the severity of the residual lesion (Table 6).

LONG-TERM OUTCOME

Although there are recognized risks and certain limitations to angioplasty, the procedure has been widely embraced by clinicians because of the prompt relief of symptoms and the apparently enduring benefit to patients with coronary artery disease. The long-term benefit of angioplasty has been examined in the NHLBI Registry for patients who had more than 5 years of follow-up (12). After hospital discharge the annual mortality rate was found to be approximately 1% per year and the rate of nonfatal myocardial infarction was 2% per year. Symptomatic improvement in the successful cases was high, with 70% of the patients pain-free at 4 years. Freedom from major cardiac events (death, myocardial infarction, need for bypass surgery) over a 5-year period of follow-up of a large series from one major center was reported to be 79% (13). These data, although they do not address the problem of restenosis and are derived from a population in which 75% of the patients had single vessel disease, do indicate that long-term clinical benefit without increased risk of death or myocardial infarction can be expected after angioplasty. Follow-up studies of patients undergoing angioplasty for multivessel disease are only now emerging. One study reporting on 605 patients undergoing angioplasty for multivessel disease (14) demonstrated that 83% of patients were free from cardiac events for a 3-year period.

A number of randomized controlled trials that have compared angioplasty to coronary bypass surgery are now nearing completion. These studies will provide very important data that will allow clinicians to better judge the relative efficacy of these two alternative forms of revascularization. The outcome of these comparisons notwithstanding, it is evident that angioplasty is increasingly being used as a clinical strategy to (a) delay the need for coronary bypass surgery in younger patients until they have extensive three-vessel coronary disease that would be best treated by coronary bypass surgery and (b) to manage elderly patients and those with severe comorbid diseases that render them high surgical risks, but who are in need of relief for intractable symptoms.

INCOMPLETE REVASCULARIZATION

The experience with surgical revascularization shows relatively convincingly that "complete revascularization," that is, graft insertion around all moderate to severe coronary stenoses, leads to a superior therapeutic result. Follow-up studies (15) suggest that complete revascularization not only relieves signs and symptoms of myocardial ischemia, but is also more effective than incomplete revascularization in protecting against future coronary events.

At present, partial revascularization after coronary angioplasty is an inherent limitation of the procedure and it can be expected to occur frequently in patients undergoing multivessel angioplasty. In addition to the extent and distribution of coronary disease and the extent of myocardial fibrosis, the likelihood of partial revascularization depends on several other factors. In large measure it relates to the specific anatomy that determines the accessibility of lesions for the procedure. The occurrence of restenosis in one or more of the dilated lesions also may result in the development of partial revascularization. Although early graft closure after bypass surgery also converts complete to partial revascularization, this is a less common phenomenon than restenosis after arterial dilation. Notwithstanding, the advocates of angioplasty in patients with multivessel disease point to the successful relief of symptoms and the elimination of objective signs of ischemia after stress tests in a high percentage of patients in whom all lesions cannot be successfully dilated. Angioplasty also allows for a strategy of performing the dilation procedure on successive days or weeks. Multiple successive interventions are feasible and, although there is some degree of cumulative risk, angioplasty differs in this regard from aortocoronary bypass graft surgery, in which the opportunity for serial repeat thoracotomies is understandably more limited.

CURRENT INDICATIONS

The approach to every angioplasty procedure requires knowledgeable judgement that can weigh the likelihood of a successful procedure against the likelihood of failure and the risk of complications that include abrupt vessel closure, morbidity, and mortality. Indications for a given procedure will vary according to anatomic (single versus multivessel disease), clinical (asymptomatic versus symptomatic patients), and physiological (presence or absence of inducible ischemia) considerations. Most importantly, the indications for angioplasty are based primarily on a multifactorial risk assessment which is weighed against expected outcome.

In identifying the indications for PTCA, the Subcommittee Report on PTCA of the American College of Cardiology/American Heart Association Task Force on Assessment of Diagnostic and Therapeutic Cardiovascular Procedures proposed three classes of indications: Class I comprises conditions for which there is general agreement that PTCA is justified; Class II comprises conditions for which PTCA is performed but where there is divergence of opinion with respect to its justification in terms of value and appropriateness; and Class III comprises conditions for which there is general agreement that PTCA is not ordinarily indicated (3). This approach is extremely useful and for a complete listing and discussion of the presently accepted indications for PTCA, the reader is referred to that document. Some of the more common indications for PTCA are presented in Table 7. In general, appropriate candidates must have significant lesions in one or more major epicardial arteries usually subtending large areas of viable myocardium, with convincing evidence of myocardial ischemia. In the optimal candidate, the likelihood of a successful dilation is expected to be over 90% with a likelihood of abrupt vessel closure of less than 4%, and a mortality rate of 0.5%. Although there are clinical conditions that may justify a lower tolerance for the risk of abrupt vessel closure, there should be no compromise on the risk for significant mortality and morbidity.

The role of angioplasty in the managment of patients during the course of an acute myocardial infarction is currently the subject of intense investigation. Evidence suggests that the role for PTCA in this setting may be smaller than anticipated. Three large randomized clinical trials have all concluded that PTCA routinely performed immediately after thrombolytic therapy not only fails to improve ventricular function or reduce reocclusion rates but can also be detrimental to the patient be-

TABLE 7. *Some common indications for percutaneous transluminal coronary angioplasty[a]*

For patients who have a significant lesion in one or more major epicardial arteries that subtend at least a moderate-sized area of viable myocardium and who

1. Have recurrent ischemic episodes after myocardial infarction.
2. Show evidence of myocardial ischemia while on medical therapy during laboratory testing (including electrocardiographic monitoring at rest, as with unstable angina).
3. Have angina pectoris that has not responded adequately to medical treatment.
4. Have been resuscitated from cardiac arrest or sustained ventricular tachycardia in the absence of acute myocardial infarction.
5. Must undergo high-risk noncardiac surgery, if angina is present or there is objective evidence of ischemia.

[a] For a complete listing and discussion of accepted indications for PTCA see reference 3.

cause of increased hemorrhagic complications (16,17, 18). A fourth study also failed to show any improvement in ventricular function or recurrent infarction rates with routine performance of PTCA 18 to 48 hr after thrombolytic therapy (19).

Although there is evidence that the procedure can be used effectively as the primary intervention (i.e., without thrombolysis) for establishing reperfusion in the very early hours of an evolving infarction, many important questions remain. These include the impact of procedural delay required for PTCA, the influence of thrombus on abrupt vessel closure, and subsequent restenosis rates. The optimal timing and long-term benefit of PTCA in the management of patients with acute infarction are questions that must await further data from ongoing investigations.

CONTRAINDICATIONS

The generally accepted contraindications to the performance of angioplasty are listed in Table 8. The presence of a significant lesion in the left main coronary artery is viewed as an absolute contraindication for balloon dilation unless this main segment is protected by at least one completely patent bypass graft to the left coronary circulation. The importance of a relative contraindication to angioplasty will vary with the symptomatic state and the general medical condition of the individual patient. For example, certain risks may be appropriate in severely symptomatic individuals who are not candidates for bypass surgery, whereas these risks would be inadvisable for an asymptomatic or mildly symptomatic individual. Clearly, because a procedure can be performed does not mean that it should be performed! Such would be the case, for example, for the patient who has advanced co-morbidity, marked depression of left ventricular function, and anoxic encephalopathy at the time of presentation with recurrent infarction.

TABLE 8. *Generally accepted contraindications to angioplasty*

Absolute	Relative
No significant obstructing lesion	Presence of a coagulopathy
Left main obstruction (>50%)	No clinical evidence for spontaneous or inducible myocardial ischemia
Severe, diffuse multivessel disease	Noninfarct-related lesions at time of acute infarction angioplasty
Abrupt vessel closure would result in cardiogenic shock	Variant angina
	Anticipated success rate < 60% (Type C lesions)
	No institutional cardiac surgery program

Inherent to the strategy of coronary angioplasty is the "price of failure." This is more than the risk of a serious complication and embraces the consideration that 5% to 10% of these procedures will be initially unsuccessful and that 3% to 6% of patients will require urgent or emergency surgery to bypass a coronary artery occluded during the procedure. Furthermore, approximately 30% of the patients who have an initially successful procedure will develop restenosis of the dilated segment over the subsequent 6 months and will require a second angioplasty or bypass surgery. Thus, there are a number of patients in whom the risk, relative to the cost and morbidity associated with angioplasty as a primary therapy, may be considerably higher than that of some patients who are treated from the outset with revascularization surgery.

TRAINING AND CREDENTIALING

It is generally acknowledged that specialized skills are required for coronary interventional techniques. Training in these procedures necessitates thorough skills in diagnostic and therapeutic cardiology and particularly cardiac catheterization and angiography. A clear and concise discussion of both the cognitive and technical skills required to perform angioplasty as well as the training requirements and the case load necessary to maintain competence, can be found in a statement for physicians from the American College of Physicians/American College of Cardiology/American Heart Association Task Force on Clinical Privileges in Cardiology (20). It basically states that

> Trainees should complete a full cardiovascular training program that meets the requirements of the American Board of Internal Medicine for certification in Cardiovascular Disease and conforms to the guidelines outlined in the American College of Cardiology 17th Bethesda Conference on Adult Cardiology Training (21). In general, this should require a minimum of twelve months of full-time experience in a cardiac catheterization laboratory. The trainee should have participated in or performed a minimum of 300 coronary angiographic procedures, with documentation of 200 performed as the primary operator. To acquire the specific technical skills required for the performance of PTCA, an additional one year of formal training in a structured fellowship program devoted to PTCA is recommended. During this time, a minimum of 125 coronary angioplasty procedures, including 75 performed as the primary operator, should be documented to attain competence in the procedure. Certification of a candidate's experience and competence should be substantiated by the supervisor or director of the training program and be documented in a procedural log book.

In discussing the maintenance of competence for performing angioplasty, this same task force recommended a minimum of 75 PTCA procedures per year performed as the primary operator.

For newly certified operators this case load should be achieved within 18 months of receiving hospital privileges to perform coronary angioplasty. If the physician's performance volume or procedure results (success and complication rates) do not meet established standards, a probationary period of closer surveillance by a recognized expert should be instituted. Since the indications for angioplasty and the technology relating to the procedure are rapidly changing, documentation of continuing education in interventional techniques is necessary. Participation in formal instruction of 30 hours at least every two years is recommended.

Maintenance of competence is important not only for physicians performing PTCA but also for the institution offering the service. A significant volume of cases per institution is essential for the maintenance of assured quality and safe care. To maintain these goals, an institution should perform at least 200 PTCA procedures annually; otherwise it should not offer, or should consider discontinuing, angioplasty as part of its health care program.

In the present climate of intense economic pressures, it should be clear that not every institution anxious to offer angioplasty as part of their health care program can be allowed to do so. Similarly, not every cardiologist desiring to perform angioplasty should perform the procedure. Credentials to perform angioplasty in hospitals should be limited to those physicians with appropriate training and demonstrated competence.

REFERENCES

1. Parisi AF. ACME Study. *N Engl J Med* 1992;326:10–16.
2. Graves EJ. Detailed diagnosis and procedures, National Hospital Discharge Survey, Hyattsville, Maryland: 1989. National Center for Health Statistics; 1991; DHHS Publication no (PHS)91–1769. (*Vital and health Statistics;* series 13; no 108).
3. Ryan TJ, Faxon DP, Gunnar RM, et al. Guidelines for percutaneous transluminal coronary angioplasty. *J Am Coll Cardiol* 1988;12:529–45; *Circulation* 1988;78:486–502.
4. Detre K, Holubkov R, Kelsey S, et al. Percutaneous transluminal coronary angioplasty in 1985–1986 and 1977–1981. The National Heart, Lung and Blood Institute Registry. *N Engl J Med* 1988;318:265–270.
5. Ellis SG, Roubin GS, King SB III, et al. In-hospital cardiac mortality after acute closure after coronary angioplasty: analysis of risk factors from 8,207 procedures. *J Am Coll Cardiol* 1988;11: 211–216.
6. Golding LAR, Loop FD, Hollman JL, et al. Early results of emergency surgery after coronary angioplasty. *Circulation* 1986;74: 26–29.
7. Talley JD, Weintraub WS, Anderson HV, et al. Late clinical outcome of coronary bypass surgery after failed elective PTCA. *Circulation* 1987;76[Suppl IV]:IV-352 (abstr).
8. Ullyot DJ. Surgical standby for percutaneous coronary angioplasty. *Circulation* 1987;76[Suppl III]:III-149–152.
9. Holmes DR, Vlietstra RE, Smith HC, et al. Restenosis after percutaneous transluminal coronary angioplasty (PTCA): a report from the PTCA Registry of the National Heart, Lung and Blood Institute. *Am J Cardiol* 1984;53:77C–81C.
10. Leimgruber PP, Roubin GS, Hollman J, et al. Restenosis after successful coronary angioplasty in patients with single-vessel disease. *Circulation* 1986;73:710–717.
11. Meier B, King SB III, Gruentzig AR, et al. Repeat coronary angioplasty. *J Am Coll Cardiol* 1984;4:463–466.
12. Kent KM, Cowley MJ, Detre KM, Delsey SF, Yeh W. Report of five-year outcome for 1977–81 and 1985–86 cohorts of the NHLBI PTCA Registry (abstr). *Circulation* 1992;86(suppl I):1–55.
13. Talley JD, Hurst JW, King SB III, et al. Clinical outcome 5 years after attempted percutaneous transluminal coronary angioplasty in 427 patients. *Circulation* 1988;77:820–829.
14. Roubin G, Weintraub WS, Sutor C, et al. Event-free survival after successful angioplasty in multivessel coronary artery disease. *J Am Coll Cardiol* 1987;9:15A (abstr).
15. Jones EL, Craver JM, Guyton RA, Bone DK, Hatcher DR Jr, Riechwald N. Importance of complete revascularization in performance of the coronary bypass operation. *Am J Cardiol* 1983; 51:7–12.
16. Topol EJ, Califf RM, George BS, et al. A randomized trial of immediate versus delayed elective angioplasty after intravenous tissue plasminogen activator in acute myocardial infarction. *N Engl J Med* 1987;317:581–588.
17. Simoons ML, Arnold AE, Betriu A, et al. Thrombolysis with tissue plasminogen activator in acute myocardial infarction: no additional benefit from immediate percutaneous coronary angioplasty. *Lancet* 1988;1:197–203.
18. The TIMI Research Group. Immediate versus delayed catheterization and angioplasty following thrombolytic therapy for acute myocardial infarction: TIMI II A results. *JAMA* 1988;260: 2849–2858.
19. The TIMI Study Group. Comparison of invasive and conservative strategies after treatment with intravenous tissue plasminogen activator in acute myocardial infarction: results of the Thrombolysis in Myocardial Infarction (TIMI) phase II trial. *N Engl J Med* 1989;320:618–627.
20. Ryan TJ, Klocke FJ, Reynolds WA, et al. Clinical competence in percutaneous transluminal coronary angioplasty. A statement for physicians from the ACP/ACC/AHA Task Force on Clinical Privileges in Cardiology. *J Am Coll Cardiol* 1990;15:1469–1474.
21. Conti CR, Faxon DP, Gruentzig AR, Gunnar RM, Lesch M, Reeves TJ. 17th Bethesda Conference: Adult cardiology training. Task Force III: training in cardiac catheterization. *J Am Coll Cardiol* 1986;7:1205–1206.

Practical Angioplasty,
edited by David P. Faxon.
Raven Press, Ltd., New York © 1993.

CHAPTER 4

Patient Preparation and Periprocedural Management

Gary R. Garber

Patient Preparation
    Patient Education/Informed consent
    Preprocedure Workup
    Surgical Backup
Preprocedural Management
    Preprocedural Medications/Orders
    Preprocedural Monitoring

Postprocedural Management
    Orders
    Sheath Removal
    Management of Post Procedural Complications

The approach to a patient about to undergo percutaneous transluminal coronary angioplasty should be a carefully orchestrated process. There are many aspects that should be well ingrained in the physician and support staff who are about to assume the responsibility for their patient. Clearly each laboratory has its own set of protocols. We will present a series of general guidelines and recommendations based upon the literature and our own experience. The exact protocols adopted by each institution will reflect the training and experience of the director of the cardiac catheterization laboratory and be colored by the recommendations prescribed by the International Society and Federation of Cardiology and the World Health Organization (1).

PATIENT PREPARATION

Patient Education and Informed Consent

In nonemergency situations, there should be a meeting with the patient, and preferably a family member, prior to the planned angioplasty. During this meeting, the attending physician should inform the patient to the exact nature of the impending procedure. The patient

needs to fully understand the potential risk for emergency bypass surgery and the long-term risks of restenosis. Table 1 lists the frequency of major complications, minor complications, and restenosis. The potential long-term event of restenosis separates this procedure from other interventional or surgical procedures and must be stressed to the patient so it is not forgotten.

In addition to the risk/benefit ratio, the patient needs to know what to expect during the procedure. Such aspects as knowing that angina will most likely occur, or that there will be sheaths left in place after the procedure, will go a long way to relieve patient anxiety and enhance cooperation during the procedure.

Patients may require varying levels of informed consent. There is ample precedent stating the physician's duty is to describe all of the important complications that would allow a reasonable person to make an informed decision. There are, however, situations where disclosure of the possible consequences in toto could so alarm the patient that it would, in fact, constitute bad medical practice (2). Therefore, knowing the emotional status of your patient is vital. Patients will provide ample clues as to how much they need to know. In general, however, it is better to err on the side of more detailed information. In this regard it is important to know to the professional standard of your region of practice, and the state laws regarding informed consent. (3,4,5)

The presence of a family member is also helpful, since

G. R. Garber: Section of Cardiology, The University Hospital, Boston University Medical Center, Boston, Massachusetts

TABLE 1. *Listing of complications and long-term events and their frequencies[a]*

Event	Frequency (%)
Major	
Death	0.2–1
Emergency bypass surgery	1.2–6.8
Myocardial infarction	4.2–4.8
Cerebrovascular event	0.1
Minor	
Surgical vascular complications (pseudoaneurysm, AV fistula, thrombosis, embolism or major bleeding)	1
Nonsurgical vascular complications (minor bleeding, hematoma)	10
Other (ectopy, allergic reactions, infection, etc.)	<0.5
Late	
Restenosis (see Chapters 2 and 20)	15–50

[a] From Dorros et al. (8) and Park et al. (55).

the patient often does not remember everything said due to the stress involved. Lastly, the conversation and people present should be documented in the medical record. The informed consent form should also be signed at the end of the meeting by either the patient or legal guardian.

Although this does not absolve the physician totally, it clearly documents that the patient was approached and that discussions did take place (5). Figure 1 shows a sample consent form. All such forms should be cleared by the hospital Institutional Review Board (IRB).

Consent to Interventional Procedure

I, _____, hereby authorize the physician in charge together with such assistants as he/she may designate to perform percutaneous transluminal coronary angioplasty and/or other interventional techniques including angiography of the heart and the coronary arteries as deemed necessary by the attending Cardiologist.

I understand that catheters (tubes) will be inserted into the arm or leg blood vessel and directed to my heart chambers and coronary blood vessels. Through a guiding catheter, a small interventional catheter (balloon, laser, atherectomy, stent or other) will be directed under x-ray guidance into the narrowing in my coronary blood vessel. The interventional device will then be utilized to reduce the narrowing within the coronary blood vessel by enlarging the artery or removing the fatty deposit (plaque). The interventional catheter will then be removed and x-ray pictures (cines) taken.

The discomfort of the interventional procedure is about the same as that associated with routine coronary angiography but will take a longer period of time to perform. The major complication of these interventional procedures is the sudden blockage of a coronary vessel (< 5% of cases). Should this complication of blockage occur during the interventional procedure and attempts to keep the coronary vessel open are unsuccessful, you will be rapidly transferred to the operating room and undergo coronary bypass surgery. Although such surgery is rarely necessary, it can become a requirement of the procedure under these special circumstances to reduce the likelihood of damage to the heart muscle (heart attack).

The nature, extent, and purpose of the procedure and the possibility of additional complications have been fully explained to me. I acknowledge that no guarantee has been made to me as to the results that may be obtained.

I certify that I have read and fully understand the above consent, that explanations have been made, and that the physicians have answered all of my questions.

_____
Date

_____
Patient

_____
Witness(Physician)

_____
Responsible relative or Guardian

_____
Relationship

FIG. 1. An example of an informed consent for angioplasty.

Preprocedure Workup

History and Physical

The evaluation of a patient prior to an interventional procedure may vary between individual institutions as far as the use of medications and postintervention care. There are, however, well-established guidelines around which individual protocols can be established (1,6).

First and foremost in the evaluation of the patient is a good history and physical examination. The history should focus on the clinical history that led to the planned intervention, issues that might effect the planned procedure, and issues that might affect emergent bypass surgery.

The presence of significant orthopnea needs to be defined since the patient will be supine for many hours during and after the procedure. A history of lumbar disc disease or sciatica will alert the angiographer to potential sources of discomfort during the procedure. Another issue often overlooked is that of prostatic hypertrophy. All men must be queried as to their ability to void, since prostatic hypertrophy may lead to an inability to void in a supine position during and after the catheterization. This would require Foley catheterization, sometimes at an inopportune time.

Any history of claudication, cerebrovascular insufficiency, or prior vascular surgery will help define vascular access and risk for vascular or neurologic complications. Knowledge of prior surgical procedures such as bypass surgery or vein stripping helps the surgeon define approach and possible sources of conduit in the event of emergent bypass.

A detailed drug history is necessary to define any allergies or adverse reactions to medications. In particular, reactions to sedatives (diazepam, demerol, or the opiates, morphine, codeine and their derivatives), antiplatelet agents (aspirin, dypyridamole), calcium channel blockers or beta blockers, and any antibiotics.

Physical examination should be complete, but again be focused upon the impending procedure. A baseline fundoscopic examination should be done in all patients. This is particularly important if the patient has subsequent cholesterol emboli (diagnosed by retinal cholesterol emboli called Hollenhorst plaques) or major cerebral event. The skin (particularly the inguinal areas and sternal region) should be carefully examined for evidence of infection or potential sources of infection. Furuncles on the sternal region could be a serious source of infection if an emergent surgical procedure is required.

The carotids need to be assessed for the presence of bruits. This may not be as important for the coronary intervention, but is important in defining the risk of the patient should emergent surgery be required. Baseline lung and cardiac exams are necessary to document the present condition of the patient as well as to help assess the hemodynamic status and risk profile. Abdominal examination should note any abnormal bruits or masses in an effort to pick up abdominal aortic aneurysms or renal artery stenosis.

The peripheral arterial exam should be taken with utmost care. All peripheral pulses need to be documented, as well as the presence or absence of thrills or bruits. If there are diminished pulses, then ankle-brachial indices should be obtained with a Doppler probe. This serves as a baseline for comparison after the procedure if the femoral route is chosen. If arm access is anticipated, listen over the supraclavicular region for subclavian bruits suggesting that there might be problems with access on that side. Lastly, a general neurological examination should be documented preprocedurally in case there are any cerebrovascular events during or after the intervention.

Laboratory Data

Complete review of the patients lab data is required. If urinalysis reveals any infection, we usually recommend delay of the procedure until this can be cleared. The risk here is not so much during the intervention, but in case the patient requires emergent surgery. There is a higher incidence of postoperative complications in anyone with a preoperative infection.

A complete blood count and coagulation parameters should be obtained as well as electrolytes and renal function indices. Chest X-ray and ECG are also required, again to document a baseline and define any concomitant disease processes.

Surgical Backup

The major risk of interventional procedures is the chance of death or myocardial infarction from vessel closure. This is usually due to arterial dissection or thrombus formation. Long experience with interventional procedures has shown that there is a small but real subset of these patients who will require emergent surgery during or immediately after their procedure. This number has been steadily falling. It was 6.8% in the early 1980s (8), fell to 3.5% in the mid-1980s (9), and at many institutions is now 1% to 2% (55). This, however, translates to somewhere between 3,000 and 6,000 patients yearly who will need emergent intervention.

In institutions without immediate surgical backup, there can be an average delay of almost 4 hr before revascularization is completed (10). Others would argue that the overall numbers are small, and that with current perfusion techniques, the amount of ischemia can be limited (11). In the United States, the requirement is that surgical backup in the hospital performing the intervention be available (1,11,12).

The level of backup varies from institution to institution. Some have suites that double as operating rooms, so that if surgery is required, the surgical team scrubs and there is no need for transport. Other institutions that have many operating rooms will bring the emergent bypass patient to the next available room. Most programs arrange backup somewhere between these two extremes (12).

Based upon the above recommendations, we have all patients undergoing interventional procedures evaluated by a cardiothoracic surgeon prior to the procedure. The surgeon's input regarding the appropriateness of the procedure is factored into the decision to treat with this modality. If a major difference in opinion occurs, the clinical case is discussed in open forum during a combined surgical–medical conference. After evaluation by the surgical team, consent is signed by the patient at that time. Obtaining consent at the time of an emergency is fraught with ethical problems.

There are very special cases where surgical backup is not required. This is in the case of patients who are not potential surgical cases for technical or medical reasons. Examples are patients with isolated coronary lesions who have no potential for conduit during surgery due to multiple prior surgeries. Another might be in the very elderly or infirm to improve their quality of life. Clearly, these patients need to know the potential implications of their procedure. These need to be fully discussed with the patient, family, and surgical team, and then clearly documented in the chart.

We do not perform lone angioplasty in patients who refuse surgical backup, who would otherwise be good candidates. In these situations, patients are dictating what they think is appropriate care, and this cannot be allowed to occur.

Jehovah's Witnesses are special cases requiring special arrangement for backup. Most Jehovah's Witnesses will not accept any blood products once outside of the body. Therefore the usual surgical backup will not suffice, since most patients will not consent to the possibility of surgery unless they can be guaranteed that no blood products will be used. There are surgical teams that will operate on these patients without transfusions, using a closed system cell-saving unit, with excellent surgical mortality statistics (7,56). If such a problem of surgical backup arises, the angioplasty should not be attempted. Transfer to an institution capable of handling "bloodless surgery" is suggested.

PREPROCEDURAL MANAGEMENT

Medications and Orders

An example of preprocedure orders is shown in Fig. 2.

General Preparation

The patient should be made NPO from midnight the night prior to the procedure. We generally allow for an evening sedative for those patients requiring extra help to sleep prior to a procedure. Transportation is notified early, so there will be no delay in the transfer of the patient to the catheterization laboratory. As mentioned above, a surgical consult is requested. No presurgical skin preparation is ordered. Antibiotics are not generally ordered either.

In general, all medications are continued the morning of the procedure. Diabetics are a particular exception. Any patients taking insulin are given half of their morning dose of long-acting insulin, and the regular insulin is withheld. This is due to the decreased oral intake the day of the procedure. The intravenous solutions in these patients is supplemented with 5% dextrose along with the electrolyte solution.

Diuretics are also generally held the morning of the procedure unless the patient absolutely requires them to stay in fluid balance. The presence of diuretics may prevent adequate volume expansion and lead to a higher incidence of contrast-induced renal failure. Diuretics will also cause the patient to void more frequently during the procedure. This often interferes with the procedure and may compromise the sterile field as well.

Sedation

In an effort to reduce allergic reactions and relieve anxiety a gentle antihistamine in combination with a sedative is prescribed for all patients. Diphenhydramine (25–50 mg, PO or IV) or promethazine (25–50 mg, PO or IV) are the usual antihistamines. Sedatives generally used are diazepam (5–10 mg, PO or IV) or secobarbital (50–100 mg, PO or IV).

Hydration

Preprocedure hydration is critical for the prevention of contrast induced renal failure (13,58). If the patient

PRE-PTCA ORDERS
1. Admit for PTCA scheduled for __/__/____
2 N.P.O. after midnight.
3. Stretcher to floor in A.M.
4. I.V. D5NS at _____ cc/hr to start at _____
5. Continue all routine meds
6. Calcium Antagonist:_____
7. Begin: Aspirin 325 mg po now
8. Begin: Persantine 75 mg po tid
9. Diazepam _____ mg P.O. on call to cath lab
10. Diphenhydramine _____ mg P.O. on call to cath lab
11. If on Insulin give half dose of NPH in AM and hold any regular insulin.
12. If Dye allergy - Prednisone 60 mg P.O. q12h * 4 doses to start the evening prior to PTCA
13. Please draw PT, PTT and platelet count; and type and screen
14. Consent Cardiovascular Surgery- Re: Pre PTCA consult

FIG. 2. An example of routine preprocedure orders for patients undergoing angioplasty.

has no evidence of congestive heart failure, orders are written for a total of one liter of normal saline over 6 to 8 hr prior to the procedure. If the patient can tolerate it (as mentioned above), any diuretics are withheld the morning of the procedure as well, to ensure an adequate volume status.

If there is evidence of congestive heart failure, the intravenous fluid order is tapered back. There is no hard and fast rule and the orders must be individualized. In all but the most severe cases, the patient should receive some preprocedure hydration.

The presence of renal failure will also modify the pre- and postprocedural hydration requirements. Use of iodinated contrast agents causes acute tubular necrosis (ATN) in a small, but significant, proportion of patients. Those at higher risk for contrast-induced ATN are those with baseline renal failure, those who are volume depleted, hypertensive patients, diabetics, and patients with proteinuria and dysproteinemias. Table 2 outlines the current recommendations for management of patients with varying degrees of renal failure.

Antiplatelet Agents

One of the major complications arising from angioplasty is acute thrombosis of the artery. This is a direct result of endothelial (and sometimes medial) injury with subsequent platelet deposition (14). Performance of angioplasty without any antiplatelet coverage has led to a detectable coronary thrombus in as many as 21% of cases (15), with a myocardial infarction (MI) rate of 6.9% to 10.7% (15,16,17). The additions of certain antiplatelet agents has reduced the periprocedural MI rate to 1.6% (16,17). Given the high event rate without such agents, angioplasty in the absence of antiplatelet agent administration within the previous 12–24 hr, in our opinion is contraindicated.

Current studies suggest that aspirin, 325 mg daily, and dipyridamole, 225 mg daily, administered for at least 24 to 48 hr prior to angioplasty is adequate therapy (1,15–18). There is some controversy as to the efficacy of dipyridamole added to aspirin, with one controlled trial (19) showing no added effect of dipyridamole and aspirin compared to aspirin alone. The general recommendation is, however, to continue to add the dipyridamole unless there are adverse effects.

If the patient is allergic to aspirin and angioplasty is necessary, the use of other agents is possible. Ibuprofen may inhibit platelet deposition (20); however, clinical trials have not been performed. Desensitization to aspirin is efficacious in patients with severe aspirin allergies (21). The desensitization period may be short (<6 months). This time frame is long enough to sustain the patient through an angioplasty procedure. To date there is no published experience with patients undergoing angioplasty who have also had aspirin desensitization, but the option is a viable one.

Low molecular weight dextran is an agent that, based upon animal studies, gained early favor in angioplasty

TABLE 2. *Management strategies for patients with renal insufficiency undergoing cardiac catheterization*

Patient group	Plan
1. Patients at high risk for contrast-induced renal failure (diabetes, hypertension, proteinuria, CHF, dysproteinurias) with serum creatinine < 1.5 mg/dl.	1. Assure adequate oral hydration prior to catheterization
2. Serum creatinine 1.5–2.0 mg/dl.	2. 1 liter NS or half-normal saline 12 hr prior to catheterization
3. a. Serum creatinine 1.5–2.0 mg/dl, in addition to diabetes or nephrotic syndrome.	3. a. 1 liter NS or half-normal saline 12 hr prior to catheterization.
b. Serum creatinine >2.0–3.0 mg/dl.	b. Mannitol, 20% (25 g/125 ml D5W), 20 ml/hr beginning immediately following catheterization, for 6 hr.
	c. Replace urine output with D5 half-normal saline + KCl 30 meq/l.
	d. If mannitol is contraindicated (i.e., CHF), 100 mg Lasix/mg creat > 1.0 immediately following catheterization; replace urine output as above.
4. Serum creatinine > 3.0 mg/dl (including patients on dialysis).	a. Renal consultation before catheterization.
	b. For patients not on dialysis management same as Group 3.

CHF, congestive heart failure; NS, normal saline.

circles as an aid in preventing arterial thrombosis (24). Repeat studies in both dogs (25) and humans (26) have failed to substantiate the initial findings in two animals. One might argue that the dextran was not given early enough prior to angioplasty to allow for its potential antiplatelet effect; however, *in vitro* platelet studies have not demonstrated that dextran prevents platelet deposition in a controlled injury model either (14,18). Based upon present studies we cannot recommend its routine use in angioplasty.

Ticlopidine, an antiplatelet agent used in Europe (22), is another promising agent. In a dose of 250 mg three times a day, it was shown to be as effective as aspirin and dipyridamole in the prevention of postangioplasty complications (23). This is contrary to experimental data that show that this agent does not prevent platelet deposition (14). We cannot recommend its use outside of clinical trials.

Other agents such as sulfinpyrazone, verapamil, nifedipine, ketanserin, and thromboxane A_2 receptor blockers are of no help in the prevention of thrombosis (14). Experimental agents such as hiruden (a thrombin antagonist) or the platelet receptor IIB/IIa inhibitor are showing promise in controlled experimental models. Several of these agents are currently undergoing clinical trials.

Calcium Channel Blockers

Mechanical intervention in the coronary artery can stimulate spasm (1,27–29). In an effort to decrease spasm, to protect the myocardium during the ischemia of an intervention (30), and as an adjunct to decrease angina (31,32), calcium channel blockers are generally recommended.

No individual calcium channel blocker (nifedipine, nicardipine, diltiazem, or verapamil) has been shown to be any better or to improve the outcome of angioplasty. The clinical situation usually dictates which blocker may be used. The agent is started prior to the angioplasty, with enough time allotted for absorption prior to the start of the procedure. Since there is no strong evidence that calcium channel blockers affect the immediate outcome, we will proceed with the procedure if for some reason the patient is unable to tolerate any calcium channel antagonist.

Nitroglycerin

Nitroglycerin is gaining in significance as an adjunct to angioplasty. There is ample evidence that it prevents the immediate postangioplasty spasm (29). Furthermore, nitroglycerin has been shown to have a significant antiplatelet effect (14,28) which would prevent further platelet-mediated spasm, as well as thrombosis.

For these reasons we use nitroglycerin in all patients undergoing angioplasty. Nitroglycerin, 100–200 micrograms, is administered directly into the coronary artery just prior to insertion of the equipment. This will be followed by another bolus immediately after the equipment is removed from the coronary. In many patients, particularly with smaller caliber arteries or in complicated cases, we will continue intravenous nitroglycerin overnight.

Anticoagulants

Heparin is clearly indicated *during* angioplasty to prevent thrombi from forming. It is usually administered at the time of instrumentation with an intravenous bolus of 100 U/kg or 10,000 U. This is supplemented by either a continuous intravenous infusion or intermittent bolus. The level of anticoagulation is usually guided by following the activated clotting time.

The presence of an intracoronary thrombus prior to angioplasty has been correlated with abrupt closure (33–35). There is ample evidence now that intravenous heparin given 1 to 5 days *prior* to angioplasty in patients with intracoronary thrombus (36–38) or with unstable angina (39,40) will have reduced abrupt closure rates. This is likely due to stabilization of the thrombus, regression of thrombogenic mass, and prevention of thrombus progression. Therefore, unless an emergent situation is present, all patients with unstable angina or intracoronary thrombus on angiogram, should receive at least 24 hr of intravenous heparin therapy prior to angioplasty.

Other Preprocedural Medications

Steroids

In patients who have a documented allergy to contrast agents, preprocedural use of steroids has been recommended. There is conflicting evidence as to whether the addition of steroids in patients with contrast reactions changes the overall incidence of further contrast reactions. Given the potential gravity of the reactions, we still recommend their use. The usual dose is prednisone, 60 mg every 12 hr for two doses prior to the procedure, and 60 mg every 12 hr for two doses after the procedure (49,50).

Medications to Prevent Restenosis

There are several medications being investigated for effectiveness in preventing restenosis. Low molecular weight heparin, cilazaparil, omega-3 fatty acids (fish oil), and colchicine are all being examined as potential agents that could be given prior to angioplasty in an effort to prevent restenosis. For a full review of these medications see the chapter on restenosis.

Preprocedural Monitoring

Preprocedural monitoring is dictated by the clinical situation. Stable patients do not require preprocedural monitoring. Patients with unstable angina, acute myocardial infarction or congestive heart failure usually come from monitored settings.

A more interesting aspect of monitoring occurs during the angioplasty procedure. We include a discussion at this particular point because it will impact on postprocedural monitoring. There is a growing body of experience with 12-lead ECG monitoring during the angioplasty. This monitoring acquires an ischemic "fingerprint" unique to that patient during balloon inflation. Then, monitoring the same leads after the angioplasty will allow the physician to separate the pain of abrupt closure from that of noncardiac pain often associated with lying supine for extended periods after angioplasty (41,42). While this technology is just being explored, we suspect it will become automated and widely used in the near future.

In the absence of 12-lead monitoring, a single or dual channel monitor should be connected to the patient while sheaths are sewn in, and for the 8 to 12 hr the patient is supine with the sand bag compression. This allows for some degree of ST segment monitoring, as well as examination of the heart rate as a clue to vagal or bleeding episodes. Furthermore, while the sheaths are in, the arterial sheath may be used for blood pressure monitoring. Again, this is helpful in maintaining adequate blood pressure during the critical early hours after angioplasty.

POSTPROCEDURAL MANAGEMENT

Orders

There are several general orders that should be routine after angioplasty (Fig. 3). Vital signs need to be checked fairly frequently early after the procedure since this is the highest risk period. Our unit checks vital measurements every 15 min for the first hour, every 30 min for the next 4 hr, hourly for 4 hr, and then every 4 hr until the patient is stable. Vital signs include not only blood pressure and heart rate, but an examination of the femoral/brachial catherization site and all distal pulses. The first meal is liquid, in case emergent catheterization for abrupt closure occurs.

Serum cardiac enzymes are routinely checked on all patients to document the presence of any myocardial damage either during or immediately after the angioplasty (43).

A routine 12-lead ECG is obtained immediately after the procedure and functions as a baseline for further comparison should the patient experience any chest discomfort. As mentioned above, if an intraprocedural 12-lead ECG was obtained during balloon inflation, then this will serve as the fingerprint for further comparison.

All patients are vigorously hydrated orally with 2 to 3 l of fluids, as well as intravenously with 1 l of normal saline over 4 to 5 hr, if the ventricular function can tolerate it. If there are risk factors for contrast-induced renal failure, we will modify the hydration orders (see Table 2).

The patient is kept at bed rest while sheaths are in place and for 12 hr after removal. The patient is kept in a supine position with the head elevated no more than 20 degrees in an effort to keep the femoral region still.

Medications

Pain medications are liberally prescribed. Often the most uncomfortable part of an angioplasty is the requirement to be supine for up to 36 hr after the procedure. Back spasm is common. Oxycodone, demerol, and morphine are usual narcotics. They are prescribed to be given every 3 to 4 hr as needed. The exact narcotic will

---

```
          POST PTCA ORDERS
1)    Resume all pre-cath orders
2)    Vital signs q1/4h x 4, q1/2h x 4 then q1h x 4 then q4h till stable
3)    Full liquid          resume pre-PTCA diet in
4)    Serum enzymes at:
5)    EKG at:
6)    Pain Med:
7)    Calcium antagonist:
8)    Persantine:
9)    Aspirin:
10)   Heparin flush to arterial sheath x _____hrs then call Cardiology to
          d/c sheaths at _____
11)   Heparin unit bolus and   unit/hr thru venous sheath. D/C at ____
12)   Force fluids to _____ liters for the next 6 hrs
13)   IV:
14)   Bedrest till 12 hours after sheath removal
15)   Do not elevate HOB 20 degrees til 8 hrs post sheath removal
16)   Sand bag to _____ groin x 8 hours p sheath removal
17)   Keep _____ leg straight x 8 hours
18)   Check _____ pedal pulses with VS
19)   IV NTG at _____ mcgm/min and adjust to BP
20)   Check _____ groin for bleeding with vital signs
21)   Call Cardiology  for systolc BP <_____ , bleeding or chest pain
```

FIG. 3. An example of routine post-PTCA orders.

vary with institutional practice but should definitely be included. Often we will write orders for the medication to be given during the first 24 hours, unless the patient refuses, thereby obviating the patient's need to ask for it.

Calcium channel blocking agents, aspirin, and dipyridamole are all continued after angioplasty. The dipyridamole is usually discontinued after five 75-mg doses, since there is little evidence to continue it long-term. The aspirin is continued long-term, usually in a dosage of 80 to 325 mg daily. This is used not only to prevent early thrombotic events but for its overall cardioprotective effect for future thrombotic events. Calcium channel blockers are continued for at least 1 month and then discontinued as the clinical situation allows.

Heparin

Heparin's use is usually divided into its use in uncomplicated cases and in complicated cases. In routine cases, heparin is continued during the period that sheaths are indwelling, and is discontinued 2 hr prior to sheath removal. We will usually pull sheaths 4 hr after the end of the procedure in completely uncomplicated single lesion cases. Some laboratories keep all patients on heparin with sheaths in overnight. There have been no studies comparing such strategies, although there has been a report of few complications in patients undergoing outpatient angioplasty with brief duration of heparinization (47).

In complex cases, where there is a dissection, thrombus, or multiple lesions, heparin may be continued for several days. We will change the heparin to half the usual dose for 2 hr prior to sheath removal, then pull sheaths and then re-treat with a bolus of 5000 U of intravenous heparin 2 hr after sheaths are removed, along with resuming the full dose heparin infusion. This is a compromise approach in a situation where one does not want to totally discontinue heparin due to the damage done to the artery, but where one must remove the sheaths prior to infection setting in.

Monitoring the adequacy of heparinization has been simplified by the use of the activated clotting time (ACT). Unlike the partial thromboplastin time (PTT), which has a significant lag time from drawing to laboratory reporting, the ACT can be done at the bedside (44–46). Usually adequate heparinization is achieved at an ACT of greater than 300. We will pull sheaths when the ACT falls below 180.

The duration of heparinization in complicated cases has also not been completely studied. It is often a reflection of the physician's concern over the level of complication incurred during the procedure. We usually use 5 days as an outer limit for heparinization. This is based loosely on the fact that in damaged arterial segments, there is evidence of near complete reendothelialization by 5 to 7 days. After continuing heparin for 5 days there is rarely thrombus formation once it is discontinued. The heparin may be discontinued in less than 5 days, again based upon the perceived level of damage and arterial patency immediately after angioplasty. As can be noted from the above discussion, there is clearly some art and luck in deciding when to discontinue such therapy. Newer intravascular imaging techniques (ultrasound and angioscopy) may help in making this decision in the near future.

In some extreme cases (such as large vein grafts with sluggish flow), the physician may want to continue anticoagulation therapy even longer. In such cases warfarin therapy may be considered. This is however an extreme case and is not usually necessary.

Nitroglycerin

As noted in the preprocedural medications, nitroglycerin has multiple salutary effects on the dilated coronary artery. It prevents platelet adhesion, thereby preventing not only thrombosis but also platelet-mediated vasoconstriction. It is also an endothelium-independent vasodilator and has been shown to cause a decrease in postangioplasty constriction. We will always give a bolus of intracoronary nitroglycerin after angioplasty. Many laboratories will even keep the patient on small doses of intravenous nitroglycerin in an effort to keep up some systemic levels of nitrates. No studies have been done examining the abrupt closure rate with and without nitroglycerin after angioplasty. We recommend that if there are any complications during the angioplasty, or if the artery dilated is of small caliber, intravenous nitroglycerin should be continued until after the sheaths are pulled.

Technique for Sheath Removal

The technique is that of Currier et al. (57).

Premedication

Sheath removal is easiest in a pain-free, relaxed, normotensive, noncoagulopathic patient. Thus, you should check that the heparin has been off for 2 hr. If there is any question, check an ACT before starting (pull the sheath if it is less than 160–180). Morphine (1 to 3 mg IV) should be given to any patient who has discomfort in the area. Atropine (0.6 mg) is also useful to prevent the vagal episodes that occur (especially with young males) in post-PTCA patients. If the patient is not completely revascularized, atropine should not be used prophylactically but should be available quickly.

Equipment

Chux, suture removal kit, two boxes of 4 in × 4 in, good gloves, sandbag, mechanical C-arm compression device disc, and strong fingers.

Preparation

The patient should be flat on the stretcher or bed, with the legs straight. The bed should be adjusted to a comfortable height for compression. The hip should be externally rotated to bring the femoral artery over the femoral head. The nurse's call bell should be given to the patient and the nurse should be there for the first few minutes. Both you and the patient should void before starting.

Venous Sheath Removal

Although techniques vary, we usually remove the venous sheath first. It is a good bioassay for the patients ability to coagulate; if hemostasis is not achieved in 10 min it is not a good idea to pull the arterial sheath without checking an ACT. Make sure that this is not the patient's only venous access. Position your first three fingers medial to the course of the artery, just proximal to the site of the sheath entry. Instruct the patient to take slow deep breaths to avoid Valsalva maneuvers. Pull the sheath in one easy motion (it is about 15 cm long). Allow a bit of back bleeding and gently compress for 5 to 10 min.

Arterial Sheath Removal—Manual

Once adequate hemostasis has been obtained on the venous side, the arterial sheath can be removed. Position the first three fingers of your left hand (for right groin) along the course of the artery such that the middle finger is over the site where the sheath enters the artery. This will usually mean that your index finger is just proximal to the skin entry site. You should be able to feel the femoral head underneath. In obese patients it will be necessary to slide the pannus up, but go by the feel of the femoral artery and femoral head, not just the site that the sheath leaves the skin. Once your left hand is in position, pull the sheath (Gruentzig sheaths are about 30 cm long) in one motion, while instructing the patient to breathe easily and not bear down. A small amount of back bleeding is allowed to prevent clot embolization and to ensure that if further bleeding does occur, it will be external and not form a hematoma. Once the torrent of blood has subsided, check the distal pulses with your other hand (or ask the nurse to do it). There is no standard technique, but most people aim to compress but not totally occlude the artery, leaving a trace distal pulse.

If your hand should fatigue there are three options: switch hands finger by finger, push down on your left hand with your right hand and relax your left, or call for someone to help you. The minimum time for compression is 20 to 30 min for a PTCA, and 30 to 40 min for an overnight PTCA or half-dose heparin pull. At the end of the allotted time, ease off over 2 to 3 min. If blood spurts out, then hold for another 20 to 30 min, think about your position, and check an ACT. If an ooze appears, reapply pressure for another 10 min and try again. If it looks good, place a sandbag and observe for several minutes prior to leaving the patient.

Arterial Sheath Removal—Mechanical C-Arm

In the old days, all sheaths were held by hand. Now we have mechanical C-arm compression devices (Compressar), but there are many cases where it should not be used. Use of the clamp requires a cooperative, nonobese person whose puncture site is correctly positioned and who has no preexisting hematoma. The venous sheath must be removed first.

Meticulous placement of the C-arm is essential for it to work well. In fact, for diagnostic catheterizations it is usually faster to pull manually. Position the clamp without the disc such that the point on the C-arm is exactly over the presumed site the sheath enters the artery. Place the disc on the C-arm and slide it down until it rests on the patient's groin. Usually the V in the disc will be just proximal to the site where the sheath enters the skin. Apply gradual pressure and pull the arterial sheath. Warn the patient that you are going to push hard and that they should not bear down. Once the sheath is out and a modicum of back bleeding has occurred, push down on the C-arm until the blood stops. This will invariably require a lot more pushing than manual holds because the area of the disc is much greater than the area of your three fingers. When the bleeding is stopped, move down to the foot and check for a pulse. As for manual holds, aim for near total compression, leaving a trace distal pulse for the duration of the hold. The time recommendations are the same as for manual holds. Leave the artery compressed for the full time before letting up over 2 to 3 min. The patient must lie absolutely still since the clamp will not move with the femoral artery like your fingers. If any evidence of a hematoma develops it is essential to remove the clamp quickly and hold it by hand. You must check the pulses and position of the clamp frequently throughout the hold. Without your finger on the pulse, you may not notice the development of a vasovagal reaction until it is too late. Hypotension from a vasovagal reaction causing abrupt closure is not a pleasant situation.

There is no reason why the clamp should not be used for larger sheaths in appropriate patients (a longer hold is probably a good reason to try the clamp). However, with a larger hole in the artery one can get into a lot of trouble a lot faster if the device is improperly positioned.

Hematoma

Despite optimal technique, these will occasionally occur. Risk factors are obesity, inability to lie flat, hypertension, and anticoagulation. If a hematoma appears during a manual hold, you are incorrectly positioned (i.e., its the same thing as if they are bleeding externally). Compression either distal to the puncture site or proximal to it can be the cause. Compression proximal to the site where the sheath enters the artery can cause bleeding because of collateral flow. Reposition your hand and call for a help if the hematoma continues to grow. If a hematoma develops during a Compressar hold, the clamp is improperly positioned. It must be quickly removed and the site held by hand.

More frequently, hematomas are noted after the patients are back in their room. As noted above, hematoma is equivalent to bleeding, so the artery should be compressed again, for at least 15 minutes. If the patient is on heparin, call the angiographer and discuss the situation (i.e., find out if the dissection was so large that the patient needs to be kept on heparin at all costs). Demarcate the extent of the hematoma and check it frequently. Check for a bruit (a new systolic bruit may reflect a newly raised flap; a continuous bruit indicates an arteriovenous fistula). If the hematoma is pulsatile, a pseudoaneurysm must be ruled out. Call for a vascular consult and arrange for an echo/Doppler.

Loss of Pulse

The mere placement of a catheter causes significant reduction of flow in normal arteries for up to 48 hr. Thus, it is not surprising that as we catheterize more people with atherosclerotic peripheral vascular disease from the leg, we see loss of distal pulses. Two keys in management are to get vascular surgery involved early, and to heparinize 2 to 4 hr after the sheaths are out. If the foot is warm, usually no acute intervention is necessary. If the foot is pulseless and cold, then urgent surgery may be needed. Doppler gradients should be checked when possible, and compared with the ones obtained and carefully documented in your precatheterization note.

Documentation

Write a brief note in the chart that you removed the sheaths, and document the presence of distal pulses and the condition of the catheter site. If a hematoma has developed, outline it with ink and check it frequently over the next few hours.

Management of Postprocedural Complications

Abrupt Closure

The most common and feared complication after angioplasty is that of abrupt closure. This occurs out of the laboratory in upwards of 5% of all angioplasties (8). In the early years of angioplasty, any patient who had abrupt closure was taken immediately to bypass surgery. It then became apparent that many patients who abruptly closed, could be managed without surgery (53).

Abrupt closure, that is recurrent chest pain *with* ECG changes, should be managed quickly. Abrupt closure represents either thrombosis at the site of angioplasty, embolization of thrombus distally, a dissection flap, subintimal hemorrhage, spasm, or a combination of the above.

There is no need in the first few minutes to bring the patient immediately back to the catheterization laboratory unless they are hemodynamically unstable. If an activated clotting time is available, it should be checked. If it is less than 300, the patient should receive an intravenous bolus of heparin, the presumption being that a thrombus has formed due to inadequate anticoagulation. Intravenous nitroglycerin should be administered for its antispasmodic effect, antiplatelet effect, and beneficial effect on ischemic myocardium. Calcium channel blockers, particularly nifedipine, may also be given to prevent spasm. Blood pressure should be maintained above 100 systolic and 60 diastolic to maintain coronary arterial perfusion pressure thus preventing further thrombosis or arterial collapse. These measures alone can restore flow and stabilize the patient in nearly 30% of abrupt closures.

If the above medical measures are unsuccessful within 30 min, then emergent repeat angioplasty is indicated. If significant thrombus is seen, then intracoronary streptokinase or rt-PA may help to debulk the volume of the thrombus. With this strategy, upwards of 80% of patients with abrupt closure may be treated nonsurgically.

Prolonged Angina

This is a relatively common complication during and after angioplasty, occurring in upwards of 7% of all patients (8). It is usually in the setting of a complicated angioplasty with a suboptimal result. Myocardial infarcts are often associated with this as well. If prolonged pain is present and the target vessel appears in good condition, the angiographer should look judiciously for small branch occlusion. Branches often overlooked are small septal branches off of the left anterior descending artery, or right ventricular branches off of the right coronary artery. Loss of these small branch vessels is usually of no consequence and they should not be rescued at the expense of risking a good result of the major vessel.

Vascular Complications

Vascular complications occur in roughly 1% of all balloon angioplasty procedures (51,52). Risk factors for vascular complications are female gender, age greater than 65, thrombolytic therapy, and postprocedural anticoagulation therapy. As the use of larger catheters for atherectomy expands, the vascular complications will most likely increase. Detection and management of several complications are discussed below.

Bleeding

This is the most common problem after angioplasty. Bleeding is usually minor and around the sheath and, therefore, easily discovered. Occasionally, the bleeding will track retroperitonealy, down the femoral sheath or, uncommonly, up the abdominal wall. It is in these cases where large amounts of blood can be lost before discovery. Always make sure that the sheath has a short dilator inserted through the hemostatic valve. This adds body to the sheath and prevents kinking which could be a source of bleeding.

Treatment of external bleeding is usually local compression with the sheaths in place. If significant bleeding continues, and it is necessary to keep the sheath in place, it may be exchanged for a slightly larger sheath to hopefully seal the bleed. An activated clotting time or partial thromboplastin time should be checked. If supratherapeutic, the heparin should be stopped, or at least withheld for a time. If the bleeding cannot be controlled, the heparin should be discontinued and the sheath pulled. This may require a prolonged femoral site hold, and one should consider the use of a clamp or rotating helpers so that one person does not tire.

Hidden bleeding does not usually respond to local compression. Treatment is always cessation of heparin and withdrawal of the indwelling sheath. The etiology of this type of bleeding is often faulty technique from puncture of the external iliac artery above the inguinal ligament, or puncture of the femoral artery distal to the bifurcation where tamponade may be difficult, due to the lack of the firm underlying femoral head. Operative drainage or repair is usually not required unless the bleeding cannot be controlled after sheath withdrawal. This usually represents arterial tear, and should be surgically treated.

Hematoma formation after sheath removal should be handled as a repeat bleeding episode. This is fully described in the section regarding sheath removal.

Pseudoaneurysms

This is the most common major vascular complication. It represents a walled off hematoma with a persistant hole in the artery. Diagnosis of a femoral pseudoaneurysm may be made on clinical grounds. There is usually a large pulsatile mass that extends outside of the normal bounds of the femoral artery. A systolic bruit may be present over the mass. Confirmation of a pseudoaneurysm is made with duplex Doppler sonography (54). There is no necessity for angiography in these cases.

If a femoral pseudoaneurysm greater than 2 cm in diameter is discovered, surgical therapy is indicated, with drainage of the hematoma and closure of the arterial puncture.

Arteriovenous Fistula

In the course of obtaining vascular access via the Seldinger technique, simultaneous puncture of the femoral artery and vein is possible. This is due to the occasional superimposition of the femoral artery and vein over each other. In the course of passing the needle, the overlying vein is occasionally perforated with passage of the needle, and occasionally the sheath, into the femoral vein. Another possible cause is lateral entry of the needle into the artery and vein (59). Once the needle or sheath is removed, there is then a communication between artery and vein. This usually closes upon removal of the needle or sheath; however, given the pressure gradient, occasionally an arteriovenous (AV) fistula may develop (52).

Diagnosis of an AV fistula is usually made on physical examination. Using a stethoscope, a continuous to and fro murmur may be heard. There may also be a palpable thrill present. Use of duplex Doppler sonography may confirm the diagnosis.

Therapy of these fistulas is expectant. They usually close within several days to weeks. Furthermore the amount of shunting is very little, given the very small size of the communication. There has been one case where a patient had congestive heart failure with a cardiac output of 7.9l/min after an aortic valvuloplasty. The symptoms resolved after correction of the fistula (59). This is an example of the potential for the formation of large fistulae with the larger sheaths being used for interventions. As noted, this is a very rare occurrence. If the fistula remains patent for more than 4 weeks, or if there are any signs of hemodynamic compromise from the shunting as noted above, then surgical repair is indicated.

Arterial Compromise

Often in the course of obtaining postangioplasty vital signs, there will be diminished pulses. The most common cause of this is the presence of a large sheath in a small artery. This is most often seen in small women, when the brachial approach is used, or in patients with peripheral vascular disease. Treatment is removal of the sheath.

Arterial thrombosis is very uncommon due to the vigorous use of heparin during and after angioplasty. The diagnosis of embolized thrombus is made after sheaths are removed (thus eliminating the sheath as a cause for loss of pulses) and the patient shows persistant loss of pulses and presence of pain associated with sensorium changes in the affected extremity. Immediate reheparinization can prevent clot propagation in small distal emboli. Occasionally, intraarterial thrombolytic therapy may be instituted to further enhance clot dissolution. Surgical thrombectomy in small distal emboli is usually not an option. Larger thrombi, compromising an entire limb are treated emergently with surgical thrombectomy, unless otherwise contraindicated.

Atheromatous embolization distally is usually due to traumatic entry of a diseased femoral artery, or dislodging of atheromatous material from a diseased distal aorta. Diagnosis of this is evident because there appears to be a shower of material distally, often to both extremities. Occasionally, if the source is high enough, renal failure or mesenteric ischemia may also be present. Treatment is rarely surgical, unless there is enough ischemia to cause compartment syndrome or limb loss distally, or bowel infarction if the embolism is more proximal.

Miscellaneous Complications

There are numerous reports of other late complications that are very uncommon. They occur at the same rate as routine cardiac catheterization (8). These are

1. Central nervous system events such as transient ischemic attacks or cerebrovascular accidents.
2. Pulmonary embolism.
3. Late allergic reactions to contrast media or to the narcotics given for pain control after the angioplasty.
4. Transient hypotension—most often occurring during the sheath pull from a vagal episode. Many centers will give 0.6 mg of intravenous atropine prior to pulling sheaths to avoid this complication.
5. Febrile episode—often from indwelling sheaths left in place longer than 24 hr.
6. Nausea. This may be due to the narcotics given for pain control, recurrent ischemia, underlying gastrointestinal pathology such as hiatus hernia or peptic ulcer disease, or to ingesting too much fluid in a supine position during the early hydration period.

REFERENCES

1. Bourassa MG, et al. Report of the Joint ISFC/WHO Task Force on Coronary Angioplasty. *Circulation* 1988;78:780–789.
2. Schroeder OC. Cardiac catheterization and informed consent: a new technic meets an old issue. *Postgrad Med* 1973:207–209.
3. Miller LJ. Informed consent: I. *JAMA* 1988;244:2100–2103.
4. Miller LJ. Informed consent: II. *JAMA* 1988;244:2347–2350.
5. Miller LJ. Informed consent: III. *JAMA* 1988;244:2556–2558.
6. Marcus ML, Schelbert HR, Skorton DJ, Wold GL. *Cardiac imaging—a companion to Braunwald's heart disease.* Philadelphia: WB Saunders; 1991:189–190.
7. Lewis CT, Murphy MC, Cooley DA. Risk factors for cardiac operations in adult Jehovah's witnesses. *Ann Thorac Surg* 1991;51:448–450.
8. Dorros G, Cowley MJ, Simpson J, et al. Percutaneous transluminal coronary angioplasty: report of complications from the National Heart, Lung and Blood Institute PTCA Registry. *Circulation* 1983;67:723–730.
9. Holmes DR, Holubkov R, Vlietstra RE, et al. Comparison of complications during percutaneous transluminal coronary angioplasty from 1977–1981 and from 1985–1986: The National Heart, Lung and Blood Institute Percutaneous Transluminal Coronary Angioplasty Registry. *J Am Coll Cardiol* 1988;12:1149–1155.
10. Parker JD. Does angioplasty need on site surgical cover? A surgeon's view. *Br Heart J* 1990;64:1–2.
11. Shaw TRD. Does angioplasty need on site surgical cover? A physician's view. *Br Heart J* 1990;64:3–4.
12. Ullyot DJ. Surgical standby for percutaneous coronary angioplasty. *Circulation* 1978;76[Suppl III]: III149–III152.
13. Eisenberg RL, Bank WO, Hedgcock MW. Renal failure after major angiography. *Am J Med* 1980;68:43.
14. Chesebro JH, Lam JYT, Badimon L, Fuster V. Restenosis after arterial angioplasty: a hemorrheologic response to injury. *Am J Cardiol* 1987;60:10B–16B.
15. Barnathan ES, Schwartz JS, Taylor L, Laskey WK, Kleaveland P, Kussmal WG, and Hirshfeld JW. Aspirin and dipyridamole in the prevention of acute coronary thrombosis complicating coronary angioplasty. *Circulation* 1987;76:125–134.
16. Bourassa MG, et al. The role of antiplatelet agents in reducing periprocedural coronary angioplasty complications. *J Am Coll Cardiol* 1988;11:238A.
17. Schwartz L, et al. Aspirin and dipyridamole in the prevention of restenosis after percutaneous transluminal angioplasty. *N Engl J Med* 1988;318:1714–1719.
18. Chesbro JH, Fuster V. Platelet-inhibitor drugs before and after coronary artery bypass surgery and coronary angioplasty: the basis of their use, data from animal studies, clinical trial data and current recommendations. *Cardiology* 1986;73:292–305.
19. Lembo NJ, et al. Does the addition of dipyridamole to aspirin decrease acute coronary angioplasty complications? The results of a prospective randomized clinical trial. *J Am Coll Cardiol* 1988;11:237A.
20. Lam JYT, Chesebro JH, Dewanjee MK, Badimon L, Fuster V. Ibuprofen: a potent antithrombotic agent for arterial injury after balloon angioplasty. *J Am Coll Cardiol* 1987;9:64A.
21. Sweet JM, Stevenson DD, Simon RA, Mathison DA. Long-term effects of aspirin desensitization treatment for aspirin sensitive rhinosinusitis asthma. *J Allergy Clin Immunol* 1990;85(1 pt 1):59–65.
22. McTavish D, Faulds D, Goa KL. Ticlopidine: an updated review of its pharmacology and therapeutic use in platelet dependent disorders. *Drugs* 1990;40:238–259.
23. White CW, Chaitman B, Lassar TA, Row ML, Khaja F, Vandormael M, Reitman M, and the Ticlopidine study group. Antiplatelet agents are effective in reducing the immediate complications of PTCA: results from the Ticlopidine Multicenter Trial. *Circulation* 1987;76[suppl IV]:IV–400.
24. Pasternak RC, Baughman KL, Fallon JT, Block PC. Scanning electron microscopy after coronary transluminal angioplasty of normal canine coronary arteries. *Am J Cardiol* 1980;45:591–598.
25. O'Gara PT, Guerrero JL, Feldman B, Fallon JT, Block PC. Effect of dextran and aspirin on platelet adherence after transluminal

angioplasty of normal canine coronary arteries. *Am J Cardiol* 1984;53:1695–1698.

26. Swanson KT, Vlietstra RE, Holmes DR, Smith HC, Reeder GS, Bresnahan JF, Bove AA. Efficacy of adjunctive dextran during percutaneous transluminal coronary angioplasty. *Am J Cardiol* 1984;54:447–448.

27. Douglas JS, King SB, Roubin GS. Influence of the methodology of percutaneous transluminal coronary angioplasty on restenosis. *Am J Cardiol* 1987;60:29B–33B.

28. Lam JYT, Chesebro JH, Fuster V. Platelets, vasoconstriction, and nitroglycerine during arterial wall injury: a new antithrombotic role for an old drug. *Circulation* 1988;78:712–716.

29. Fischell TA, Derby G, Tse TM, Stadius ML. Coronary artery vasoconstriction routinely occurs after percutaneous transluminal coronary angioplasty: a quantitative arteriographic analysis. *Circulation* 1988;78:1323–1334.

30. Knabb RM, Rosamond TL, Fox KAA, Sobel BE, Bergmann SR. Enhancement of salvage of reperfused ischemic myocardium by diltiazem. *J Am Coll Cardiol* 1986;8:861–871.

31. Schreiner G, Erbel R, Henkel B, Pop T, Meyer J. Improved ischemic tolerance during percutaneous coronary angioplasty (PTCA) by antianginal drugs. *Circulation* 1983;63[Suppl III]:98.

32. Serruys PW, Van den Brand M, Brower RW. Regional cardioplegic and protective effect of nifedipine during PTCA. *Circulation* 1983;68[Suppl III]:142.

33. Surgrue D, Holmes DR, Smith HC, Reeder GS, Lane GE, Vlietstra RE, Bresnahan JF, Hammes LN, Piehler JM. Coronary artery thrombus as a risk factor for acute vessel occlusion during percutaneous transluminal coronary angioplasty: improving results. *Br Heart J* 1986;56:62–66.

34. Ellis SG, Ropubin GS, King SB, Douglas JS, Weintraub WS, Thomas RG, Cos WR. Angiographic and clinical predictors of acute closure after native vessel coronary angioplasty. *Circulation* 1988;77:372–379.

35. Mabin TA, Holmes DR, Smith HC, Vliestra RE, Bove AA, Reeder GS, Chesbro JH, Bresnahan JF, Orszulak TA. Intracoronary thrombus: role in coronary occlusion complicating percutaneous transluminal coronary angioplasty. *J Am Coll Cardiol* 1985;5:198–202.

36. Lukas Laskey MA, Deutsch E, Hirshfeld JW, Kussmal WG, Barnathan E, Laskey WK. Influence of heparin therapy on percutaneous transluminal coronary angioplasty outcome in patients with coronary arterial thrombus. *Am J Cardiol* 1990;65:179–182.

37. Mooney MR, Mooney JF, Goldenberg IF, Almquist AK, Van Tassel RA. Percutaneous transluminal coronary angioplasty in the setting of large intracoronary thrombi. *Am J Cardiol* 1990;65:427–431.

38. Douglas JS, Lutz JF, Clements SD, Robinson PH, Roubin GS, Lembo NJ, King SB. Therapy of large intracoronary thrombi in candidates for percutaneous transluminal coronary angioplasty. *J Am Coll Cardiol* 1988;11:238A.

39. Lukas Laskey MA, Deutsch E, Barnathan E, Laskey WK. Influence of heparin therapy on percutaneous transluminal coronary angioplasty outcome in unstable angina pectoris. *Am J Cardiol* 1990;65:1425–1429.

40. Pow TK, Varricchione TR, Jacobs AK, Ruocco NA, Ryan TJ, Christelis EM, Faxon DP. Does pretreatment with heparin prevent abrupt closure following PTCA? *J Am Coll Cardiol* 1988;11:238A.

41. Krucoff MW, Jackson YR, Kehoe MK, Kent KM. Quantitative and qualitative ST segment monitoring during and after percutaneous transluminal coronary angioplasty. *Circulation* 1990;81[suppl IV]:IV20–IV26.

42. Bush HS, Ferguson JJ, Angelini P, Willerson JT. Twelve-lead electrocardiographic evaluation of ischemia during percutaneous transluminal coronary angioplasty and its correlation with acute reocclusion. *Am Heart J* 1991;121(6 part 1):1591–1599.

43. Klein LW, Kramer BL, Howard E, Lesch M. Incidence and clinical significance of transient creatine kinase elevations and the diagnosis of non-Q wave myocardial infarction associated with coronary angioplasty. *J Am Coll Cardiol* 1991;17:621–626.

44. Ogilby DJ, Kopelman HA, Lkein LW, Agarwal JB. Adequate heparinization during PTCA: assessment using activated clotting times. *Cathet Cardiovasc Diagnosis* 1989;18:206–209.

45. Barah N, Smith J, Baugh RF. Heparin monitoring in the coronary care unit after percutaneous transluminal coronary angioplasty. *Heart Lung* 1990;19:265–270.

46. Rath B, Bennett DH. Monitoring the effect of heparin by measurement of activated clotting time during and after percutaneous transluminal coronary angioplasty. *Br Heart J* 1990;63:18–21.

47. Cragg DR, Friedman HZ, Almany SL, Gangadharan V, Ramos RG, Levine AB, LeBeau TA, O'Neill WW. Early hospital discharge after percutaneous transluminal coronary angioplasty. *Am J Cardiol* 1989;64:1270–1274.

48. Skillman JJ, Kent KC. Arterial complications of transfemoral cardiac procedures. *Counterpulse* 1991;2:4–8.

49. Kelly JF, Patterson R, Liebeman P, et al. Radiographic contrast media studies in high-risk patients. *J Allergy Clin Immunol* 1978;62:181.

50. Lasser EC, Berry CC, Tolner LB, et al. Pretreatment with corticosteroids to alleviate reactions to intravenous contrast material. *N Engl J Med* 1987;317:845.

51. Skillman JJ, Kim D, Baim DS. Vascular complications of percutaneous femoral cardiac interventions: incidence and operative repair. *Arch Surg* 1988;123:1207–1212.

52. Oweida SW, Roubin GS, Smith RB, Salam AA. Postcatheterization vascular complications associated with percutaneous transluminal coronary angioplasty. *J Vasc Surg* 1990;12:310–315.

53. Hollman J, Gruentzig AR, Douglas JS, King SB, Ischinger T, Meier B. Acute occlusion after percutaneous transluminal coronary angioplasty—a new approach. *Circulation* 1983;68:725–732.

54. Helvie MA, Rubin JM, Silver TM, Kresowik TF. The distinction between femoral artery pseudoaneurysms and other causes of groin masses: value of duplex Doppler sonography. *Am J Roentgenol* 1988;150:1177–1180.

55. Park DD, Laramee LA, Teirstein P, Ligon RW, Giorgi LV, Hartzler GO, McCallister BD. Major complications during PTCA: an analysis of 5413 cases. *J Am Coll Cardiol* 1988;11:237A.

56. Olsen JB, Alstrup P, Madsen T. Open-heart surgery in Jehovah's Witnesses. *Scand J Thorac Cardiovasc Surg* 1990;24:165–169.

57. Currier JC, Jacobs AK, Faxon DP. Interdepartmental communication.

58. Berkseth RO, Kjellstrand CM. Radiologic contrast-induced nephropathy. *Med Clin North Am* 1984;68:351.

Practical Angioplasty,
edited by David P. Faxon.
Raven Press, Ltd., New York © 1993.

CHAPTER 5

Vascular Approaches

Nicholas Ruocco

FEMORAL APPROACH—TECHNICAL CONSIDERATIONS

With the advent of preformed Judkins catheters the vast majority of coronary angiography and angioplasty is performed from the groin approach. Thus, knowledge of the correct technique and possible risk of percutaneously accessing the femoral vessels is particularly important to any angiographers training (1–3). A clear understanding of the anatomy is the first priority (4). Figure 1 details the landmarks of the groin. In a nonobese patient the inguinal crease and the line formed between the anterior superior iliac spine and the pubic tubercle, where the inguinal ligament lies, provide reliable landmarks as to the safe area from which to access the femoral artery and vein. The recommended point of entry into the femoral vessels is approximately 2 cm above the inguinal crease, bisecting the line formed by the bony landmarks. The dangers of accessing the femoral artery too low include entering the smaller profunda femoris or superficial femoral artery, which might dissect and cause a hematoma or pseudo-aneurysm. Also, the more caudal the point of entry, the more the femoral artery and vein overlap, increasing the chances of creating an arteriovenous fistula. The major complication of accessing either vessel too high is very serious, the danger being invasion of the peritoneal cavity and exposing the patient to the risk of a large intraperitoneal bleed if adequate hemostasis is not obtained after the sheath is pulled (3,5,6).

In an obese patient, identifying the appropriate area to access can be much more difficult. External landmarks are generally misleading and tend to shift your access site falsely low. A helpful practice in this situation is to lay the Potts needle on the patient's groin at the site that appears appropriate, then to fluoroscope the groin, visu-

alizing where the tip of the needle overlaps the head of the femur (Fig. 2). The femoral vessels cross the head of the femur below the inguinal ligament at the appropriate site for access. It is important to envision the needle entering the femoral vessel approximately 1 to 2 cm superior to the point where it enters the skin, since the needle is advanced at a 45-degree angle. The other advantage of localizing access in this manner is that, when the sheaths are removed, the femoral head provides a stable support for compression of the vessel when applying pressure to obtain hemostasis (Fig. 3).

Once the access site has been identified, adequate anesthesia is paramount to patient comfort. Most of the patient's sensation comes from enervation of the skin and, therefore, the amount of superficial lidocaine is very important. After warning the patient, approximately 5 cc should be injected through a 25-gauge needle to produce a significant bleb in the patient's skin. This should be done relatively slowly since it can be painful if injected too fast. Another 5 to 10 cc should be injected, through a 21-gauge needle, into the deeper tissues surrounding the femoral vessels. The adequacy of anesthesia can then be tested by touching the #11 scalpel blade to the patient's skin prior to making the incision. If a sharp sensation is still present more lidocaine is necessary. A shallow incision is then made through the epidermis. One should avoid deep incisions, particularly in thin patients, to avoid puncturing a relatively superficial femoral artery. A hemostat is then used to form a tract through the deeper tissue in the direction that your needle will proceed. The purpose of making the tract is twofold. One is that it minimizes the resistance one will perceive as the needle is advanced towards the vessel and allows the pulsations of the artery or the "pop" of entering the vein to be perceived in the fingers. The second reason is to provide a communication to the outside should the patient bleed after sheath removal. This potentially limits the amount of occult blood that may accumulate undetected.

N. R. Ruocco: Section of Cardiology, The University Hospital, Boston University Medical Center, Boston, Massachusetts

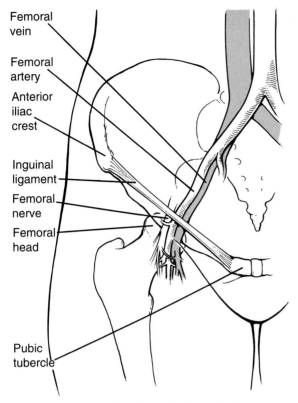

Femoral
vein

Femoral
artery

Anterior
iliac
crest

Inguinal
ligament

Femoral
nerve

Femoral
head

Pubic
tubercle

FIG. 1. The anatomy of the femoral triangle is shown, demonstrating the relationships between the femoral vein, artery, and nerve, and the inguinal ligament.

The sensation perceived in the fingers cannot be overemphasized. Although access is a visually blind procedure, it is not one without important tactile input. When accessing the vein from the right side of the patient your left index or middle finger should be on the arterial pulse. The tip of the needle is placed 1 cm medial to the pulse, parallel to the patient and advanced at a 45-degree angle. The needle should be advanced sufficiently slowly that if you feel arterial pulsations you still have not punctured the vessel and can withdraw, flush the needle and reapproach more medially. If you do puncture the artery, make sure you have excellent return before advancing the guidewire, since your approach is more medial than desired and may be in a branch vessel, or more seriously may have punctured both the artery and vein thus placing the patient at risk for an arteriovenous (AV) fistula. It is often safest to withdraw the needle, hold pressure for 5 to 10 min, and then reapproach.

Puncturing the vein should be perceived as a "pop" similar to a spinal tap. This sensation is not nearly as reliable as the arterial pulsation present when accessing the artery. Even if you do not feel a pop, the needle should be advanced until you hit bone (femoral head). A non–Luer-lok syringe should be placed on the needle and negative pressure should be applied as you withdraw. Correct access should allow vigorous blood return on aspiration. The syringe is removed and the J wire

supplied with the sheath is advanced through the needle. It is at this point that significant trauma to the vessel may occur. The wire should pass easily through the needle into the vessel. You should never push or force the wire as it is very easy to puncture a vein or dissect an artery. If the wire does not go easily, a novice should surrender the needle and allow a more experienced operator to perform some gentle manipulation, such as slight withdrawal or altering the angle of the needle. You should observe these maneuvers before attempting them for the first time. It is often possible to advance the wire atraumatically in these situations, but it is also easy for experienced hands to determine when one should surrender and start over. The first maneuver is often to just withdraw the wire and establish that you still have adequate blood return. If blood return is less than optimal it is not worth even attempting wire placement, since it will either be unsuccessful or result in a complication. Once the wire exits the needle, if there is any question about placement it is always safest to fluoroscope the wire to document appropriate position. The wire is then advanced into the vein and the needle is withdrawn while applying pressure to the groin to avoid bleeding. The sheath is then advanced over the wire. It is obviously very important to have control of the guidewire before you advance the sheath into the vein. A good 10 cm of the wire should extend beyond the sheath when the tip of the sheath is in contact with the patient. Making sure that the sheath is firmly attached to the dilator, you then smoothly and firmly advance the sheath over the wire. This is another point of potential morbidity. If there is resistance to sheath advancement and you have not fluoroscoped the wire to this point then fluoroscopy should be performed. The wire can often go retrograde atraumatically, and advancing the sheath will meet resistance that should not be present. In a patient with a history of multiple procedures, a large amount of scar tissue can cause resistance. If blood return was excellent and wire advancement and placement appropriate, then this patient may require gradual dilation with smaller dilators before the desired sheath can be placed. Any crimping of the sheath should prompt predilation with the dilator alone before attempting to pass a new sheath.

The procedure for accessing the artery is very similar in principle to accessing the vein. The most important difference is detecting arterial pulsations during needle advancement. If you are positioned correctly it is rare not to appreciate arterial pulsation prior to entering the artery. A common mistake is to advance the needle too quickly to appreciate the vessel. Access then becomes more of a random stab than a skilled maneuver. In thin females with small arteries and little connective tissue, although pulsations may be appreciated, the vessel often rolls as one advances the needle. In these cases once the arterial pulse is detected the needle may have to be advanced quickly to impale the vessel before it rolls.

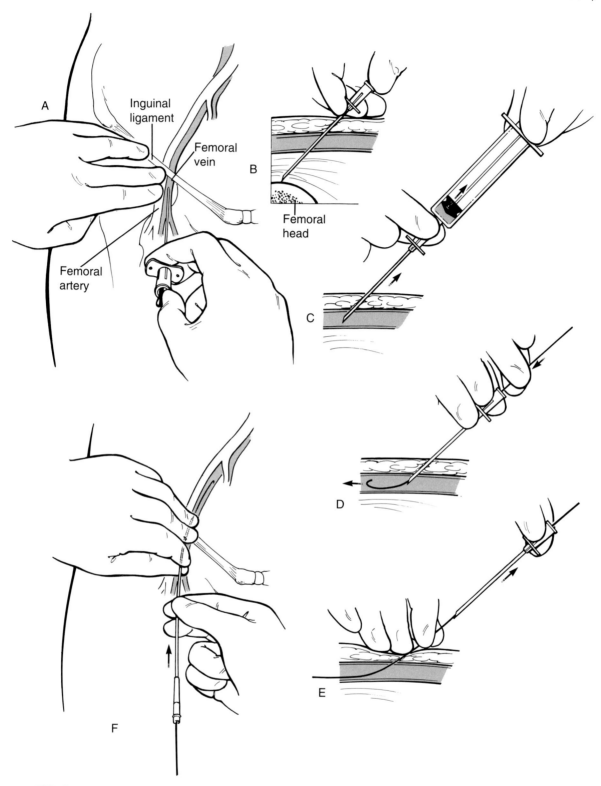

FIG. 2. The technique used to access the femoral vein (shown) or femoral artery (not shown) is illustrated. The artery is palpated at the inguinal ligament (**A**), the needle is advanced into or beyond the vessel (**B**) and the needle is aspirated for vein access only (**C**). When blood returns freely, a guidewire is advanced through the needle into the vessel (**D**), the needle is removed (**E**) and an introducer sheath and dilator are inserted over the guidewire (**F**).

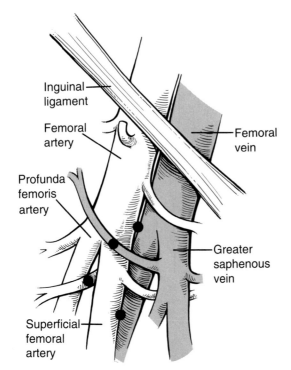

FIG. 3. The femoral artery and vein are in close proximity to one another with multiple points where branches cross. These areas indicated by a black dot can be the site of potential arteriovenous (AV) fistulas. Entry into the femoral vessels just below the inguinal ligament decreases the chance of a formation of an AV fistula.

Once the needle is freely in, the arterial lumen blood return should be vigorous. As with venous access, advancement of the wire should not even be attempted unless a good stream of blood, consistent with the patient's arterial pressure, is obtained. If there is resistance to wire advancement in the presence of good blood return, gentle manipulation by an experienced person similar to that described for venous access can be performed. The use of the short wire for arterial access is an issue with some operators. The rationale for using the 120-cm J wire is that you know early on if you are going to have difficulty advancing your catheters. Other operators prefer the short wire, since once the sheath is in place, many options are available for traversing a stenotic or tortuous aortoiliac system. It is easier and safer to change wires and catheters through a stable sheath as opposed to manipulating or exchanging a #35 wire through a needle. The downside to sheath placement with the short wire in this situation is that one might not be able to traverse the iliac and thus a sheath has been placed unnecessarily. If you anticipate this problem and downsize your sheath (5French) until you traverse the anatomy, the procedure results in minimal trauma and inconvenience to the patient and the groin holder person.

Once the sheath is placed it should be double flushed via the side arm. Proper flushing of the sheath is para-

mount in avoiding the development and embolization of thrombus. The sheaths should be flushed with each catheter exchange to avoid embolizing potential thrombus with the introduction of a new catheter.

Although severe aortoiliac disease is a contraindication to catheterization via the femoral artery, one often encounters unsuspected disease in patients with good femoral pulses. If the disease is so severe that sufficient wire cannot be advanced to allow sheath placement, or if the patient complains of significant pain while attempting to advance the wire (a sign of intimal dissection), one should withdraw the needle and hold pressure for 5 to 10 min before going to the other groin. If the wire can be advanced atraumatically for 15 to 20 cm, then the sheath can be placed and other techniques can be used to traverse the aortoiliac vessels. Before trying these techniques one should make sure that blood returns freely from the sheath. Arterial pressure is obtained by hooking the side arm on the sheath to a pressure transducer standard procedure, and comparing it to the patient's cuff pressure is a way to determine if you are dealing with a severe stenosis or occlusion, versus a tortuous vessel. Also, if blood return and pressure are adequate an injection of contrast can delineate the anatomy. With a stable sheath in place, the operator has a number of approaches available to traverse the iliac. Frequently, just switching from the standard J wire to an atraumatic Benston wire or slippery Terumo wire is successful. The Benston wire is coreless and able to traverse extremely tortuous vessels atraumatically, while the Terumo glide wire has a hydrophilic coating which makes it very slippery and able to traverse stenotic, diseased vessels. Both of these wires are usually advanced through a right Judkins coronary catheter which also allows for repositioning of the wire as one is advancing. An aggressive approach for patients with limited access is to use an .018 gauge floppy angioplasty wire guided by occasional touches of contrast, essentially using angioplasty like wire manipulation to traverse the iliac. Once the right Judkins is central, subsequent catheter exchanges should be done over an exchange wire in patients with complicated anatomy. For patients with particularly tortuous iliac vessels, it is sometimes useful to exchange the standard sheath, which is 11 cm long, for a Grüntzig sheath, which is 23 cm long. The long sheath will help straighten out the vessel, avoids renegotiating tortuous vessels, and provides some support for catheter manipulation.

Other considerations particular to sheathes include leaving them in for prolonged periods. It is not uncommon in complicated angioplasty patients to leave sheathes in overnight in order to maintain systemic anticoagulation therapy. We try to avoid durations longer than 24 hr, since morbidity directly correlates with duration. Sheathes are now available which are particularly compliant and allow the patient to elevate the head of the bed slightly without causing local trauma. In some patients, systemic anticoagulation during overnight sheath placement is associated with significant local oozing of blood. If this occurs one should first make sure that the heparin dose is within the therapeutic range. If it is, then it is sometimes effective to upsize the sheath by one French size to obtain hemostasis. Finally, if sheathes are going to stay in after a particularly long and difficult case it is common practice to administer prophylactic antibiotics until they are removed.

BRACHIAL ACCESS—TECHNICAL CONSIDERATIONS

Vascular access via brachial cut-down is a dying art. In the days when catheterization was done primarily via the arm with a Sones catheter, brachial cut-down could be done quickly and safely. Now that the procedure is done only on rare occasions in most labs, it tends to take a long time and is associated with an increased morbidity, due to inexperienced people accessing and repairing the brachial vessel. This is not to say that access via brachial artery cut-down is not a useful technique to know. On the contrary, it can often be the only available access. The issue is how to train individuals to perform a technique that is only rarely used. I think the first axiom is that if you have not done a significant number and don't feel proficient, then don't do them. The patient can always be referred to an operator or institution that has experience with the technique. If there is a person who is proficient within your institution then make the effort to assist on a number of cases and to be observed by her during your first few.

Although only a few of us continue to do brachial cut-downs, our lab does use the brachial approach frequently. With the improvement in percutaneous sheathes, the brachial artery can be accessed safely and effectively with a percutaneous approach (7,8). As in femoral access, the most important element is a good understanding of brachial anatomy and the potential complications that can occur (Fig. 4). Because the brachial compartment is smaller it cannot tolerate the small hematomas that are asymptomatic in the groin. Hematomas can lead to brachial nerve compression and damage. Other important considerations include the duration of brachial access. Overnight heparin is not uncommon after angioplasty via the femoral approach but is not an option via a percutaneous brachial approach.

The patient's arm is prepared, in the same manner as for a brachial cut-down, on an arm board with the palm up. The location for entry of the needle is approximately 2 to 3 cm above the brachial crease. After the area is anesthetized the needle is positioned at a 45-degree angle, parallel to the arterial path, which runs a little medial. It is advanced slowly in the same manner as for femoral artery access. Single-wall arterial sticks are desir-

able to lower potential bleeding complications. Once a good arterial return is obtained, a short J wire is advanced through the needle into the brachial artery. Again, the same caution used during femoral access is required for percutaneous brachial access. If there is any resistance to sheath placement the wire should be visualized using fluoroscopy to document correct positioning. Once the sheath is in place, it should be double flushed with a heparinized solution and repeatedly flushed after each catheter exchange to avoid the development of even small thrombi within the sheath. The margin for error is smaller when using the brachial approach and extra caution must be emphasized.

When using the brachial approach, catheter options are limited by which arm is used. Standard Judkins catheters can often be used from the left arm. This is not possible from the right arm and if the operator is not proficient with a Sones catheter, Amplatz catheters can be used.

HIGH-RISK PATIENTS

Peripheral Vascular Disease

The most common factor increasing the risk of vascular access and, therefore, the morbidity of cardiac catheterization is peripheral vascular disease. Indeed, lack of acceptable access is a definite, although rarely used, contraindication to cardiac catheterization. The patient population undergoing catheterization is likely to have some degree of peripheral vascular disease. It is the obligation of the angiographer to do a careful physical exam to assess the severity and extent of peripheral vascular disease prior to catheterization. This baseline evaluation will allow selection of the safest route, the one least likely to be associated with morbidity. It will also establish a baseline for comparison after the procedure so as to allow early detection of problems precipitated by the catheterization.

The evaluation clinically involves the documentation of a history of claudication or prior peripheral vascular surgery. On physical exam the intensity of all pulses should be documented, as well as the presence of bruits. Blood pressures should be taken in both arms and, if any disease is suspected in the lower extremities, in both legs. This allows comparison of an arm : leg index which is more sensitive for detecting disease than simple palpation of pulses. Also, an awareness of unequal blood pressures in a patient's upper extremities, along with possible subclavian bruits, is extremely important in patients facing coronary bypass surgery, since internal mammary arteries are commonly used today. If this situation exists, selective angiography of the innominate or left subclavian artery during catheterization is indicated, to rule out subclavian stenosis.

In the absence of any problems, the right groin is commonly the first choice for access because of the physical layout of most labs. However, if claudication is present in the patient's right leg and on physical exam there is a bruit which is not present on the left, it makes sense to do the catheterization through the left groin. Similarly, if the patient has severe peripheral vascular disease in the lower extremities, with bruits and absent pulses on physical exam, then the safest route may be via the brachial artery. With the exception of having had a recent peripheral angiography performed which is available for analysis there are no objective criteria to prohibit attempting access, even in the presence of disease. One reason for this is that, even in the absence of palpable distal pulses, the aorto-iliac-femoral system may be intact and the absent pulses due to distal disease. Therefore, in some labs the presence of a femoral pulse is all that is required to attempt femoral access. The margin for error will be smaller in these patients and the local complication rate higher. As always, one has to assess the risk to benefit ratio and to make sure the benefits of performing the catheterization and obtaining the information out weigh the potential risk. The purpose of a careful evaluation and selection of the access route is to lower this risk as much as possible.

Catheterization of Venous and Prosthetic Vascular Grafts

As indicated in the above discussion, the safest route for peripheral access should always be selected. A history of prior peripheral vascular surgery involving a femoral bypass is a relative contraindication for access. However, when necessary, and with minor modifications of standard technique, catheterization either through the vein or prosthetic vascular grafts can be done safely (9–12). When evaluating access through a graft, the same issues involving native vessels need to be assessed. The intensity of the pulse should be particularly strong in a graft with good runoff, since they tend to be superficial. The pulses and blood pressure distal to the graft should also be evaluated.

The modifications of standard technique revolve around sheath placement and removal. When placing a sheath into a prosthetic graft which is less compliant than normal tissue it is useful to gradually dilate the graft with successive dilators. If a 7 French sheath is being placed it is useful to predilate with a 6 French dilator followed by both a 7 and 8 French dilator before placing the 7 French sheath. This allows for more gradual dilation of the noncompliant graft material, and thus avoids crimping the sheath and preventing excessive compressive forces on the sheath, which might hinder guide manipulation.

Removal of a sheath from a prosthetic graft is very similar to removing it from a native vessel. However, as is sometimes recommended with a native vessel, a brief period of compression which totally eliminates the distal pulse should be avoided. The goal is to establish hemostasis while maintaining some degree of forward flow. Over a period of 15 to 20 min this pressure should be gradually withdrawn. The use of the hemostatic clamp or compressor should be avoided since they often initially result in complete occlusion of blood flow and one loses the tactile input available when the groin is held by hand.

COMPLICATIONS

Fortunately, in carefully selected patients undergoing angiography by experienced physicians, the risk of vascular complications are low. There is evidence that the likelihood of complications rises as the experience level of the operator falls, and this has led to recommendations regarding the minimum number of angiograms necessary to maintain proficiency (13). There is also evidence that as the severity of the patient's illness increases the likelihood of serious complications increases (3). These findings suggest that the sickest, most complicated patients should undergo catheterization at high-volume centers by the most experienced operators. It also suggests that the average patient can be treated safely in the community by an operator who maintains a volume of at least 50 cases a year (13).

An important aspect of any laboratory is careful attention to quality assurance. All aspects of patient care revolving around the catheterization procedure should be tracked. Indications, findings, outcome, and especially the incidence of complications compared to accepted thresholds need to be followed on a quarterly and yearly basis. This approach fosters early detection and correction of potential problems. Major vascular complications and accepted thresholds based on large series of coronary angiograms are outlined in Table 1 (3,5). Other infrequent complications include the development of arteriovenous fistula, nerve damage, and infection. Minor hematomas occur not infrequently, but major bleeding requiring transfusion should be rare. Meticulous attention to detail will minimize complications related to access, while early detection and involvement of vascular surgeons will minimize the morbidity associated with complications.

TABLE 1. *Major vascular complications and accepted thresholds for coronary angiograms*

Vascular complications	Threshold (%)
Arterial thrombosis	0.49–0.68
Arterial dissection and/or aneurysm	0.17–0.25
Embolization	0.05–0.09

REFERENCES

1. Seldinger S-I. Catheter replacement of the needle in percutaneous arteriography: a new technique. *Acta Radiol Diagn* 1953;39:368.

2. Barry WH, Levin DC, Green LG, Bettman MA, Mudge GH, Phillips D. Left heart catheterization and angiography via the percutaneous femoral approach using an arterial sheath. *Cathet Cardiovasc Diagn* 1979;5:401–409.

3. Bourassa MG, Noble J. Complication rate of coronary arteriography; a review of 5250 cases studied by a percutaneous femoral technique. *Circulation* 1976;53:106.

4. Boileau Grant JC: *Grant's atlas of anatomy.* Baltimore: Williams & Wilkins; 1972.

5. Davis K, Denedy JW, Kemp HG, Judkins MP, Gosselin AJ, Killip T. Complications of coronary arteriography from the collaborative study of coronary artery surgery (CASS). *Circulation* 1979;59:1105–1111.

6. Adams DF, Abrams LH. Complications of coronary arteriography: a follow-up report. *Cardiovasc Radiol* 1979;2:89–96.

7. Maouad J, Herbert JL, Fernandez F, Gay J. Percutaneous brachial approach using the femoral artery sheath for left heart catheterization and selective coronary angiography. *Cathet Cardiovasc Diagn* 1985;11:539–546.

8. Pepine CJ, VonGunten C, Hill JA. Percutaneous brachial catheterization using a modified sheath and new catheter system. *Cathet Cardiovasc Diagn* 1984;10:637–642.

9. Eisenbert RL, Mani RL, McDonald EJ. The complication rate of catheter angiography by direct puncture through aorto-femoral bypass grafts. *AJR Am J Roentgenol* 1976;126:814–816.

10. Wade GL, Smith DC, Mohr LL. Follow-up of 50 consecutive angiograms obtained utilizing puncture of prosthetic vascular grafts. *Radiology* 1983;146:663–664.

11. Smith, DC. Catheterization of prosthetic vascular grafts: acceptable technique [Editorial]. *AJR Am J Roentgenol* 1984;143:1117–1118.

12. Zajko AB, McLean GK, Freiman DB, Oleaga JA, Ring EJ. Percutaneous puncture of venous bypass grafts for transluminal angioplasty. *AJR Am J Roentgenol* 1981;137:799–801.

13. Pepine et al. ACC/AHA Guidelines for Cardiac Catheterization and Cardiac Catheterization Laboratories, *Circulation* 1991;84:2213–2247.

Practical Angioplasty,
edited by David P. Faxon.
Raven Press, Ltd., New York © 1993.

CHAPTER 6

Selection of Guiding Catheters

Alice K. Jacobs

Since the advent of percutaneous transluminal coronary angioplasty (PTCA), the rapid expansion in technology has resulted in a dramatic increase in the number of available guiding catheters used to perform the procedure. With various sizes and shapes of guides to choose from, it is important to select the catheter which is most likely to result in a successful procedure and least likely to result in an associated complication. This selection process should be based upon a specific set of guidelines and principles and the information obtained from the diagnostic angiogram.

FUNCTION OF THE GUIDING CATHETER

The early guides were hollow tubes made of Teflon, tended to buckle, were difficult to manipulate, and had little ability to hold a specific shape. Therefore, they functioned only as a conduit. The overall trend in guides has gone from the larger French and stiffer catheters to smaller size, softer catheters, with larger internal lumens. With the expansion and change in equipment, the basic functions of the guiding catheter have evolved. Currently, guiding catheters form an integral part of the dilatation system.

First, to perform adequately, the guiding catheter must be able to selectively engage the ostium of the coronary artery without occluding arterial inflow. Although catheter damping is less frequently an issue in the left coronary artery, it can be problematic in the ostium of the right coronary artery. The introduction of side holes in the catheter shaft which allow continuous perfusion despite wedged engagement of the catheter has provided a partial solution to this problem.

Second, the guiding catheter functions to deliver contrast agent into the coronary artery so as to visualize the target lesion as well as side branches. With the use of selective digital angiography to provide a "road-map" of the artery, guiding catheter contrast injection can be used less frequently. However, with the trend toward smaller-profile balloon dilatation catheters and fixed-wire dilatation catheters which preclude the use of distal contrast injections, guiding catheter injections are essential. The smaller balloon catheters and larger lumen guides optimize the angiography.

Perhaps the most important function of the guiding catheter is to provide adequate support for advancement of the dilatation catheter across the lesion. This support is obtained by deep engagement of the guiding catheter into the coronary ostium, buttressing of the catheter against the opposite aortic wall and from the intrinsic stiffness of the guiding catheter material. Although steerable guidewires and low-profile dilatation catheters have made guiding catheter support less critical in some situations, the expansion of the practice of PTCA to include distal lesions in tortuous and calcified vessels necessitates optimal support from the guiding catheter. The features of an ideal guiding catheter are listed in Table 1.

STRUCTURE OF THE GUIDING CATHETER

The guiding catheters consist of a shaft; a soft tip, which may be tapered; a radiopaque tip marker; and a hub which connects the catheter to the manifold system. The shaft of the catheter is composed of three layers: an inner Teflon lining to reduce friction between the guiding and the dilatation catheters; a mid-layer made of either epoxy and fiber braid, or a wire braid, to permit torque control; and an outer layer of polyethylene or polyurethane to provide stiffness and ability to retain preformed shape (memory) (1). In general, the "stiffer" the catheter, the better is the support, the faster is the torque response, and the more difficult is the deep seating in the coronary ostium. A longitudinal section of a representative guiding catheter is illustrated in Fig. 1.

A. K. Jacobs: Section of Cardiology, The University Hospital, Boston University Medical Center, Boston, Massachusetts, 02118

TABLE 1. *Ideal guiding catheter characteristics*

Easy to seat
Large lumen to deliver adequate contrast for visualization
  with multiple balloon systems
Coaxial engagement to maximize backup and flow, and to
  direct balloon into artery
Deliver accurate pressure readings
Atraumatic to coronary arteries
Small enough to subselect coronary arteries
Nonthrombogenic
Radiopaque for accurate placement
Lubricious lumen for easy balloon/wire movement
Curve retention for back-up support

TYPES OF GUIDING CATHETERS

Almost all of the coronary catheters used for diagnostic angiography (both femoral and brachial approach) are available as guiding catheters. The more commonly used catheter shapes are shown in Fig. 2. The femoral guiding catheter is 100 cm long and has a 7, 8, or 9 French outside diameter. The brachial catheter is 90 cm long and has a 9 or 8.3 French outside diameter. The inner diameter of these catheters ranges between 0.066 and 0.092 in. The soft (and occasionally tapered) tip permits larger body catheters with increased support and flow to be combined with softer tips which reduce the risk of trauma at the coronary ostium and allow deeper intubation. The guiding catheters in routine use are shown in Table 2.

Overall, there has been a trend toward reducing the size of the guiding catheters (2). The rationale for performing coronary angioplasty with smaller diameter catheters is based on the potential advantages. Smaller

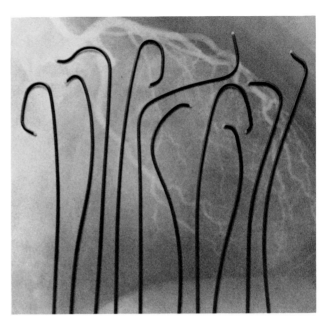

FIG. 2. The most frequently used guiding catheter curves. From left to right: left Judkins, left internal mammary, left Amplatz, left Judkins (smaller size), Arani, right bypass, left short-tip Judkins, right Judkins, hockey stick, right Amplatz.

catheters provide less pressure damping and injury to the coronary ostium, reduce the risk of vascular complications, especially in patients with peripheral vascular disease, and increase the possibility of early ambulation and hospital discharge (3). In addition, patient discomfort and arterial bleeding may be minimized due to the smaller arterial punctures. With the trend toward

TABLE 2. *Femoral guiding catheters*

Manufacturer	Available sizes			
	(Inner diameter, in)			
	9F	8F	7F	6F
ACS				
E.T. Hi-Flow		0.076		
Powerguide		0.080	0.070	
USCI				
Super 7			0.070	
Illumen - 8		0.080		
Illumen with flex guard		0.080		
Super 9	0.090			
Cordis				
XL Brite Tip		0.084		0.062
Brite Tip		0.078	0.072	
Medtronic				
Sherpa	0.092	0.079	0.070	
Giant Lumen	0.088	0.079	0.066	
Peak Flow		0.083		
SciMed				
Triguide		0.079	0.072	
Schneider				
Standard	0.080	0.076	0.063	
Visiguide		0.079		
Superflow	0.092	0.082	0.072	

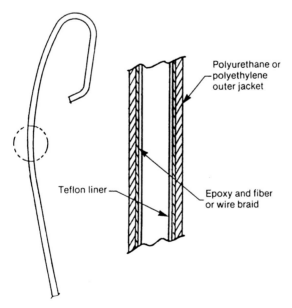

FIG. 1. Diagram of a longitudinal section of a representative guiding catheter. From Patterson et al. (7), with permission.

Polyurethane or polyethylene outer jacket

Teflon liner

Epoxy and fiber or wire braid

smaller profile balloon dilatation catheters and fixed wire systems, the use of smaller guiding catheters is a logical and feasible strategy.

The concept of using small diagnostic catheters (5 and 6 French) for PTCA was first reported in 1989 (4). In a small series (5), early success rate was relatively low (79%). More recently, Feldman and colleagues (6) reported a 94% success rate in 154 patients using 6 French (6F) guiding catheters with 0.051-in lumens and 1.5 to 3.5-mm fixed-wire balloon dilatation catheters. These small guiding catheters have overcome some of the limitations of the diagnostic catheters used as guides. Resistance along the preformed curves, which is high in diagnostic catheters, is reduced in the Teflon- or silicon-coated guide. In addition, the catheter tip is not tapered, facilitating balloon-catheter movement and balloon removal.

However, the potential disadvantages of smaller size guiding catheters must be carefully considered. The lumen of these catheters is too small to permit optimal visualization or to permit the use of specialized equipment, such as stents or bail-out catheters which are necessary to manage procedure-related complications. When using a fixed-wire system which must be changed, access to the distal vessel cannot be maintained by use of a 4 French soft probe sheath since it will not pass through a 6 French guiding catheter. The ability to measure accurate pressure as well as to provide backup support is also reduced.

CATHETER SELECTION

General Considerations

There are several major anatomic determinants of the optimal approach to the procedure (brachial or femoral artery) and thereby the optimal guiding catheter. These include the degree of rotation of the ascending aorta and valve plane, the angulation of the proximal vessel from the ascending aorta, the origin of the innominate artery on the aortic arch, and the length of the aortic arch. There are three basic anatomic variations of the plane of the aortic valve, based on the angle of the valve plane with the horizontal plane. When viewed in the 30° left anterior oblique projection of the ascending aorta, the valve plane is either 0 to 30° (type I), 30 to 60° (type II),

or 60 to 90° (type III) (7), as shown in Fig. 3. In type II and III aortas, the brachial approach may be more advantageous because of a greater likelihood of a coaxial backup with a soft Stertzer brachial guiding catheter rather than with preformed guides from the femoral approach. Rarely, the angulation of the proximal vessel from the ascending aorta will influence the decision to use the brachial approach. Superior takeoff to the right coronary artery is best handled by the brachial approach, whereas inferior takeoff of the left main trunk is better approached from the femoral artery. When the innominate artery inserts more distally on the aortic arch, such as in long-standing hypertension, the advantages of the brachial approach are negated. In general, as the length of the aortic arch increases, so does the ease of femoral coaxial guiding catheter intubation.

In general, the major advantages of the brachial approach include (i) vascular access when limited by peripheral vascular disease or previous vascular surgery, (ii) improved ability to deal with specific anatomic variants (ostial left internal mammary artery stenoses, anomalous coronary artery location), (iii) improved control at the ostium of the vessel by easier torque control from the arm, particularly in the right coronary artery, and (iv) early removal of the catheter at completion of the procedure with early ambulation and potential hospital discharge. Currently, it is estimated that approximately 10% of angioplasty procedures are either more easily performed or can only be performed via the brachial approach. Most femoral guiding catheters can be used via the brachial artery.

The selection of a specific guiding catheter should be based upon several factors, the most important of which are listed in Table 3. When studying the diagnostic angiogram, careful consideration should be given to the takeoff of the proximal coronary artery from the ascending aorta and to the relationship between the diagnostic catheter and the coronary orifice. The coronary guiding catheters in general, however, can be expected to have a more gentle curve and have a shorter tip than their diagnostic counterparts.

In addition, the size and shape of the aorta, the amount of backup support needed, the length of the left main trunk, and the location of the coronary ostium are important considerations. In general, the more dilated the aorta, the more potentially problematic adequate guide support will be. The need for backup support in-

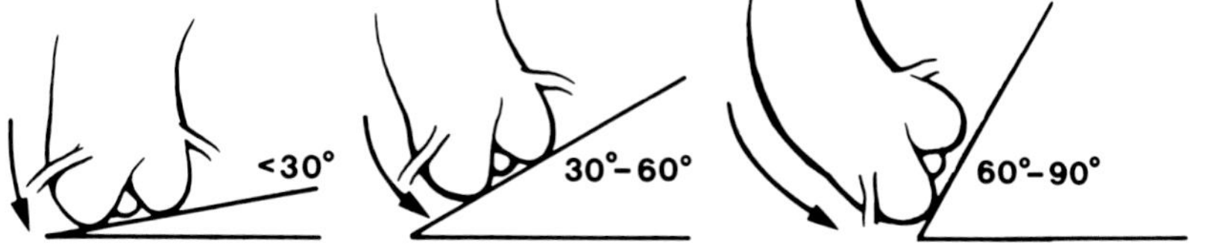

FIG. 3. Diagram of the three aortic valve plane orientations. From George et al. (7), with permission.

TABLE 3. *Guiding catheter selection factors*

Size and/or shape of aorta
Location of ostium
Angle of takeoff
Amount of backup support needed
Length of left main

creases in small, diffusely diseased vessels, calcified lesions, distal lesions, and lesions distal to vessel tortuosity. Backup support is facilitated by larger and stiffer guiding catheters. Short left main trunks enhance selective left coronary circumflex (LCX) or left anterior descending (LAD) coronary artery intubation whereas long left main trunks may necessitate Amplatz-type guides for lesions located in the left circumflex artery, depending on the angle of take-off from the aorta. Anomalous origins of the coronary ostia are best served by non–Judkins-type guides.

Insignificant ostial coronary artery lesions, particularly when not intended for dilatation, can be especially problematic. In either the right or left coronary artery, it is preferable to use smaller guiding catheters so as to decrease the chance of occluding arterial inflow. In addition, it is wise to choose a system which is less likely to require any backup support, such as a fixed-wire balloon dilatation catheter. In the right coronary artery, arterial inflow can be enhanced and pressure damping can be reduced with the addition of side holes to the shaft of the catheter. Side holes, however, impair adequate visualization. In the left coronary artery, although theoretically side holes would provide the same benefit, the risk of decreasing flow to the left coronary system despite maintaining normal guiding catheter pressure, may substantially increase the risk of the procedure. With any approach, it should be recognized that ostial lesions may significantly increase the risk of a major complication. This risk should be carefully considered when choosing angioplasty as the revascularization strategy.

Once the catheter is chosen, it is also important to manipulate the guide in the coronary ostium to ensure proper fit, position, and potential for backup support prior to moving the balloon and wire system into the coronary artery. After the wire and balloon are manipulated, if the guiding catheter easily disengages from the ostium, and the necessity of guide support is anticipated, it is appropriate to change the guiding catheter prior to crossing the lesion with the wire. Once the wire traverses the lesion, and if the guiding catheter does not provide the support necessary for the balloon catheter to cross the lesion, there are several alternatives. First, exchanging the dilatation catheter for a smaller balloon catheter with a lower profile may be effective. Second, it is possible to exchange the guiding catheter for one with a different shape, but this is technically difficult (it is best to change the balloon catheter and guiding catheter together because the smaller dilatation catheter can more effectively track the wire) and usually requires two operators. Third, the wire may be withdrawn and the entire system changed, but the chance of abrupt vessel closure (particularly in a stenosis greater than 90% ± thrombus) is increased.

Specific Considerations

Use of the Left Judkins Catheter

The left Judkins guiding catheter is most often used for PTCA of the left coronary artery. Depending on the size of the catheter and the maneuvers used, this guide can be used to approach lesions located in the LAD as well as in the LCX. To select the LAD, it is necessary to push the catheter forward in the ascending aorta, moving the secondary curve inferior and the tip superior. Once engaged in the ostium, rotation of the hub in a counterclockwise direction will direct the tip anterior and superior toward the LAD (Fig. 4). A slightly smaller catheter ($L_{3.5}$ French in a normal size root or an $L_{4.0}$ French in a dilated root) will help to orient the catheter tip toward the LAD as well (8).

The Judkins catheter, with its tip pointing superior, is not ideally suited for approach to the LCX, which is directed posterior and inferior at its bifurcation from the left main trunk. If the diagnostic study was performed with a Judkins catheter, the angiogram should be carefully reviewed with attention toward the direction of the

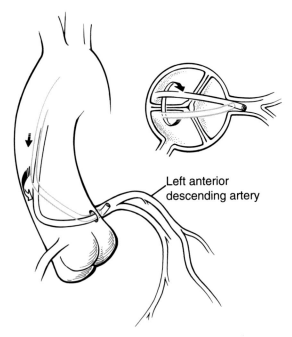

FIG. 4. Schematic view of the maneuver used to select the left anterior descending (LAD) artery with a Judkins catheter once the left main trunk is engaged. Counterclockwise rotation brings the heel of the catheter posterior and the tip anterior into the LAD.

catheter tip. To select the LCX, once the catheter is engaged in the left main trunk, it is necessary to pull the catheter back, directing the tip inferior. Rotation of the hub clockwise will direct the secondary curve anterior and the tip posterior toward the LCX ostium. A slightly larger guide (an $L_{4.5}$ for a normal size root) or a short tip Judkins guide (Fig. 5) will also facilitate movement of the tip toward the LCX. Again, it is important to remember that the tips of the guiding catheters are slightly more relaxed in curve when compared to the same size diagnostic catheter. It is also possible to deep seat (or "Amplatz") the left Judkins catheter by a clockwise hub rotation and catheter advancement over the dilatation system (Fig. 6). This maneuver will provide backup support as well as facilitate entry into the LCX.

Use of the Right Judkins Catheter

As with the use of diagnostic catheters, seating of the right Judkins guide in the ostium of the right coronary artery (RCA) is performed by advancement of the catheter over the arch followed by clockwise hub rotation, which moves the tip anterior and inferior. As the tip drops, the catheter is pulled back, while rotating to engage the ostium. The R_4 French is the most frequently used catheter; occasionally R_5 French catheters are used in a dilated aorta or in an elongated arch. The advantages of the right Judkins catheter are that it is easy to seat and broadly applicable. However, unless deeply seated within the artery, it provides poor backup support (Fig. 7). It also provides poor cannulation of a superior takeoff from the sinus of Valsalva.

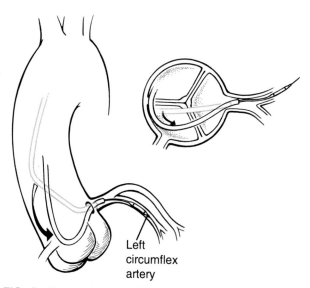

FIG. 6. Schematic view of the maneuver to "Amplatz" or selectively intubate the LCX with a Judkins guide. Once the guide is engaged in the left main trunk, clockwise rotation and advancement over the balloon dilatation system will turn the Judkins guide over into the left coronary circumflex artery.

Use of the Amplatz Catheter

The Amplatz curve can be used in the right or left coronary artery. When seated, the tip points inferiorly, making it suitable to select the LCX and to cannulate inferior takeoffs coaxially (Fig. 8). The guiding catheter

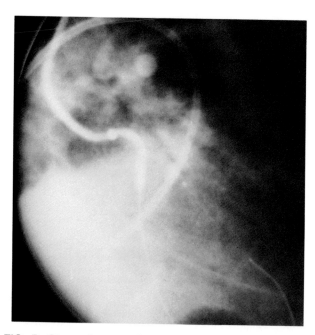

FIG. 5. Cineangiogram of a short-tip left Judkins catheter used to selectively engage the left coronary circumflex artery during PTCA.

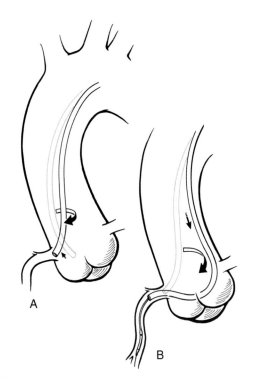

FIG. 7. Schematic view of the right Judkins guide engaged in the right coronary artery (left anterior oblique projection). Note the potential to actively intubate the proximal artery but the poor potential to buttress along the aortic wall.

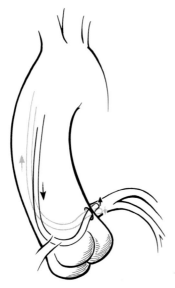

FIG. 8. Schematic view of the left Amplatz guide selectively engaged in the left coronary circumflex artery.

also has the potential to provide excellent support. The catheter is removed by advancing the shaft until the tip disengages the ostium into the aortic root. The catheter is then rotated and withdrawn. However, removal of the guiding catheter can be associated with risk; withdrawal of the catheter when the tip is engaged in the ostium facilitates movement into the coronary artery. In addition, deep intubation can create wedging and damping problems.

Technique of Deep Seating for Backup Support (Active Support)

Often, it is necessary to deep seat the guiding catheter in order to provide the necessary support (active support) to cross the lesion with the balloon dilatation catheter. This is known as "active support", whereby the guiding catheter facilitates balloon passage by advancing deeply into the coronary artery. Since this maneuver has the potential to injure the ostium of the coronary, it should be performed with soft-tip guiding catheters if possible. It is important that (i) the coronary be large enough to accept the guide, (ii) the proximal vessel be free of disease as well as excessive tortuosity, (iii) the coronary blood flow be maintained, and (iv) there be minimal resistance to the passage of the guide (9). Pressure should be monitored at the tip of the guiding catheter continuously. Pressure may damp for brief periods, but deep intubation should be performed with speed and caution. The guiding catheter should be advanced over the leading dilatation catheter to afford stabilization and tracking, in a push-pull fashion. The guidewire alone is less likely to provide support for advancement of the guiding catheter and the risk of injury to the coronary

intima would be higher. After the lesion is crossed with the balloon catheter, and following inflation of the balloon, the guide should be withdrawn. When effectively performed, deep seating of the guiding catheter provides optimal support (Fig. 9).

Buttressing the Catheter for Backup Support (Passive Support)

It is also often necessary to "bank" the guide along the opposite wall of the aorta to stabilize the catheter and provide optimal guide support (passive support with or without deep coronary intubation). This buttressing of the catheter may be facilitated by choosing a slightly oversized guide. Alternatively, a broad loop in the guid-

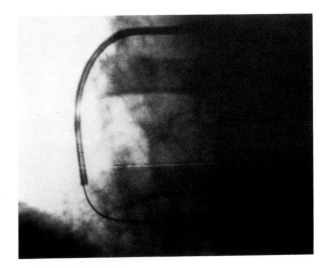

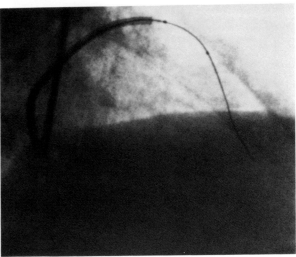

FIG. 9. Cineangiogram of active guiding catheter support. **A:** Note the deep intubation of the right coronary artery with the guiding catheter in the left anterior oblique projection. **B:** Note the deep intubation of the guiding catheter in the left anterior descending artery (over the dilating system) in the right anterior oblique projection. From George et al. (7), with permission.

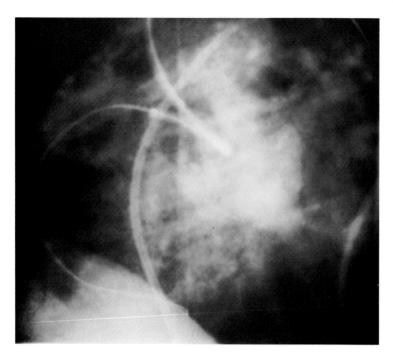

FIG. 10. Cineangiogram illustrating passive support of the guiding catheter in the right coronary artery ostium by buttressing it along the wall of the aorta.

ing catheter can be formed so as to support it against the opposite aortic wall or coronary sinuses. Once a stable loop has been formed, more pressure can be applied to the balloon catheter. This maneuver can be performed by using the Judkins (Fig. 10) or occasionally the Amplatz catheter by forceful rotation and simultaneous advancement of the guide over the dilatation catheter. However, it is more effectively performed by using a special catheter such as the Arani guide (Fig. 11).

Management of Damping

Pressure damping occurs when engagement of the guiding catheter into the ostium results in a reduction of arterial inflow. This occurs most often in the right coronary artery and in the setting of small caliber arteries or ostial lesions. If prolonged, the flow reduction can result in hypotension, bradycardia, and ventricular arrhyth-

mias. Management consists of using smaller guiding catheters (7 French), choosing a catheter with side holes to maintain coronary perfusion, and using a balloon dilatation system with a low profile so as to reduce the chance that backup support and deep seating of the guide will be necessary. If possible, once the coronary artery is instrumented with the guidewire and balloon catheter, the guiding catheter should be withdrawn and placed just outside the coronary ostium as often as possible throughout the procedure. It should be remembered, however, that pressure damping significantly increases the risk of the procedure.

APPROACH TO THE LEFT CORONARY ARTERY

The length of the left main coronary artery and the angle with which it takes off from the aorta are important factors in guiding catheter selection. The horizontal

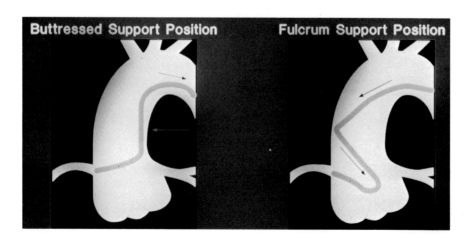

FIG. 11. Diagram of the Arani guiding catheter. Note both the fulcrum and buttress positions.

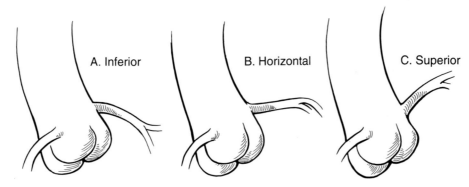

FIG. 12. A: Schematic view of an inferior takeoff of the left main trunk. **B:** Schematic view of a horizontal takeoff of the left main trunk. **C:** Schematic view of a superior takeoff of the left main trunk.

or lateral takeoff is most frequently encountered and is the least problematic (Fig. 12B). The horizontal takeoff can easily be approached with the Judkins or Amplatz guides appropriately sized for the aortic root. The Judkins guide is easy to engage and can be deep seated to provide active support. The Amplatz catheter provides excellent passive support and in a short left main, facilitates entry into the LCX. Even in a long left main where the LCX cannot be selectively cannulated, the inferior directed tip of the catheter (as opposed to the superior directed tip of the Judkins guide) is more favorable for

instrumentation of the LCX. Similarly, a short-tip left Judkins guide may be effective in this situation.

For upward takeoff of the left main coronary artery (Fig. 12C), engagement of the ostium is facilitated by using a slightly smaller Judkins catheter such as an $L_{3.5}$ French in a normal-sized root, particularly when the target lesion is located in the LAD. The most superiorly directed tip in the Judkins series is the interventional medical guiding catheter and it may be advantageous in this situation. Cannulation of a superiorly directed left main can also be accomplished with an Amplatz cath-

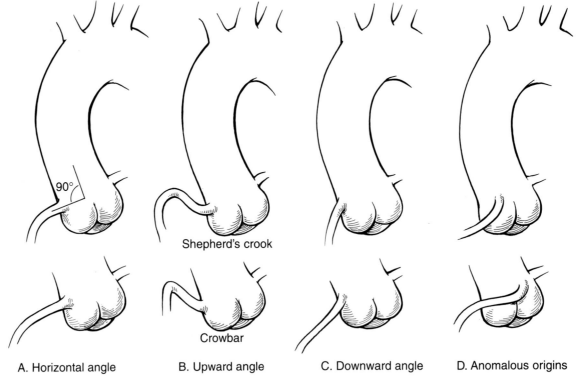

A. Horizontal angle   B. Upward angle   C. Downward angle   D. Anomalous origins

FIG. 13. A: Schematic view of a horizontal takeoff of the right coronary artery. **B:** Schematic view of an upward takeoff of the right coronary artery. Note both the ''shepherd's crook'' and ''crowbar'' configurations. **C:** Schematic view of a downward takeoff of the right coronary artery. **D:** Schematic view of an anomalous takeoff of the coronary artery.

eter, particularly if the catheter is advanced against the aortic sinus so as to allow the tip of the catheter to rise. In this situation, passive backup support may be less optimal. Superiorly directed catheter tips, such as the El Gamal (10) may be useful in this situation as well.

Inferior takeoff of the left main trunk (Fig. 12A) can be approached using an Amplatz guide (tip points inferior when engaged) or an inferiorly directed guide such as a multipurpose catheter. The latter guide, however, provides suboptimal passive backup support unless a loop is created in the catheter to buttress it against the aortic wall.

APPROACH TO THE RIGHT CORONARY ARTERY

Approach to the RCA poses a different set of problems due to the multiple variations of the RCA origins and proximal segments. Most of these problems can be managed with a wide selection of available guiding catheters (11). There are several factors which can be examined when reviewing the angiogram prior to selection of the guiding catheter. These include the size and shape of the ascending aorta, the location of the RCA orifice in the sinus of Valsalva, the degree of anterior or posterior orientation, and the location and severity of the target lesions. Perhaps the most important factor determining guiding catheter selection, however, is the angle of the origin of the RCA and the length of the proximal segment.

Horizontal Angle

The horizontal or right-angle takeoff from the sinus of Valsalva is most frequently encountered (Fig. 13A). Since the distal tip of the right Judkins catheter is directed horizontally upon engagement of the RCA ostium, there is a favorable coaxial relationship between the catheter and the proximal coronary artery. However, if backup support is necessary or if the proximal segment is long, an alternative guiding catheter curve may be required. The Judkins catheter may, however, be deeply seated in the proximal segment so as to increase its ability to provide the active support needed. The Arani 90° (Fig. 11) guiding catheter provides excellent support in this setting, from either the buttressed or fulcrum positions (12). The Amplatz catheter also provides good passive support, and various sizes are available to fit the aortic root. Both the Arani and Amplatz guides are problematic in the setting of ostial disease since they are more difficult to engage.

Upward Angle

The upward angle of takeoff (<90° from aorta) often referred to as a shepherd's crook (13) or a crowbar may

be more difficult to cannulate in a coaxial position (Fig. 13B). In this situation, a Judkins catheter is rarely effective, unless minimal guide support is required. The shepherd's crook configuration is characterized by a very short horizontal proximal segment followed by a superiorly directed segment. The guiding catheters that best cannulate the proximal segment coaxially and provide backup support necessary to negotiate the turn inferiorly within the artery are the 90° Arani and the Amplatz curves. Both catheters aggressively cannulate the ostium.

The crowbar configuration has no proximal horizontal segment and has an immediate upward takeoff. A smaller-sized Judkins catheter ($R_{3.5}$ French) may point superior, but provides little backup support. Amplatz left curves (more superior orientation than Amplatz right curves) and 75° Arani guides are both potentially effective in this situation. Occasionally left bypass graft guides or left internal mammary artery guides (14) (most superior orientation) are effective for coaxial cannulation, but they provide little backup, which is almost always necessary to transverse the turn inferiorly.

The Arani catheter is especially effective in the upward takeoff RCA (15). The double loop design permits the primary curve (75° or 90°) to be positioned either against the opposite aortic wall or against the sinus of Valsalva providing excellent backup support. The tip of the catheter may seat in the ostium or be advanced into the proximal vessel. However, the Arani is difficult to engage and aggressively cannulates the ostium.

Downward Angle

The downward takeoff (greater than 90° from the aorta) is less frequently encountered and tends to be less problematic (Fig. 13C). The downward takeoff facilitates crossing of the lesion, especially when an inferiorly oriented guiding catheter is selected. Often, the Judkins

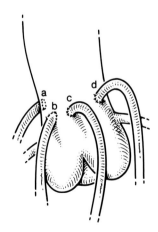

FIG. 14. Schematic view of the variable takeoff of saphenous vein grafts along the wall of the aorta. From Douglas (17), with permission.

catheter may be used, but lateral projection of the tip may be undesirable. It is sometimes possible to rotate the tip (turnover) so that it points inferiorly. However, right bypass graft, multipurpose, and right Amplatz guides all have the potential to effectively cannulate the ostium in a coaxial position due to the inferior orientation. If backup support is required, these guiding catheters need to be deeply seated, a maneuver which is usually readily performed.

Anomalous Origin

A RCA with an anomalous origin may require a significant amount of catheter manipulation prior to engaging the ostium (Fig. 13D). Origins high in the sinus (and anteriorly located) may be approached with left Amplatz curves (16). The El Gamal catheter may also be useful in this setting.

APPROACH TO CORONARY BYPASS GRAFTS

Percutaneous transluminal coronary angioplasty of conduit lesions (left internal mammary artery and saphenous vein graft) is associated with technical considerations similar to those of native coronary artery angioplasty. It is important to engage the ostium of the graft with as much coaxial alignment as possible and with a guiding catheter shape that will provide enough support to reach the lesion with the dilatation system through the long graft.

In general, saphenous vein bypass grafts have a variable and less predictable location on the aorta than the native arteries (Fig. 14) (17). Several guiding catheters have the potential to be effective, and the selection of the guide is most dependent upon the angle with which the vein meets the aorta.

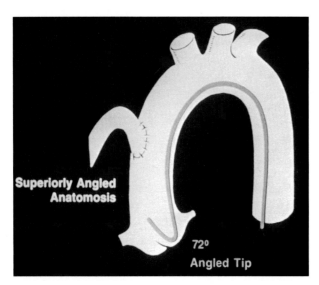

FIG. 15. Diagram of an El Gamal guide used to approach a superior takeoff of a saphenous vein graft.

Horizontal takeoff grafts can be approached with right venous bypass or right Amplatz guides. Superior takeoff is most easily cannulated with an El Gamal (Fig. 15), left venous bypass, left Amplatz or multipurpose guiding catheter. Inferior takeoff can be approached with a right Judkins, right bypass, or small right Amplatz catheter.

During PTCA of the left internal mammary artery, special care should be taken to avoid trauma to the fragile origin of the artery. Using the femoral or ipsilateral brachial approach, successful cannulation of the ostium is usually achieved with a left internal mammary artery guiding catheter.

REFERENCES

1. Patterson JA, Tilkian AG. Coronary angioplasty. In: Tilkian AG, Dailey EK, eds. *Cardiovascular procedures: diagnostic techniques and therapeutic procedures.* St. Louis, MO: CV Mosby; 1986: 328–378.
2. Kern MJ. Small-diameter guiding catheters for coronary angioplasty. Cardio Intervention 1992;20–24.
3. Kern MJ, Talley JD, Deligonul U, et al. Preliminary experience with 5 and 6 French diagnostic catheters as guiding catheters for coronary angioplasty. *Cathet Cardiovasc Diagn* 1991;22:60–63.
4. Salinger MH, Kern MJ. First use of a 5 French diagnostic catheter as a guiding catheter for percutaneous transluminal coronary angioplasty. *Cathet Cardiovasc Diagn* 1989;18:276–278.
5. Kern MJ, Cohen M, Talley JD, et al. Early amubation after 5 French diagnostic cardiac catheterization: results of a multicenter trial. *J Am Coll Cardiol* 1990;15:1475–1483.
6. Feldman R, Glemser E, Kaizer J, Standley M. Coronary angioplasty using new 6 French guiding catheters. *Cathet Cardiovasc Diagn* 1991;23:93–99.
7. George BS, Stertzer SH. Brachial technique to intervention. In: Topol EJ, ed. *Textbook of interventional cardiology.* Philadelphia: WB Saunders; 1990:515–534.
8. Baim DS. Percutaneous transluminal coronary angioplasty—analysis of unsuccessful procedures as a guide toward improved results. *Cardiovasc Intervent Radiol* 1992;5:186.
9. Carr ML. The use of the guiding catheters in coronary angioplasty: the technique of manipulating catheters to obtain the necessary power to cross tight coronary stenoses. *Cathet Cardiovasc Diagn* 1986;12:189–197.
10. El Gamal MIH, Bonnier JJRM, Michels HR, van Gelder LM. Improved success rate of percutaneous transluminal graft and coronary angioplasty with the El Gamal guiding catheter. *Cathet Cardiovasc Diagn* 1985;11:89–96.
11. Myler RK, Boucher RA, Cumberland DC, Stertzer SH. Guiding catheter selection for right coronary artery angioplasty. *Cathet Cardiovasc Diagn* 1990;19:58–67.
12. Arani DT. A new catheter for angioplasty of the right coronary artery and aorto-coronary bypass grafts. *Cathet Cardiovasc Diagn* 1985;11:647–653.
13. Gossman DE, Tuzcu EM, Simpfendorfer C, Beck GJ. Percutaneous transluminal angioplasty for shepherd's crook right coronary artery stenosis. *Cathet Cardiovasc Diagn* 1988;15:189–191.
14. Kulick DL. Use of the internal mammary artery guiding catheter for percutaneous transluminal coronary angioplasty of the Shepperd's crook right coronary artery. *Cathet Cardiovasc Diagn* 1989;16:190–192.
15. Arani DT, Bunnell IL, Visco JP, Conley JG. Double loop guiding catheter: a primary catheter for angioplasty of the right coronary artery. *Cathet Cardiovasc Diagn* 1988;15:125–131.
16. Mooss AN, Heintz MH. Percutaneous transluminal angioplasty of anomalous right coronary artery. *Cathet Cardiovasc Diagn* 1989;16:16–18.
17. Douglas JS Jr. Angioplasty of saphenous vein and internal mammary artery bypass grafts. In: Topol EJ, ed. *Textbook of interventional cardiology.* Philadelphia: WB Saunders; 1990;327–343.

Practical Angioplasty,
edited by David P. Faxon.
Raven Press, Ltd., New York © 1993.

CHAPTER 7

Selection of Balloon Catheters and Guidewires

David P. Faxon

INTRODUCTION

The growth of angioplasty, its improved success and the reduction in complications can be in large part attributed to the development of improved angioplasty catheters, guidewires, and guiding catheters. The initial fixed guidewire systems had unacceptable profiles given today's standards. In addition they were minimally directable and manipulation of the balloon catheter required aggressive rotation of the guiding catheter. While dramatic improvements in catheters have occurred, the understanding of the selection and use of the balloon catheter, guidewire, and guiding catheter is essentially in achieving a successful dilation and is as important today as it was when the procedure initially began. This chapter will discuss balloon catheters and guidewires but will also integrate the use of guiding catheters where appropriate. The extremely rapid developments in new catheters and the competitive commercial environment make it impossible for all of the data in this chapter to be completely up to date.

BALLOON CATHETER SYSTEMS

Fundamentals of Construction

Most coronary angioplasty balloons are made of four materials: polyvinyl, polyolelin copolymers, polyethylene, or polyethylene terphthalate (PET) (1). The balloon materials have distinctive inflation characteristics, ranging from moderately compliant with polyvinyl to least compliant with the PET material (Table 1). In addition to variations in compliance, the various balloons achieve a nominal size (e.g., 3.0 mm) at different inflation pressures. These two aspects are very important in the use, as

well as the choice, of balloon catheters (2). Figure 1 shows the reported compliances for various balloon catheters and illustrates the differences in performance (3–5). For instance, with a 3.0-mm PET balloon (e.g., USCI sprint) the nominal pressure to achieve 3.0 mm is 5 atmospheres, while at 10 atmospheres of pressure the diameter is only 3.16 mm. In contrast, a polyolelin catheter (e.g., SciMed skinny) has a nominal inflation pressure of 7 atmospheres increasing to 3.29 mm in diameter at 10 atmospheres. While this compliance characteristic can be used to upsize a balloon catheter by as much as 0.24 mm without the need to change to a larger balloon, it also can present potential problems. In a rigid stenosis that requires a high pressure to dilate, a compliant balloon will "dog bone" around the stenosis increasing its size proximal and distal to the stenosis, thus potentially overstretching and dissecting the adjacent normal vessel wall. In this setting an initial choice of a noncompliant balloon material would be advantageous. In addition, some investigators have reported that PET conforms better to angulated lesions, and one recent report suggests a lower dissection rate as a consequence (6). However, these observations are anecdotal and a clear clinical difference has not yet been demonstrated.

Another important characteristic of balloon material is profile, a characteristic that is independent of the catheter construction as well as balloon materials. Table I lists the deflated profiles of many of the currently available catheters. In general, the smaller the profile the easier it will be to pass a high-grade stenosis. However, other factors such as pushability and tractability also play important roles in crossing a severe stenosis. If the stenosis is not severe (e.g., <70%), then the profile is not a significant factor since the minimal lumen diameter in this circumstance is 0.8 or 0.9 mm, considerably bigger than the profile of most balloon catheters. A recent report indicated that deflated balloon profiles reported by the manufacturers are not always accurate and that the method of measurement is not uniform (7). In addition,

D. P. Faxon: Section of Cardiology, The University Hospital, Boston University Medical Center, Boston, MA 02118

TABLE 1. Physical characteristics of balloon catheters

Over-the-Wire Systems

Product	Company	Shaft diameter	Balloon Profile (inches) 1.5	2.0	2.5	3.0	3.5	4.0	Balloon material	Nominal size	Coating	Maximum guidewire	Lumen design	Rated burst (atm)	Marker placement
ACS OMEGA™	ACS®	2.9–3.0F	.022	.023	.025	.028	.030	.034	PE600®	6	MICROGLIDE®	.010	Coaxial	8	Middle
ACS PRISM™	ACS®	3.3F	.029	.031	.032	.034	.035	.037	PE600®	6	MICROGLIDE®	.014	Coaxial	8	Middle
ACS SPECTRUM™	ACS	3.3F	.033	.034	.036	.037	—	—	PE	12	MICROGLIDE	.014	Coaxial	18	Middle
ACS TEN™ .010	ACS	2.8F	.024	.026	.027	.028	.030	.033	PE600	6	MICROGLIDE	.010	Coaxial	8	Middle
HARTZLER ACX®	ACS	3.4–3.7F	—	.031	.032	.035	.037	.038	PE600	6	MICROGLIDE	.014	Coaxial	8	Middle
HARTZLER ACX II®	ACS	3.3F	.029	.031	.032	.034	.035	.037	PE600	6	MICROGLIDE	.014	Coaxial	8	Middle
PINKERTON™ .018	ACS	3.6F	.034	.035	.037	.039	.040	.042	PE600	6	MICROGLIDE	.018	Coaxial	6	Middle
SULP II®	ACS	3.7F	—	.037	.044	.047	.051	.054	PE	6	MICROGLIDE	.014	Coaxial	6	Middle
INTREPID™	BAXTER®	3.2–3.5F	Not commercially released						POC	6	MDX Silicon™	.018	Coaxial	8–9.3	Middle
SLINKY™	BAXTER	3.0–3.2F	—	.028	.031	.032	.036	—	POC	6	MDX Silicon	.014	Coaxial	6–9	Middle
HELIX™	CORDIS®	3.0–3.5F	—	.031	.031	.032	.033	.035	DURALYN	6–8	None	.018	Coaxial	8	Middle
NITECH SLIDER™	Mansfield®	2.9F	—	.029	.033	.035	.039	—	HDPE	6	GLIDECOAT™	.014	Dual	10–12	Middle
SLIDER™ .014	Mansfield	3.4F	—	.029	.033	.035	.039	.040	PE	6	GLIDECOAT	.014	Triple	10	Middle
SLIDER™ .018	Mansfield	3.4F	—	.032	.035	.039	.041	.044	HDPE	6	GLIDECOAT	.018	Triple	10	Middle
SLIDER ST™	Mansfield	2.7F	—	.029	.033	.035	.039	—	HDPE	6	GLIDECOAT	.014	Triple	10–12	Middle
14 K™	Medtronic®	2.8F	Not commercially released						PE	5	ENHANCE™	.014	Coaxial	N/C/R	Middle
THRUFLEX II™/18K™	Medtronic	3.5F	—	.034	.038	.042	.048	—	PE	5	ENHANCE	.018	Coaxial	6	Middle
MICROSOFT TRAC®	Schneider®	4.3F	.031	.034	.036	.038	.042	.046	PET	4	Silicon	.014	Coaxial	16	Middle
MICROSOFT TRAC® XLP™	Schneider	3.0–3.5F	.025	.027	.029	.031	.034	—	PET	10	EXPRESSCOAT™	.014	Coaxial	16	Middle
MIRAGE™	SCIMED®	2.9–3.8F	.032	.034	.035	.038	.040	.044	POC	6	XTRA™	.018	Coaxial	8–10	Middle
SHADOW™	SCIMED	2.7–3.5F	.030	.031	.033	.037	.039	.042	POC	6	XTRA	.014	Coaxial	8–10	Middle
SKINNY™ .014	SCIMED	2.7–3.5F	.027	.031	.033	.037	.040	.042	POC	8	XTRA	.014	Coaxial	9–10	Middle
SKINNY™ .018/MVP	SCIMED	2.7–3.5F	.031	.034	.037	.039	.040	.044	POC	8	XTRA	.018	Coaxial	9–10	Middle
STRONG™	SCIMED	4.3F	—	.036	.038	.043	—	—	POC	6–7	None	.014	Coaxial	11.6–12.2	Middle
FORCE™/MINI-PROFILE™	USCI®	3.5F	—	.031	.033	.035	.037	—	PET	5	PRO/PEL™	.018	Dual	9	Middle
PROFILE PLUS™	USCI	4.3F	—	.033	.038	.039	.040	.041	PET	5	None	.018	Dual	5	Middle
SOLO™	USCI	3.0F	—	.029	.030	.032	.034	.036	PET	5	PRO/PEL	.014	D & O	12	Middle
SPRINT™	USCI	3.5F	—	.031	.033	.035	.037	.039	PET	5	PRO/PEL	.018	Coaxial	8	Middle

Integrated Systems

Device	Mfr	Shaft (F)							Material		Coating	Guidewire	Design		Location
HARTZLER EXCEL®	ACS	2.9F	—	.023	.024	.029	—		PE600	6	MICROGLIDE	N/A	fixed wire	8	Middle
HARTZLER LPS®	ACS	3.5F	.026	.026	.032	.033	.038		PE600	6	MICROGLIDE	N/A	fixed wire	8	Middle
HARTZLER MICRO 600 S®	ACS	3.0F	.025	.025	.027	.039	.031		PE600	6	MICROGLIDE	N/A	semi-movable	8	Middle
HARTZLER MICRO II®	ACS	3.7F	.033	.035	.042	.045	.050		PE	6	MICROGLIDE	N/A	semi-movable	8	Middle
SLALOM™	ACS	1.9–2.5F	—	.023	.025	.029	—		PE600	6	MICROGLIDE	N/A	fixed wire	8	Middle
ORION™	Cordis	2.4F	—	.028	.028	.030	—		Duralyn	8	XTRA	N/A	fixed wire	12	Middle
ACE™	SCIMED	1.8F	—	.022	.030	.032	.036		POC	7	None	N/A	fixed wire	8	Proximal
DGW™ (1.5 mm)	SCIMED	1.7F	.018	—	—	—	—		POC	7	None	N/A	Coaxial	10	N/A
PROBE III™	USCI	1.7F	—	.019	.021	.026	—		PET	5	None	N/A	fixed wire	10.6	Proximal

Rapid Exchange Systems

Device	Mfr	Shaft (F)							Material		Coating	Guidewire	Design		Location
ACS RX® .014	ACS	3.3F	—	.032	.034	.037	.039	.041	PE600	6	MICROGLIDE	.014	Modified D	8	Middle
ACS RX® .018	ACS	3.7F	.034	.035	.038	.040	.042	.046	PE600	6	MICROGLIDE	.018	Modified D	8	Middle
ACS RX ALPHA® .014	ACS	2.3–3.3F	.029	.030	.031	.033	.034	.035	PE600	6	MICROGLIDE	.014	Modified D	8	Middle
ACS RX ALPHA® .018	ACS	2.3–3.7F	—	.034	.035	.037	.038	.039	PE600	6	MICROGLIDE	.018	Modified D	8	Middle
ACS RX STREAK™ .014	ACS	2.3–3.3F	.029	.030	.031	.033	.034	.035	PE600	6	MICROGLIDE	.014	Modified D	8	Middle
PICCOLINO FORTE™	Schneider	3.0–3.2F	.025	.027	.028	.031	.034	.036	PET	10–12	EXPRESSCOAT	.014	Coaxial	16	Middle
EXPRESS™	SCIMED	1.8–2.7/3.0F	.028	.029	.031	.035	.039	.040	POC	6	XTRA	.014	Coaxial	8–10	Middle

Perfusion Systems

Device	Mfr	Shaft (F)							Material		Coating	Guidewire	Design		Location
ACS RX PERFUSION™	ACS	3.7–4.2F	—	—	.054	.055	.056	.059	PE600	6	MICROGLIDE	.018	Dual	8	M/D/P
STACK 40-S™	ACS	3.9F	—	—	.052	.053	.054	.055	PE600	6	MICROGLIDE	.018	Dual	8	M/D/P
STACK PERFUSION®	ACS	3.9–4.5F	—	.056	.057	.058	.060	.062	PE600	6	MICROGLIDE	.018	Dual	8	M/D/P

Long and Short Balloons

Device	Mfr	Shaft (F)							Material		Coating	Guidewire	Design		Location
HARTZLER ACX II®-L&S	ACS	3.3F	—	.031	.032	.034	.035	.037	PE600	6	MICROGLIDE	.014	Coaxial	8	Middle
PINKERTON™-L&S	ACS	3.6F	—	.035	.037	.039	.040	.042	PE600	6	MICROGLIDE	.018	Coaxial	8	Middle
STACK® LONG-25 mm balloon	ACS	3.9–4.5F	—	—	.057	.058	.060	.062	PE600	6	MICROGLIDE	.018	Dual	8	M/D/P
SULP II®-L&S	ACS	3.7F	—	.037	.044	.047	.051	.054	PE	6	MICROGLIDE	.014	Coaxial	6	Middle
LONG SKINNY™	SCIMED	3.2–3.5F	—	.031	.034	.038	.040	.044	POC	8	XTRA	.014	Coaxial	9–10	Middle
LPS™	USCI	4.3F	—	.039	.047	.050	.051	.053	PVC	5	None	.018	Dual	5	Middle

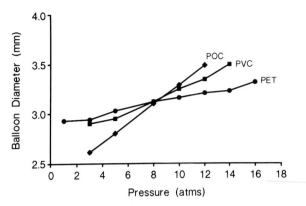

FIG. 1. Typical balloon compliance characteristics for a 3-mm angioplasty balloon. Polyolelin copolymer (POC) has the greatest change in the balloon diameter over a range of inflation pressures. While polyethylene terphthalate (PET) has the least, and polyvinyl chloride (PUC) has intermediate characteristics.

profiles can change significantly once the balloon is inflated as some balloon materials do not readily refold down to a minimal size. This is particularly true for the PET material. In order to facilitate profiles, some catheters such as the USCI sprint or probe are packaged with a small tube which is used to further reduce the profile of the catheter following debubbling. More recently balloon catheters have been made with memory in order to allow the balloon to return to the optimal deflated profile (e.g., ACS sprint).

The stiffness and size of the shaft, as well as the shaft material, influence the pushability and trackability of the catheter. The shaft is often extruded to include numerous lumens, one for the balloon lumen, one for a through lumen for the guidewire, and, in some settings, an additional lumen for perfusion or a stiffening wire. Catheters can also be made in a coaxial form (tube in a tube) where the central lumen serves as the wire lumen and the intermediate lumen serves as a balloon inflation lumen. The pushability can be further increased by the fabrication of the catheter and the use of stiffer plastic polymers. In addition, use of stiffening guidewires braids or stainless steel reinforcement have also been effective in increasing the stiffness of the catheter shaft, for example, the Stack perfusion catheter, (stiffening wires), the Medtronic Thruflex (braids and coils), and the ACS Rx alpha (stainless steel reinforcement).

Trackability is the force required to push a catheter through a tortuous vessel. It is a difficult aspect of balloon catheter performance to measure since it depends upon shaft size and flexibility, the friction against the atherosclerotic vessel wall, the balloon profile, and pushability. Recently, most manufacturers have developed coatings for their balloon catheters to reduce friction. These coatings are usually made of silicon or a similar material (e.g., microglide for the ACS catheter, propel

for USCI). Bench testing indicates a 30% reduction in friction with coatings (3).

Types of Balloon Catheters

There are four basic types of catheters: Over-the-wire, fixed-wire, monorails, and perfusion catheters (Figs. 2–6). In addition, there are a series of specialty balloon catheters for use in unusual circumstances. Each type of catheter has particular advantages and disadvantages, as listed in Table 2.

Although fixed-wire systems are the oldest catheter type, they have been completely redesigned and do not resemble their ancestors. The catheters most commonly used of this type are the USCI probe, the SciMed ACE, and ACS Slalom. The catheters are constructed with an inner guidewire that extends through the balloon catheter and beyond for a length of 2 to 2.5 cm (Fig. 2). The guidewire at the tip is usually intermediate in flexibility, ranging in size from 0.014 to 0.016 in, and the balloon is mounted directly on the outer shaft. The profile of these catheters is significantly smaller than that of the over-the-wire catheter systems (0.020—0.036 in). This smaller profile permits passage through a tighter stenosis than can be achieved with over-the-wire systems. In addition, the smaller shaft allows them to be placed into smaller guiding catheters, including the recently developed 6 French guiding catheters (8). In standard 8 French guiding angioplasty guiding catheters, the small

TABLE 2. Advantages and disadvantages of various balloon catheter types

Advantages	Disadvantages
Fixed-wire Systems	
Small profile	Cannot easily be exchanged
Excellent visualization	Fixed guidewire at tip
Conform well to bends	Wire movement less
Easier to use	responsive than
	independent wires
Over-the-Wire Systems	
Larger selection of balloons	Larger profile
Exchange easier	Poorer visualization
Can measure pressure	More complicated to use
gradient	than fixed wire
Distal contrast injection	
possible	
Can use a variety of	
guidewires	
Monorail Systems	
Rapid lesion access	Back-bleeding
Rapid exchange	Wire and balloon can tangle
Improved visualization	
Improved pushability	

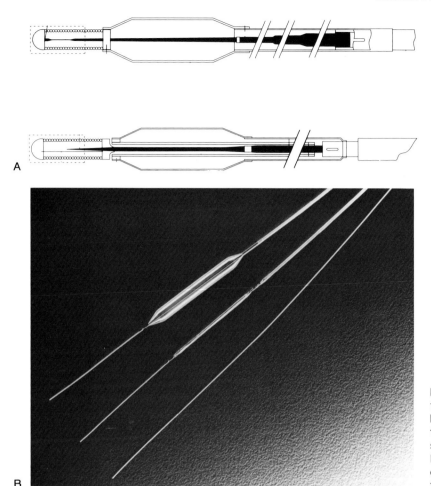

A

B

FIG. 2. Fixed-wire catheters have a central fixed guidewire that extends beyond the balloon and is attached proximally and distally to the catheter shaft. **A:** Two examples of construction, the SciMed ACE (*top*) and the USCI-Probe (*bottom*). **B:** The USCI-Probe inflated and deflated in comparison with a 0.14-in guidewire to illustrate its low profile.

profile of these catheters result in superb contrast injections and coronary visualization. One particular advantage of the fixed-wire systems is the ease with which bifurcation lesions can be dilated. Often they are coupled with one over-the-wire system in order to allow more flexibility in balloon catheter choice, as well as to permit upsizing if necessary. The disadvantages of fixed-wire catheter systems is that they cannot be easily exchanged for a larger balloon size without the necessity of recrossing the vessel. Alternatively, the balloon can be left across the stenosis and another fixed wire system passed alongside it, down into the stenosis, with removal of the initial balloon. This, however, is more cumbersome than the usual exchange process described later in this chapter. In general, however, straightforward lesions can be easily dilated with a fixed-wire system and can often be recrossed without limitations if upsizing is necessary. One alternative to exchanging with a fixed-wire system is the use of a 5 French probe sheath. Prior to introduction into the guide the fixed-wire catheter is placed within the probe sheath and extends beyond the tip. Once dilation has occurred the probe sheath can be passed through the stenosis using the fixed-wire system as a guidewire. If exchange is necessary, repassage of a larger balloon cath-

eter can be done without removal of the sheath. However, the probe sheath adds significant rigidity to the catheter and it can often kink in the exchange process. For this reason it is not routinely used. In addition, it needs to be placed over the balloon catheter prior to its insertion, making preprocedural planning important. Another limitation of fixed-wire systems is that they are less steerable and manipulatable than an independent guidewire. Finally, the 2.5-cm length to the wire beyond the tip of the balloon can often pose problems in small vessels where there is not enough room to park the tip of the guidewire while placing the balloon within the stenosis. Despite these limitations, fixed-wire systems continue to be frequently used and constitute 12% of current catheter sales (ACS, personal communications). The most commonly used balloon type is the over-the-wire catheter system. There are seven manufacturers currently in the United States, and the balloon sizes range from 1.5 to 4 mm in diameter, with a balloon length ranging from 15 to 40 mm (Fig. 3). The primary advantage of over-the-wire systems is their flexibility in the choice of guidewires and balloon sizes and types. The independent movement of both the guidewire and balloon permit enhanced tractability around tortuous

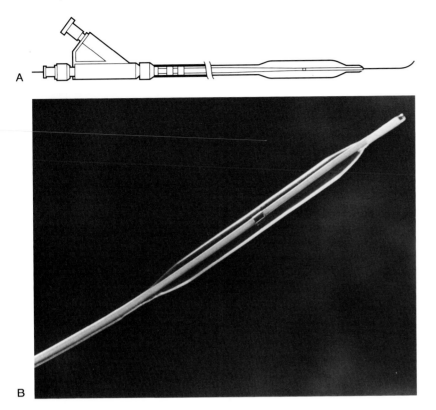

A

B

FIG. 3. Over-the-wire systems have a central lumen to allow independent movement of the wire. Various sizes and constructions are shown in Table 3. **A:** Typical balloon catheter design. **B:** ACS ACX catheter.

turns, using the so-called "push-pull" technique described later. The larger lumen also allows for distal pressure measurements and contrast injections in certain catheters (e.g., ACS Pinkerton). This may be particularly useful in approaching chronic total occlusions, where distal dye injections can assure that there is proper placement of the wire and balloon within the lumen prior to angioplasty. The major disadvantages include the somewhat cumbersome exchange process, and the difficulty in visualization due to the larger shaft of the catheter which is necessary to accommodate a central guidewire. Also, the large shaft size limits the use of two balloon catheters simultaneously for bifurcation lesions unless extremely large lumen guiding catheters (e.g., Schneider 9F superflow) (0.092-in ID) are used. The balloon profile, material, trackability, and pushability are important in selection of over-the-wire systems. The details of these factors have been previously discussed (Table 1).

Monorails were first introduced by Doctor Bonzel in Europe and have since been introduced in the United States by a number of manufacturers (9). They are rapidly gaining popularity and now comprise 40% of the angioplasty market. They possess some of the characteristics of both the fixed-wire and over-the-wire systems. The distal 17 to 25 cm of the catheter has a central lumen, but this lumen exits the catheter so that the wire and shaft of the catheter are separate (Fig. 4). This permits a smaller catheter shaft, and consequently there is a larger guiding catheter lumen for injecting contrast medium and improving visibility. In addition, the smaller

shaft can be strengthened, permitting better pushability. The distal end of the catheter, where the central guidewire is placed, is similar in most aspects to the over-the-wire system and permits good tracking of the balloon over the guidewire. The main advantages of the monorail system are rapid lesion access, maximum visualization by use of a bare-wire approach, the ability to rapidly exchange the balloon, and improved pushability and trackability. Exchange can be easily done by pulling the catheter back to the entry point into the guiding catheter and then, by holding the guidewire, gradually removing the portion of the catheter with the central lumen (Fig. 5). Since the central lumen section is shorter than the length of the guidewire, addition of an exchange wire or an add-on wire is not necessary. It also permits very rapid advancement of the catheter, since the guidewire can be externally fixed in one hand while the balloon is pushed rapidly with the other. Some manufacturers have provided a peel-away central lumen which allows the guidewire to be pulled away from the catheter up to the balloon itself, further facilitating removal by shortening the distance to the catheter tip. This rapid exchange system is of some advantage when exchange of balloon catheters is anticipated, for instance, when dilating tandem lesions that require separate balloons of different sizes. It is also useful if one cannot accurately measure the diameter of the vessel prior to dilation and, therefore, exchange is anticipated. However, since the guidewire exits the back-bleeding device at the hub of the guiding catheter, wire movement is only possible when the

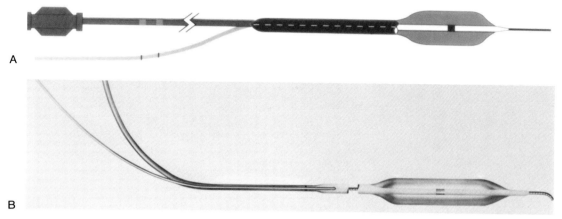

FIG. 4. The monorail systems are similar to the over-the-wire systems except that the guidewire exits the catheter 15 to 20 cm distal to the tip, a feature allowing for rapid exchange of the catheter. **A:** Design of the catheter showing the tapering of the shaft after the wire exits the catheter. The smaller more proximal shaft facilitates contrast injections during angioplasty. **B:** Exterior appearance of the monorail catheters.

adapter is open. This results in back-bleeding of blood and inaccurate measurement of blood pressure during wire motion. However, this is considered only a minor inconvenience by most operators.

Perfusion balloon catheters are over-the-wire or monorail systems that have larger central lumens with 10 proximal and 4 distal side holes to permit passage of blood through the distal end of the catheter (Fig. 6). Passive perfusion occurs during balloon inflation. With the ACS Stack perfusion balloon catheter, blood flow is approximately 60 cc/min at a blood pressure of 80 mmHg (10). Since blood flow is dependent upon blood pressure, use of these catheters in hypotensive patients may not supply a sufficient amount of blood to the ischemic territory to prevent myocardial ischemia. To achieve a large enough lumen, the profile of these catheters is the largest of all over-the-wire systems (0.053 to 0.067 mm), and the tip is significantly longer than a standard balloon catheter in order to permit sufficient side holes for perfusion.

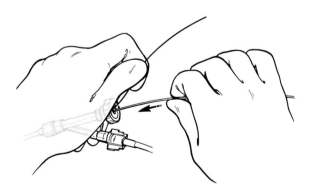

FIG. 5. Exchange of the monorail catheter can easily be accomplished by holding the guidewire in place with one hand, while advancing and withdrawing the catheter with the other. Exchange can take place without fluroscopy, eliminating radiation exposure.

In addition, the tip often has a separate wire marker which also increases the profile of the distal tip. These factors severely limit the use of these balloon catheters to proximal stenoses in large vessels. As a result, most operators use perfusion balloon catheters as a bail-out catheter for the treatment of abrupt closure or significant dissections. Currently, smaller diameter perfusion balloon catheters with shorter tips are under development and should be available shortly. One such catheter is the ACS Stack 40-S catheter which is smaller in profile (0.052–0.055 in); however, it provides only 40 cc/min of blood perfusion at a blood pressure of 80 mmHg. This may in fact be sufficient in smaller vessels. The use of prolonged balloon inflations in order to prevent or treat coronary dissections, as well as to prevent restenosis, has undergone considerable recent investigation. Anecdotal studies have demonstrated that the Stack perfusion balloon can reduce the incidence of significant dissections requiring surgery by from 50% to 70% (11). In one recently published randomized trial of perfusion balloon angioplasty versus routinely angioplasty, a 15-min perfusion balloon inflation significantly reduced the initial incidence of dissection. However, overall there was no difference in success rate nor in the incidence of subsequent restenosis (12).

Specialty catheters also include long balloons (30–40 mm in length), angled balloons, and short balloons (10 cm). The latter two are infrequently used today but were developed primarily to prevent dissection in lesions on severe bends or extremely discrete lesions. The long balloon catheters however have been shown to be helpful in long diffuse coronary disease (e.g., >2 cm) (13). Long and diffuse disease has been associated with a two- to four-fold increase in the risk of dissection and abrupt closure (14). Several recent studies suggest that long balloons can significantly reduce this dissection rate from

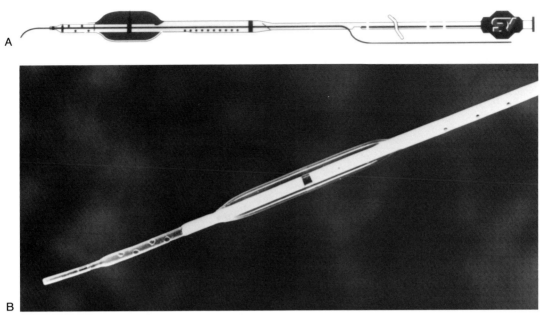

FIG. 6. Perfusion catheters allow passage of the blood to occur during balloon inflation through small holes proximal to the balloon and distal to the balloon. The need for four distal holes results in a longer tip extension beyond the balloon and a larger shaft of the catheter. **A:** The construction of currently available perfusion balloons. The catheter design can be a monorail design as shown or an over-the-wire design. **B:** An example of a Stack perfusion balloon catheter demonstrating the side holes.

18% to 9% while maintaining a high overall success rate of 90% to 95% (15).

Guidewires

Proper selection of guidewires is as important as balloon catheter selection. It needs to be integrated with the balloon catheter used as well as the lesion and vessel anatomy attempted. The guidewire is composed of three main elements: a central core wire, a shaping ribbon, and an outer spring coil (Fig. 7). The central core usually does not extend to the tip and is tapered to allow gradual decrease in wire stiffness. The shaping rhythm extends from the central core to the tip of the spring wire and is welded to the tip, both to allow shaping of the tip and also to prevent separation of the tip from the shaft of the wire. The coil is sometimes graduated in size, and the spacing between the coils can also be altered to change the stiffness of the wire. These aspects impart varying degrees of stiffness, torqueability, and shapeability to the guidewires. Most guidewires are also coated with silicon or Teflon to facilitate passage through the balloon catheter and coronary vessels.

Guidewires range in diameter from 0.10 to 0.18 in. The larger guidewires are stiffer, and more torqueable and tractable than smaller guidewires. Most current systems utilize a 0.14-in wire. The ACS 10 system is a specially designed balloon and guidewire system that utilizes a 0.010-in guidewire. The wires are 175 cm in

length, except for exchange wires which are 300 cm in length. Most standard wires are extendible, with a separate wire which is attached to the distal end in order to extend the length of the wire to the length of an exchange wire (e.g., 320 cm). The USCI system employees a distal hypotube with a crimped wire that is inserted into the hypotube. The extension wire is slightly larger than the primary wire and this can create some resistance in exchanging low profile balloons. The ACS Doc system is similar to the hypotube system made by USCI except that the hypotube is contained on the wire that is added to the primary wire. The ACS wire is slightly smaller than the USCI wire and often passes through low profile balloons and new interventional devices with greater ease.

Another difference between the USCI and ACS systems is that the distal 25 cm of the USCI wire is radiopaque, compared to only 3 cm of the ACS guidewire. However, the ACS system can be specially ordered to have a longer opaque segment. The wire stiffness is likewise variable. The very flexible or hyperflex wire from USCI or the high torque floppy wire from ACS are soft at the tip, and this allows for less traumatic passing of the guidewire through the coronary artery. However, because of the increased softness they are likewise less steerable. One exception is the 0.018-in high-torque floppy that has both flexibility and steerability but can only be used in a few balloon catheters due to its size. The mostly commonly used wires are intermediate in stiffness and include the flexwire by USCI or the Hi-

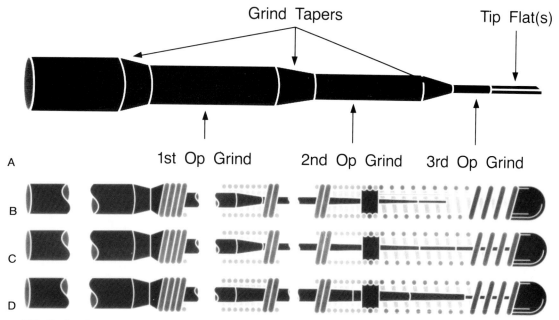

FIG. 7. A guidewire is composed of a coiled spring wire over a central wire that is gradually tapered to the tip (**A**). If the central core does not extend to the tip, a shaping ribbon extends from the core to the end of the spring wire (**B**). This type of construction results in a soft-tipped wire. If the core wire does extend to the tip, the degree of taper can influence the wire stiffness ranging from moderately stiff (**C**) to very stiff (**D**).

torque intermediate wire by ACS. These wires are intermediate in both torque control and stiffness and thus are the workhorses for most operators. The stiff guidewires are the steerable USCI or the high-torque standard by ACS. The increased stiffness is achieved by extending the core wire to the tip. While increased torque control is achieved, the increased stiffness does increase the risk of trauma to the vessel. The stiffest wire is the USCI 0.16-in standard guidewire. We reserve this guidewire for failures of the 0.014-in guidewires and primarily restrict it to vessels that are chronically totally occluded. A disadvantage of the standard steerable wires are that they tend to hold their shape less well and require frequent reshaping if extreme bends on the tip of the wire are necessary. A general rule of thumb is that a soft, very flexible wire will be able to negotiate one 90° turn. A wire with stiffness in the mid range will be able to negotiate a 90° turn and a 45° turn, and only the stiff steerable wires will be able to negotiate two 90° turns. The one exception to this rule is a very large and undiseased vessel where floppy and flexible wires often work quite well in negotiating tortuosity.

SELECTION AND USE OF BALLOON CATHETERS

General Considerations

One of the most important aspect of balloon selection is the detailed review of the cineangiogram prior to be-

ginning the procedure. The anticipated position of the guiding catheter in the coronary ostium, the type and flexibility of the guide, and the size and tortuosity of the vessels leading to the stenosis need to be carefully assessed, as well as to lesion morphology and distal vessel anatomy. The devising of a predilation strategy is best done by review of the cine film prior to the case and is often less optimally done on-line in the catheterization lab, despite the availability of high-resolution video or digital road mapping. In straightforward cases, decision can usually be made in the lab, with a high success rate. However, in more complex cases a careful review is necessary. One alternative is to develop the cineangiograms while the patient is still in the catheterization lab and to review the films prior to initiating the procedure. It is a good practice to use one type of balloon, wire, and guide for routine cases as the staff and physicians become extremely well versed in the strengths and weaknesses of a particular balloon catheter system.

In the selection of a balloon catheter it is our general practice to chose a balloon that closely approximates the adjacent nondiseased segment of the vessel. This may be difficult if the vessel tapers or has no clearly normal segment. It is also difficult to size the balloon properly at a bifurcation point, since the distal vessel is often considerably smaller than the proximal lesion. Our practice is to average the proximal and distal segments and to measure these carefully on the angiogram using a digital caliper system. Alternatively, measurements can be made with digital angiography on-line in order to properly size the

TABLE 3. *Dimensions of balloons and guide*

Balloon name	Max OD		Device outer											
	(French)	(Inch)	.022	.023	.024	.026	.030	.031	.032	.033	.035	.036	.038	.039
USCI Probe-III (2.0 mm–2.5 mm)	1.7	.022	.050	.051	.052	.054	.058	.059	.060	.061	.063	.064	.066	.067
ACE (1.5–2.0 mm)	1.8	.023	.051	.052	.053	.055	.059	.060	.061	.062	.064	.065	.067	.068
Long ACE (2.0 mm)	1.8	.024	.052	.053	.054	.056	.060	.061	.062	.063	.065	.066	.068	.069
USCI Probe-III (3.0 mm)	2.0	.026	.054	.055	.056	.058	.062	.063	.064	.065	.067	.068	.070	.071
ACE (2.5 mm)	2.3	.030	.058	.059	.060	.062	.066	.067	.068	.069	.071	.072	.074	.075
Orion	2.4	.031	.059	.060	.061	.063	.067	.068	.069	.070	.072	.073	.075	.076
ACE (3.0 mm), Long ACE (2.5 mm)	2.5	.032	.060	.061	.062	.064	.068	.069	.070	.071	.073	.074	.076	.077
Slalom	2.5	.033	.061	.062	.063	.065	.069	.070	.071	.072	.074	.075	.077	.078
Slider-ST (2.0 mm–3.0 mm), Express (1.5 mm–3.0 mm), Long ACE (3.0 mm)	2.7	.035	.063	.064	.065	.067	.071	.072	.073	.074	.076	.077	.079	.080
Ten, ACE (4.0 mm), Cobra-10	2.8	.036	.064	.065	.066	.068	.072	.073	.074	.075	.077	.078	.080	.081
Excel, Omega (1.5 mm–3.5 mm), NiTech (2.0 mm–3.0 mm), 14K (1.5 mm–3.0 mm), F-14 (1.5 mm–3.0 mm)	2.9	.038	.066	.067	.068	.070	.074	.075	.076	.077	.079	.080	.082	.083
Cobra-14 (1.5 mm-3.0 mm), Express (3.5 mm), F-14 (3.5 mm), Long ACE (3.5 mm), Micro-600, NiTech (3.5 mm), Omega (4.0 mm), Slider-ST (3.5 mm), Solo	3.0	.039	.067	.068	.069	.071	.075	.076	.077	.078	.080	.081	.083	.084
F-14 (4.0 mm), Express (4.0 mm)	3.1	.040	.068	.069	.070	.072	.076	.077	.078	.079	.081	.082	.084	.085
14K (3.5 mm)	3.2	.041	.069	.070	.071	.073	.077	.078	.079	.080	.082	.083	.085	.086
Reach-14, Slinky, Cobra-14 (3.5 mm–4.0 mm), Piccolino & Forte	3.2	.042	.070	.071	.072	.074	.078	.079	.080	.081	.083	.084	.086	.087
ACX-II, Prism, Long-Prism, RX-Alpha .014″, RX-.014″, Streak	3.3	.043	.071	.072	.073	.075	.079	.080	.081	.082	.084	.085	.087	.088
Synergy, Slider, .014″ & Slider .018″ (2.0 mm–3.5 mm)	3.4	.044	.072	.073	.074	.076	.080	.081	.082	.083	.085	.086	.088	.089
Slider-.014″ (4.0 mm)	3.5	.045	.073	.074	.075	.077	.081	.082	.083	.084	.086	.087	.089	.090
Intrepid, Helix, 18K, MVP, Skinny, Long Skinny, XLP, Sprint, Force	3.5	.046	.074	.075	.076	.078	.082	.083	.084	.085	.087	.088	.090	.091
Pinkerton, Mirage (P-18), Shadow (P-14)	3.6	.047	.075	.076	.077	.079	.083	.084	.085	.086	.088	.089	.091	.092
Long ACX, RX-Alpha-.018″, RX-.018″, Slider .018″ (4.0 mm)	3.7	.048	.076	.077	.078	.080	.084	.085	.086	.087	.089	.090	.092	.093

Shaded region indicates incompatibility with all guide catheters.

for determining balloon combinations

diameter in inches

.040	.041	.042	.043	.044	.045	.046	.047	.048	.052	.053	.054	.055	.056	.059	.060	.062
.068	.069	.070	.071	.072	.073	.074	.075	.076	.080	.081	.082	.083	.084	.087	.088	.090
.069	.070	.071	.072	.073	.074	.075	.076	.077	.081	.082	.083	.084	.085	.088	.089	.091
.070	.071	.072	.073	.074	.075	.076	.077	.078	.082	.083	.084	.085	.086	.089	.090	.092
.072	.073	.074	.075	.076	.077	.078	.079	.080	.084	.085	.086	.087	.088	.091	.092	.094
.076	.077	.078	.079	.080	.081	.082	.083	.084	.088	.089	.090	.091	.092	.095	.096	.098
.077	.078	.079	.080	.081	.082	.083	.084	.085	.089	.090	.091	.092	.093	.096	.097	.099
.078	.079	.080	.081	.082	.083	.084	.085	.086	.090	.091	.092	.093	.094	.097	.098	.100
.079	.080	.081	.082	.083	.084	.085	.086	.087	.091	.092	.093	.094	.095	.098	.099	.101
.081	.082	.083	.084	.085	.086	.087	.088	.089	.093	.094	.095	.096	.097	.100	.101	.103
.082	.083	.084	.085	.086	.087	.088	.089	.090	.094	.095	.096	.097	.098	.101	.102	.104
.084	.085	.086	.087	.088	.089	.090	.091	.092	.096	.097	.098	.099	.100	.103	.104	.106
.085	.086	.087	.088	.089	.090	.091	.092	.093	.097	.098	.099	.100	.101	.104	.105	.107
.086	.087	.088	.089	.090	.091	.092	.093	.094	.098	.099	.100	.101	.102	.105	.106	.108
.087	.088	.089	.090	.091	.092	.093	.094	.095	.099	.100	.101	.102	.103	.106	.107	.109
.088	.089	.090	.091	.092	.093	.094	.095	.096	.100	.101	.102	.103	.104	.107	.108	.110
.089	.090	.091	.092	.093	.094	.095	.096	.097	.101	.102	.103	.104	.105	.108	.109	.111
.090	.091	.092	.093	.094	.095	.096	.097	.098	.102	.103	.104	.105	.106	.109	.110	.112
.091	.092	.093	.094	.095	.096	.097	.098	.099	.103	.104	.105	.106	.107	.110	.111	.113
.092	.093	.094	.095	.096	.097	.098	.099	.100	.104	.105	.106	.107	.108	.111	.112	.114
.093	.094	.095	.096	.097	.098	.099	.100	.101	.105	.106	.107	.108	.109	.112	.113	.115
.094	.095	.096	.097	.098	.099	.100	.101	.102	.106	.107	.108	.109	.110	.113	.114	.116

TABLE 3.

Balloon name	Max OD (French)	(Inch)	.022	.023	.024	.026	.030	.031	.032	.033	.035	.036	Device outer .038	.039
Stack 40-S (2.5 mm)	4.0	.052	.080	.081	.082	.084	.088	.089	.090	.091	.093	.094	.096	.097
Stack 40-S (3.0 mm)	4.1	.053	.081	.082	.083	.085	.089	.090	.091	.092	.094	.095	.097	.098
Stack 40-S (3.5 mm)	4.2	.054	.082	.083	.084	.086	.090	.091	.092	.093	.095	.096	.098	.099
RX Perfusion (2.5 mm–3.0 mm), Stack 40-S (4.0 mm)	4.2	.055	.083	.084	.085	.087	.091	.092	.093	.094	.096	.097	.099	.100
RX Perfusion (3.5 mm)	4.3	.056	.084	.085	.086	.088	.092	.093	.094	.095	.097	.098	.100	.101
RX Perfusion (4.0 mm), Stack Perfusion (2.0 mm–3.0 mm)	4.5	.059	.087	.088	.089	.091	.095	.096	.097	.098	.100	.101	.103	.104
Stack Perfusion (3.5 mm)	4.6	.060	.088	.089	.090	.092	.096	.097	.098	.099	.101	.102	.104	.105
Stack Perfusion (4.0 mm)	4.8	.062	.090	.091	.092	.094	.098	.099	.100	.101	.103	.104	.106	.107

Guide	ID.	Guide	ID.	Guide
ACS PowerGuide 8F	.080″	Cordis Brite-tip 8F	.079″	Medtronic Sherpa 8F
Baxter Marathon 7F	.070″	Cordis Brite-tip XL 8F	.084″	Medtronic Sherpa 9F
Baxter Marathon 8F	.079″	Medtronic Sherpa 6F	.054″	Medtronic Sherpa 10F
Cordis Brite-tip 7F	.072″	Medtronic Sherpa 7F	.072″	Medtronic PeakFlo 8F

balloon catheter. The absence of careful measurement of the vessel size results in use of multiple balloons and significantly increases the cost of the procedure. We try to size the balloon catheter so that the ratio between the balloon diameter and the vessel diameter is 1:1 to 1:1.2. In an effort to optimize the match between the balloon and the vessel diameters one should have a full selection of balloon catheters with size increments of 0.25 mm. When working between two balloon sizes, we usually round up to the next quarter size since the balloon is often not fully expanded at usual dilating pressures. An exception to this rule is in settings where the lesion is in a extreme bend, where undersizing may be desirable. A moderately compliant balloon material allows further adjustment of the balloon size by taking advantage of the change in balloon diameter at high pressures and obviates the need for a balloon exchange. However, as previously mentioned, if the stenosis is heavily calcified inflation of a compliant balloon can result in "dog boning" around the stenosis.

Setup

The balloon are packaged sterile and instructions on preparation are included. Most systems use an aspiration preparation. The ACS ACX system and Stack are prepared using a positive preparation system. This is best done by mixing equal volumes of x-ray contrast medium and saline in a beaker and then drawing up 20 cc of the mixture in a 50-cc syringe. Negative pressure is applied directly to the hub of the balloon lumen for 1 to 2 min. A double negative preparation, which involves aspiration for 30 sec, release of pressure, and then reaspiration can also help reduce the size of the residual air bubble seen after an aspiration prep. The ACS positive preparation system is done by attaching the inflation device directly to the balloon and inflating up to 6 atmospheres. The tip of the balloon is held so that the distal lumen faces the ceiling and gradually the column of contrast is seen to enter the balloon and to expel the air through a small hole at the tip of the balloon. Pressure is continued until a small drop of contrast is evident or until 30 sec have passed, at which time the balloon is placed on neutral pressure. One disadvantage of a positive preparation is that the balloon is distended prior to its use in the patient; this alters the profile of the balloon, as well as changing the size of the balloon if the balloon material is compliant. Studies have demonstrated that the balloon size can change as much as 0.002–0.003 mm (7). Newer catheters such as the ACX Verbatum system have balloons that are molded to fold back to their previous shape and avoid the formation of wings, which characterize some balloon materials. Most commonly, balloons are prepared by the angioplasty assistant or a technician during the early stages of the angioplasty procedure,

Continued.

diameter in inches

.040	.041	.042	.043	.044	.045	.046	.047	.048	.052	.053	.054	.055	.056	.059	.060	.062
.098	.099	.100	.101	.102	.103	.104	.105	.106	.110	.111	.112	.113	.114	.117	.118	.120
.099	.100	.101	.102	.103	.104	.105	.106	.107	.111	.112	.113	.114	.115	.118	.119	.121
.100	.101	.102	.103	.104	.105	.106	.107	.108	.112	.113	.114	.115	.116	.119	.120	.122
.101	.102	.103	.104	.105	.106	.107	.108	.109	.113	.114	.115	.116	.117	.120	.121	.123
.102	.103	.104	.105	.106	.107	.108	.109	.110	.114	.115	.116	.117	.118	.121	.122	.124
.105	.106	.107	.108	.109	.110	.111	.112	.113	.117	.118	.119	.120	.121	.124	.125	.127
.106	.107	.108	.109	.110	.111	.112	.113	.114	.118	.119	.120	.121	.122	.125	.126	.128
.108	.109	.110	.111	.112	.113	.114	.115	.116	.120	.121	.122	.123	.124	.127	.128	.130

ID.	Guide	ID.	Guide	ID.
.079″	Schn. SoftTip 8F	.076″	Schn. SuperFlow 10F	.107″
.092″	Schn. VisiGuide 8F	.079″	USCI Super-7	.070″
.108″	Schn. SuperFlow 8F	.082″	USCI Illumen-8	.080″
.083″	Schn. SuperFlow 9F	.091″	USCI Super-9	.092″

when access and screening angiography views are obtained.

Manipulation

Angioplasty operators manipulate the equipment, using either a single- or double-operator technique. In the single-operator technique the primary operator manipulates the guiding catheter, the balloon catheter and the guidewire. The secondary operator assists in contrast injection and balloon inflation. In a double-operator technique the manipulation is divided between two operators. Usually the operator closest to the catheter entry site manipulates the guiding catheter and balloon catheter while the second operator manipulates the guidewire. This latter technique requires greater coordination between the two operators in order to avoid the inadvertent movement of one of the three components. However, the single operator technique is more difficult to learn as one needs to become facile in moving two and three components of the system simultaneously.

When using the over-the-wire or monorail systems, the guidewire is initially passed with a balloon up to the tip of the guiding catheter. Proper guiding catheter position and stability are important prior to initially crossing the lesion. The guidewire should be moved slowly forward using a still video image or digitized image as a road map. Intermittent contrast injections guide in correct passage of the wire down the vessel and through the stenosis. The use of biplane imaging or frequent movement of the imaging tube for optimal working positions in orthogonal views is also advantageous. The feel and torqueability of the various wires must be learned in order to understand when undue pressure is being placed on the wire and vascular damage can occur. Jerking or darting motions are usually not helpful. Instead careful, slow torqueing and forward motion of the wire is most effective. Many operators move the guidewire by holding the end of the balloon catheter and moving the torqueing device to within 2 to 3 cm of the end of the back-bleeding device and then reposition the torqueing device again back on the wire each time the wire is moved forward. An alternative technique, less frequently used, is to torque the guidewire with the right hand while moving the balloon catheter through the guiding catheter with the left in order to advance the guidewire. Prior to insertion, the distal tip of the wire should be bent in order to approximate the turns necessary to traverse the vessel proximal to the lesion, as well as to cross the lesion. If these angles differ greatly, then it is best to chose an angle that is halfway between the largest and smallest angle. Too great a turn at the tip of the wire can make passage difficult, as the wire will undoubtedly select most of the side branches proximal to the lesion. On the other hand, too small a bend may make it difficult to selectively choose the branch that needs to be assessed. For instance if there is a sharp 90° turn between the left main and the circumflex, a 90° turn will help in accessing the circumflex. However, if the lesion is concentric, then the 90° bend will make it difficult to pass through the stenosis. In this setting, a 45° bend may be optimal for both.

Once the guidewire is past the stenosis, it then should be moved to as distal a position as possible. In general, the wire should be passed at least one full balloon length beyond the lesion, or approximately 2 to 3 cm. It is best to leave the wire in the largest vessel or the vessel that you would want to salvage if a severe propagating dissection occurred. Small side branches should be avoided as these often can cause ectopy and can inadvertently bend the wire. The balloon should then be passed over the guidewire by holding the guidewire stationary, and the balloon should be on negative pressure as it advances over the guidewire into the stenosis. Again, contrast injections can facilitate proper placement. Often use of the stiffer balloon catheter causes injection of the balloon catheter from the ostium of the coronary artery and, if this occurs, the guidewire should be immediately pulled over the balloon catheter to reinsert it into a firm, stabilized position. With the balloon catheter in the coronary artery, the chance of dissecting the coronary artery, even with aggressive intubation of the coronary artery, is much less likely; but aggressive intubation should only be done if necessary to establish a firm guiding position. Care clearly needs to be made in this maneuver if the vessel tapers significantly or has proximal disease that might be inadvertently dissected by the guidewire. Once the balloon is passed into the stenosis the guidewire should then be removed to a safe and less occlusive position, if it was advanced to obtain stability. The balloon is then inflated and various inflation strategies have been used by various operators. In general most operators inflate the balloon to 2 atmospheres in order to determine that it is properly placed within the stenosis by visualization of a dumbbell. Pressure is gradually increased then to a minimal inflation pressure, namely 4 atmospheres, and then increased to the nominal pressure for the balloon size, most often 6 atmospheres. Balloon inflation times on average range from 60 to 90 sec, but longer inflations may be possible when good collaterals exist or when one is dilating a chronic total occlusion. It is currently unclear whether longer inflations result in an improved angioplasty result. More than one inflation is necessary to minimize elastic recoil. The balloon should be reinflated if there is any defect in the balloon, or if a mild defect occurs after the balloon is reinflated at very low pressure, as these signs indicate that some degree of stenosis or elastic recoil still exists. After each balloon inflation, contrast injections can help identify the change in stenosis. However, if the balloon is partially obstructing the artery and good visualization is not possible, then

the balloon should be removed and optimal views obtained in order to access the success of the procedure. We routinely obtain repeat angiographic views with the guidewire across the stenosis but the balloon withdrawn into the guiding catheter; if these views show a residual stenosis of 20% or less, without the occurrence of an intimal tear, then the guidewire is removed and the view is again repeated. It is important to repeat the views following the guidewire removal since the guidewire can partially stent significant dissections which may not be visible with it in place.

Special Anatomical Situations

Bifurcation Lesions

A detailed description of the technique for approaching and dilating bifurcation lesions is contained in Chapter 9. This situation demands careful planning in the choice of equipment. While initially bifurcation lesions were approached using two separate guiding catheters and balloon catheters, the larger lumen guiding catheters (0.80- to 0.94-in ID) will accommodate two low-profile balloon catheters. A chart of potential balloon combinations is shown in Table 3. Three potential combinations are possible: two fixed-wire systems, two over-the-wire systems or monorails, or one fixed wire and one over-the-wire. As with single lesions, the fixed-wire and monorails offer the advantages of better steerability and easier upsizing or exchange if necessary. Bifurcation lesions are associated with an increased risk of abrupt closure and dissection, and the safety of a guidewire across the lesion is an advantage. However, fixed-wire systems are easy to use and greatly speed up the time of the procedure. Thus the use of a fixed-wire system in a relatively easy straightforward lesion and an over-the-wire system in a more complex lesion are most common. The need for a double wire depends upon the takeoff and the size of the side branch. Two balloons can be inflated simultaneously if the proximal vessel is of large enough size, and the two distal vessels are at least one-third smaller than the proximal. More often, however, each individual lesion is dilated separately. If the side branch itself is not diseased and does not arise directly out of the stenosis, then it has been our practice not to place the guidewire in the side branch unless flow is reduced following initial dilation of the primary lesion. In order to be ready for this possibility a double back-bleeding device needs to be used.

Tandem Lesions

If the tandem lesions are located close to one another then a long balloon (3–4 cm) is advantageous. If the stenoses are separated by more than 4 cm, then it is advisable to dilate the proximal lesion before the distal lesion in order to provide continuous flow to the proximal lesion while the distal is being dilated. An alternative strategy is to use two balloons, one for the proximal lesion and one for the distal, where both are inflated at the same time. This is a particularly advantageous strategy when using fixed-wire systems, since multiple recrossing of the lesions is not necessary.

Heavily Calcified Lesions

Very low profile balloons facilitate passes through heavily calcified lesions; however, because of the high pressures required (e.g., 12–25 atmospheres) high-pressure balloon catheters should be used. The USCI probe offers a balance between very low profile and relatively high pressure tolerances. However, when even higher pressures may be anticipated, the use of a SciMed Strong balloon or other high pressure balloons that can be inflated to 20 atmospheres may be necessary.

Total Occlusions

A detailed description to the approach to total occlusions is contained in Chapter 10.

Diffuse Disease

Diffuse disease is most commonly defined as presentation of a 2-cm long segment showing at least 50% narrowing. These lesions have a significantly higher risk of abrupt closure and dissection, as well as restenosis, than discrete lesions. The use of long balloons can significantly improve the success relative to complications. Alternatively, devices such as the rotoblater and excimer laser have been used effectively in this setting.

Very Large Vessels

Two different techniques have been used to tackle this problem. First, large peripheral angioplasty balloon catheters (5–7 mm in diameter) can be used to dilate straight, large vessels, particularly saphenous vein grafts. However, their flexibility and trackability are less than optimal, and an alternative technique of "kissing balloons" can be used effectively. Here, two balloons are inflated simultaneously in a fashion similar to that used in a bifurcation lesion. One disadvantage of the technique is that the two balloons result in a twice diameter in one direction but one diameter change in the other resulting in asymmetric dilations of the artery. Despite

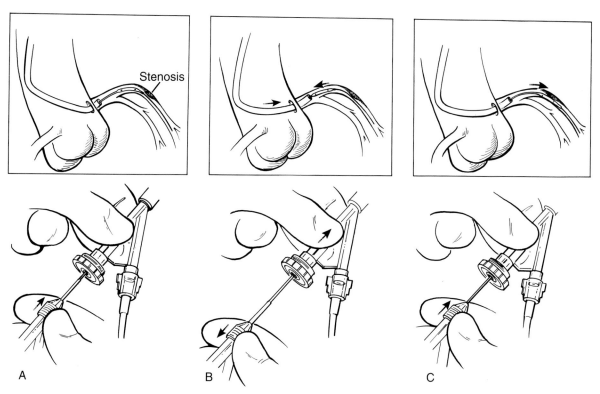

FIG. 8. The push-pull maneuver is illustrated. In order to provide a firm guide position when attempting to cross a severe stenosis (**A**), the guide is advanced over the balloon while pulling gently on the balloon (**B**). This will pull the guiding catheter into the coronary artery. Then, holding the guide catheter firmly in place, the balloon can be further pushed through the stenosis (**C**).

this, however, the technique is usually effective when encountering this situation.

Catheter and/or Wire Manipulation

Push-Pull Technique

Passage of the balloon through a tortuous vessel or tight stenosis can often be difficult. In this setting the guiding catheter should be pulled into the coronary ostium over the balloon and wire by placing slight tension on the balloon catheter and gently pushing forward the guiding catheter. Then, by holding the guiding catheter in place, the balloon can be moved forward while gently pulling back on the guidewire. Gradual intubation of the guiding catheter down the coronary artery and into a

firm, stable position can be sequentially done until the proper amount of force is achieved in order to cross the lesion (Fig. 8).

Wire Shaping

The tip of the guidewire should be reshaped to the size and the degree necessary to negotiate the stenosis (Fig. 9). This can be done by using a hemostat that is gently pulled over the tip of the shaping ribbon. This method, however, usually results in a large gentle curve that is often not short enough for routine use. A preferable technique is to hold the guidewire in one hand and catch the tip of the other wire between the first finger and thumb, squeezing the wire in order to create the small curve. The fingers can be rolled backward in order to make a small

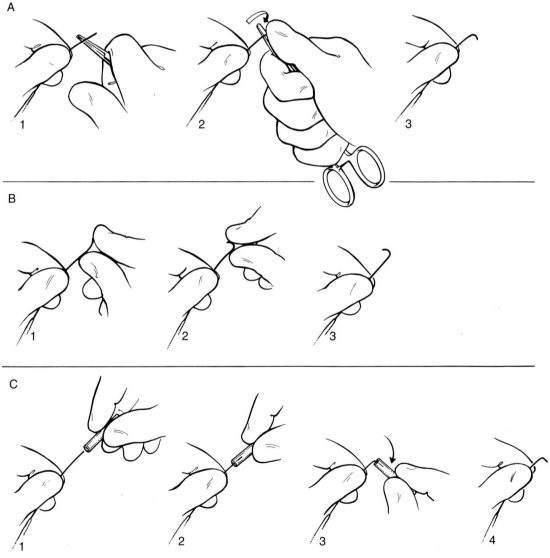

FIG. 9. The various methods commonly used to shape the guidewire are illustrated. **A:** Use of a hemostat or needle to shape the tip. **B:** Pinching the tip of the wire between the fingers. **C:** Use of a small plastic tube to hold the tip while it is bent.

tip at the end and, when at least some curve is generated, further bending is easier. An alternative method is to use a small plastic tube placed over the tip of the wire which then can be bent in order to trap the wire and facilitate its shaping (Fig. 9C). In some circumstances two bends are necessary; one at the tip and one 2 cm back. This secondary bend is very helpful in turning the wire into the circumflex artery or to a superiorly directed left anterior descending artery. The distance between the primary and secondary bend should be tailored to match the degree of turn and the location of the tip of the guiding catheter.

Retrieval

Rarely, guidewires or tips of balloon catheters can break off and become lodged in coronary vessels (15–17). Several techniques have been used to retrieve these fragments (Fig. 10). One technique involves use of a very flexible guidewire which is bent back and then sutured to the tip of a balloon catheter or probing sheath. The wire passing through the center of the catheter then can move either forward or backward in order to form a snare which can trap the broken fragment and pull it out. Alternatively a 300-cm exchange wire can be bent in the middle and the two wires can be passed through a larger probing sheath to form a snare. Alternatively, a high torque floppy guidewire can be placed through a probing sheath, and the tip can be bent back and wedged into the probing sheath, likewise forming a snare in order to remove foreign material. Another technique that can be used is a passage of two separate guidewires than can be tied together at their tip to form a basket and which, once across the pertaining material, can be twisted in order to trap the material between the two wires and pull it out. Finally, material can be removed by inflating the balloon catheter at extremely low pressure (e.g., 1–2 atmospheres) and gradually pulling back. The friction of the balloon across the retained balloon or wire can help draw it back into the guiding catheter. It is essential with any of these techniques that the guiding catheter remain firmly in place in the coronary artery to avoid embolization of the material into the aorta. Once the fragment is within the guiding catheter than the entire catheter can be removed from the patient.

A more common situation is the breakage of an angioplasty wire due to entrapment of the tip within a small branch. Initially, the wire is still attached to itself through the outer coil wire. This can be recognized by a gap in the radiolucent part of the wire. In addition, it should be appreciated that this has occurred if pulling back on the wire results in no change in the tip of the guidewire within the coronary artery. Rather than continuing to pull back on the wire and further uncoil the

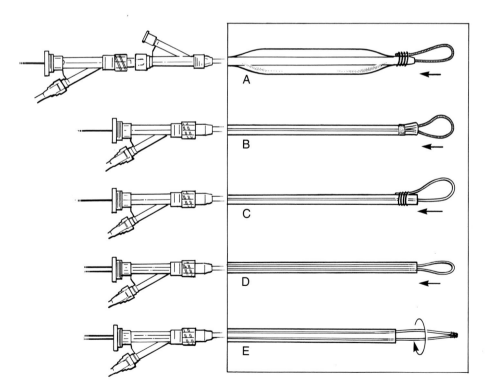

FIG. 10. The various snare devices used to retrieve broken guidewires and catheters from within the coronary system. **A:** A guidewire sutured back onto the balloon catheter. **B:** A commercially available guidewire snare catheter (retriever-18; Target Therapeutics, Freemont, CA). **C:** A wire is sutured to the tip of a probe sheath. **D:** An exchange wire is looped through the probe sheath. **E:** Two guidewires are sutured at the tips to create a wire basket which can be rotated and used as a snare.

outer wire risking the possibility of breakage, it is safer to gradually push the balloon catheter back over the broken wire and down over the tip of the wire. The entire balloon and wire within it can then be removed together. This method allows the tip of the balloon to help dislodge the wire and free it as well.

References

1. Avedissian MG, Kileavy EC, Garcia JM, Dear WE. Percutaneous transluminal coronary angioplasty: a review of current balloon dilation systems. *Cathet Cardiovasc Diagn* 1989;18:263–275.
2. Jain J. Effect of balloon pressure on angioplasty balloon. *Am J Cardiol* 1986;57:26–28.
3. USCI Product Information, USCI Division of BARD, Billnea, MA.
4. ACS Product Information, Advanced Catheter Systems, Clara, CA.
5. SciMed Product Information, SciMed Corp., Maple Grove, MN.
6. Berry KJ, Drew TM, McKendal L, Sharaf BL, Thomas ES, Williams DO. Balloon material as a risk factor for coronary angioplasty procedural complications. *Circulation* 1991;84:II-130.
7. Ferguson JJ, Parnis SM, Fuqua JM. Inaccuracies in manufacturer-reported PTCA balloon profiles. *Cathet Cardiovasc Diagn* 1992;25:101–106.
8. Cordis Product Information, Cordis Corp, Miami, FL.
9. Fincin L, Meier B, Roy P, Steffenino G, Rutinhauser W. Clinical experience with a monorail balloon catheter for coronary angioplasty. *Cathet Cardiovasc Diagn* 1988;14:206–212.
10. Stack RS, Quigley PJ, Collins G, Phillips HR. Perfusion balloon catheter. *Am J Cardiol* 1988;61:77g–80g.
11. Leitschuh MA, Mills RM, Larosa D, Jacobs AK, Ruocco NA, Faxon DP. Outcome after major dissection during coronary angioplasty using a perfusion balloon catheter. *Am J Cardiol* 1991;67:1056–1060.
12. Ohman EM, Marquis JF, Ricci DR, Brown R, Knudston ML, Kereiakes DJ, Samaha JK, Margolis JR, Niedermann A, Dean L, Gurbel P, Sketch M, Wilderman N, Lee K, Califf R. The effect of gradual prolonged inflation during angioplasty on inhospital long-term outcome: the results of a multicenter randomized trial. *J Am Coll Cardiol* 1992;19:33A.
13. Savas V, Puchrowciz S, Williams L, Grines C, O'Neill W. Angioplasty outcome using long balloons and high risk lesions. *J Am Coll Cardiol* 1992;19:34A.
14. Zider J, Tenaglia A, Jackman J, Fortin D, Frid D, Chung T, Cheng J, Royal S, Krucoff M, O'Conner C, Stack R. Improved acute results for PTCA of long coronary lesions using long angioplasty balloon catheters. *J Am Coll Cardiol* 1992;19:34A.
15. Hartzler S, Rutherford BD, McCohaham DR. Retained percutaneous transluminal coronary angioplasty equipment components and their management. *Am J Cardiol* 1987;60:1260–1264.
16. Serota H, Deligonul U, Lew B, Kern M, Aquire F, Vandormael M. Improved method for transcatheter retrieval of intercoronary detached angioplasty guidewire segments. *Cathet Cardiovasc Diagn* 1989;17:248–251.
17. Crone J, Morgan MJ. Complications of cardiac catheterization and angiography: prevention and management. New York: Futura Publishing Company; 1989.

Practical Angioplasty,
edited by David P. Faxon.
Raven Press, Ltd., New York © 1993.

CHAPTER 8

Dilation Strategies in Patients with Multivessel Disease

Peter B. Berger and David R. Holmes, Jr.

Percutaneous transluminal coronary angioplasty (PTCA) was initially described in 1977 for the treatment of proximal, discrete, noncalcified, subtotal stenoses in patients with preserved left ventricular function (1). Following the introduction of PTCA, its application has increased greatly to include patients with unstable angina, complex lesions, reduced ventricular function, and a growing number of patients with multivessel disease. The purpose of this chapter is to review the use of PTCA in patients with multivessel disease. Analysis of the reported results of angioplasty among patients with multivessel disease requires careful analysis of many factors, including the different definitions of multivessel disease, the relative importance of completeness of revascularization, the different ways in which initial success and complications have been defined, and the long-term benefits among successfully treated patients. All of these factors have important implications for patient selection.

MULTIVESSEL DISEASE

The definition of multivessel disease has varied between different studies. It has generally been defined in one of three ways; (i) stenosis greater than or equal to 70% of the diameter in two or more coronary arteries (70%-70%), (2,3,4) (ii) 70% or greater stenosis in one coronary artery and a 50% or greater stenosis in a second coronary artery (70%-50%), (5,6) or (iii) 50% or greater stenosis in two or more coronary arteries (50%-50%) (7–11). Regardless of which definition is used, multivessel disease is present in the majority of patients undergoing coronary angioplasty. Whereas the initial National Heart, Lung, and Blood Institute (NHLBI) PTCA Re-

gistry study indicated that 25% of patients who underwent PTCA between 1977 and 1981 had multivessel disease (applying the 70%-70% definition), the proportion of patients with multivessel disease undergoing PTCA during 1985–1986 had increased to 53% percent in the second NHLBI PTCA Registry (2). At the Mid-American Heart Institute, 47% of patients undergoing PTCA between 1986 and 1988 had multivessel disease using the 70%-70% criteria (3). At the Mayo Clinic, between January 1 and December 31, 1990, the proportion of patients with multivessel disease undergoing PTCA was 51% using the 70%-70% criterion, and 70% using the 70%-50% criterion. In contrast, among surgical patients in the Coronary Artery Surgery Study (CASS), the proportion of patients with multivessel disease was 73% using the 70%-70% criterion, and 82% using the 50%-50% criteria (12). At the Mayo Clinic, the percentage of patients with multivessel disease undergoing bypass surgery in 1989 was 90.6% and 94.7% applying these two definitions, respectively. These data emphasize the difficulty in comparing different patient series when using different definitions, but indicate that multivessel disease is more common among patients undergoing coronary artery bypass than PTCA. Such differences have important implications in comparing published data on patient outcome following bypass surgery and angioplasty.

The majority of patients with multivessel disease undergoing PTCA have two-vessel disease (2,6,13), whereas the majority of patients undergoing coronary artery bypass surgery with multivessel disease have three-vessel disease (Fig. 1) (14–16). Other important differences between patients with multivessel disease undergoing PTCA and those undergoing coronary artery bypass surgery include a greater frequency of significant left main coronary disease and reduced left ventricular function in the latter group (2,15).

P. B. Berger and D. R. Holmes, Jr.: Division of Cardiovascular Diseases, Mayo Clinic, Rochester, Minnesota

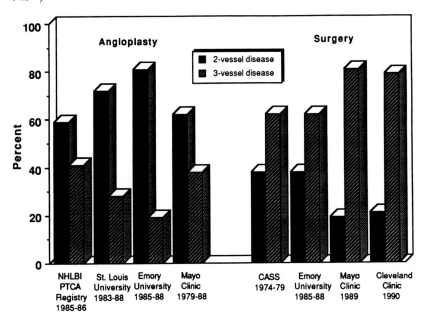

FIG. 1. The proportion of multivessel disease patients with two- versus three-vessel coronary disease undergoing percutaneous transluminal coronary angioplasty and coronary artery bypass surgery in several large patient series. Patients with left main lesions of 50% or more were included in the three-vessel disease group in the Mayo Clinic surgical series, but were analyzed separately in the Emory University surgical series.

Several prospective randomized trials are being performed to directly compare the clinical outcome of patients with multivessel disease undergoing PTCA and coronary artery bypass surgery (Table 1). Some of these trials have already completed enrollment, and one of them, the Randomized Interventional Treatment of Angina (RITA), has reported the initial and follow-up results of 1,011 patients in the trial with single or multivessel coronary artery disease randomized to either PTCA or CABG (17). After a median 2.5 years of follow-up, there was no difference in the pre-defined combined primary endpoint of death or myocardial infarction between the two treatment groups (8.6%, 43 of 501 PTCA patients vs 9.8%, 50 of 510 CABG patients, $p = 0.47$). Importantly, there was no difference in these adverse outcomes between the two treatments when stratified for the number of vessels diseased. Repeat revascularization was performed more frequently among patients in the PTCA group, as would be expected; 189 PTCA patients (37%) required repeat revascularization compared to 20 CABG patients (4.0%, $p = 0.0001$). The prevalence of angina at last follow-up was also more common in the PTCA group (31% vs 22% in the CABG group, $p = 0.007$). Early data from the Bypass Angioplasty Revascu-

TABLE 1. *Ongoing prospective randomized trials comparing percutaneous transluminal coronary angioplasty with coronary artery bypass surgery in patients with multivessel disease*

Trial	Angiographic criteria	Follow-up schedule	Major end points
BARI	2 or 3 vessels ≥ 50% stenotic	6 weeks; 1, 3, and 5 years	Mortality, MI, anginal class, exercise performance, heart failure, LV function, subsequent revascularization procedures, quality of life; subgroup with coronary angiographic assessment
RITA	1, 2, or 3 vessels ≥ 50% stenotic	1 and 6 months; 1, 2, 3, 4, and 5 years	Mortality, MI, anginal class, exercise capacity, LV function, return to work, subsequent revascularization procedures
EAST	2 or 3 vessels ≥ 50% stenotic	1 and 3 years	Mortality, MI, angiographic revascularization status, thallium 201 perfusion, subsequent revascularization procedures, quality of life
GABI	2 or 3 vessels ≥ 70% stenotic	3, 6, and 12 months	Mortality, MI, anginal class, exercise capacity
CABRI	2 or 3 vessels ≥ 50% stenotic	6 months and 2 years	Mortality, MI, anginal class, exercise capacity with thallium imaging, heart failure, angiographic assessment

BARI, Bypass Angioplasty Revascularization Investigation; RITA, Randomized Interventional Treatment of Angina; EAST, Emory Angioplasty Surgery Trial; GABI, German Angioplasty Bypass Trial; CABRI, Coronary Angioplasty Bypass Revascularization Investigation; MI, myocardial infarction; LV, left ventricular.

larization Investigation (BARI) trial provide insight into the proportion of patients with multivessel disease eligible for coronary angioplasty. Enrollment in this trial was completed in June, 1991 and included 1,827 patients. Of the 12,526 patients with multivessel disease who met the clinical inclusion criteria for the BARI trial, only 40% were anatomically suitable for coronary angioplasty. By comparison, 97% of patients who were eligible for inclusion in the trial were suitable for bypass surgery (Bourassa et al, submitted for publication). Therefore, more patients with multivessel disease requiring revascularization were suitable for surgery than for coronary angioplasty. This disparity reflects the presence of chronic total occlusions and of subtotal coronary lesions with features that remain problematic for PTCA.

EXTENT OF REVASCULARIZATION

The anticipated extent of revascularization is an important consideration when selecting patients with multivessel disease for coronary angioplasty, but the need to achieve complete revascularization remains a subject of controversy. The importance of complete revascularization initially arose from early surgical series in which patients with complete revascularization had improved morbidity and survival compared to patients with incomplete revascularization (18,19). Complete revascularization among angioplasty patients has been defined in two different ways: either as the successful dilation of all lesions of 50% or more (3,9,20), or as the successful dilation of all lesions of 70% or more in the coronary circulation (6). However, assessment of the completeness of revascularization has been unevenly applied to patients following coronary angioplasty and coronary artery bypass grafting. In surgical series, patients in whom a bypass graft is anastomosed to each of the major epicardial coronary arteries that had significant stenosis have generally been described as having had complete revascularization, even though major branches may have been left ungrafted (18,21,22), or significant disease may be present in the grafted vessel beyond the anastomosis site. Revascularization of left ventricular segments that are akinetic or dyskinetic has not always been necessary for it to be considered that complete revascularization had been achieved (22). Others have considered revascularization to be complete when the number of grafts placed is the same or greater than the number of diseased coronary arteries, even though grafts may be anastomosed to the distal segment of a major vessel and its major branch, and a diseased vessel left ungrafted (19,23). There is also variability in the way complete revascularization is defined in PTCA patient series. In general, patients undergoing PTCA in whom any lesion of 50% or more remains in the coronary circulation are considered to have incomplete revascularization, even though revasculariza-

tion may have been as complete as would have been achieved with coronary bypass surgery. Few surgical studies have used this rigorous definition of complete revascularization (24).

Notwithstanding the difficulty in determining the true frequency of completeness of revascularization equivalently between surgery and angioplasty patients, it appears that complete revascularization is probably achieved in a greater proportion of patients with multivessel disease undergoing coronary bypass surgery than PTCA. Complete revascularization following PTCA, defined as the absence of lesions greater than or equal to 50% following the procedure, was reported by Deligonul et al. to have been achieved in 34% of patients with two-vessel disease and 26% of patients with three-vessel disease (8). Applying the same definition, Vandormael et al. reported complete revascularization in 47% of patients with two-vessel disease and 21% of patients with three-vessel disease (13). However, in view of the fact that stenoses of less than 70% usually do not produce ischemia and may not progress for years, such lesions are generally not dilated, and it may be more appropriate to define complete revascularization as the dilation of all lesions greater than or equal to 70%. When one applies this definition of complete revascularization to these same angioplasty series, complete revascularization was actually achieved in 50% of patients with two-vessel disease and 47% of patients with three-vessel disease in the Deligonul series, and in 48% of patients with multivessel disease in the Vandormael series (Table 2). Using this same definition, data from the NHLBI PTCA Registry indicate that complete revascularization was achieved in 44% of patients (127 of 286) with multivessel disease in the first NHLBI PTCA Registry (5), and in 41% of patients (356 of 867) in a recent series reported by Bell et al. (6). The most common reason that complete revascularization is not achieved among patients with multivessel disease is the presence of a chronic total occlusion (5,8). By comparison, complete revascularization, applying the various definitions for surgical patients described above, is achieved in approximately 60% to 70% of patients with multivessel disease undergoing coronary artery bypass surgery (18,21,22,25).

Whether the inability to achieve complete revascularization is a significant limitation of coronary angioplasty remains controversial. The belief that incomplete revascularization may be associated with a greater risk of adverse outcome is an extrapolation from several early surgical series, in which adverse outcomes occurred more commonly among patients with incomplete surgical revascularization (18). However, subsequent analyses have revealed that important baseline anatomic and clinical differences exist among surgical patients in whom complete and incomplete revascularization was achieved (19,26). When multivariate analyses have been performed in which left ventricular function and other im-

TABLE 2. *Percentage of patients with multivessel disease undergoing percutaneous transluminal coronary angioplasty in whom complete revascularization was achieved*[a]

Series	Year	Patients	Definition of Complete Revascularization		References
			No remaining lesion ≥ 50% (%)	No remaining lesion ≥ 70% (%)	
Deligonul et al.	1988	397	32	49	(8)
Vandormael et al.	1985	97	37	48	(13)
Reeder et al.	1988	286	NA	44	(5)
Bell et al.	1990	867	NA	41	(6)

NA, not available.
[a] Utilizing two different definitions of complete revascularization.

portant variables were included, survival among patients with complete and incomplete revascularization has been found to be related to differences in baseline characteristics between the two groups and not to the degree of revascularization achieved (23,27), although incomplete revascularization remained an important risk factor for mortality in one study (19).

There are several additional reasons why the data from early surgical series suggesting greater benefit from complete revascularization may not be applicable to coronary angioplasty. Complete revascularization is the goal of coronary artery bypass surgery in part because of the increased risk of reoperation among patients who have undergone prior bypass surgery. However, repeat angioplasty is not associated with an increased risk among patients who have undergone prior angioplasty, and in fact the procedure can be easily repeated. Another reason that angioplasty is not performed on all coronary lesions in order to achieve complete revascularization relates to concern about restenosis. Since one-third of dilated lesions will recur and may then be more severe than the original atherosclerotic lesions, moderately stenotic lesions (<70%) are usually not dilated. In addition, such moderate stenoses may not progress (28,29).

Despite these reasons showing that a strategy of complete revascularization may not be as important following coronary angioplasty as it initially appeared following bypass surgery, early analyses of patient series undergoing coronary angioplasty found that adverse outcomes occurred more commonly among patients with incomplete revascularization (30). However, subsequent analyses suggest that, as in the case of bypass surgery, adverse outcomes may be principally due to differences in baseline characteristics (5). Incomplete revascularization was not associated with an increased risk of mortality in those studies in which multivariate analyses including important baseline characteristics have been performed (3,5,6). Therefore, among carefully selected patients, incomplete revascularization appears to be an acceptable strategy. The degree of ischemia and extent of left ventricular dysfunction appear to influence the need for complete revascularization, however. In patients

with severe ischemia and left ventricular dysfunction, the need to achieve complete revascularization appears to be the greatest (19,27).

How can one identify those patients with multivessel disease in whom coronary angioplasty is likely to provide substantial benefit? First, it is important to identify the reasons for which coronary angioplasty are most commonly performed. The most common indication for coronary angioplasty is relief of symptoms. Numerous reports provide strong evidence that the majority of patients undergoing coronary angioplasty have a reduction in the frequency and severity of anginal symptoms. The second most common indication is in an attempt to prolong survival. It is well documented that subsets of patients have improved survival with coronary artery bypass surgery compared to medical therapy; these include patients with three-vessel disease and reduced left ventricular function with mild (class 1 or 2) angina (Fig. 2) (31); patients with severe (class 3 or 4) angina, two-vessel disease and severely reduced ventricular function (Fig. 3) (32); and patients with multivessel disease and an early positive stress test, regardless of ventricular function (Fig. 4) (33). Many believe these same subsets of patients may also derive survival benefit from coronary angioplasty, particularly if a similar degree of revascularization can be achieved. Although patients with left

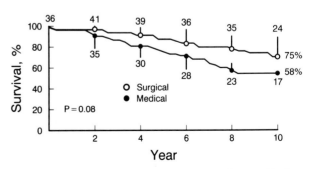

FIG. 2. Cumulative survival rates among patients with Canadian Cardiovascular Society class 1 or 2 angina, an ejection fraction less than 50% and three-vessel disease, randomized to medical and surgical therapy in the Coronary Artery Surgical Study.

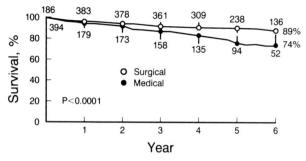

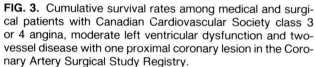

FIG. 3. Cumulative survival rates among medical and surgical patients with Canadian Cardiovascular Society class 3 or 4 angina, moderate left ventricular dysfunction and two-vessel disease with one proximal coronary lesion in the Coronary Artery Surgical Study Registry.

FIG. 4. Cumulative survival rates among medical and surgical patients with a high-risk exercise test in the Coronary Artery Surgical Study Registry. An exercise test was considered high risk if there was a ST-segment depression of 1 mm or more and a final exercise stage of 1 or less.

main lesions greater than or equal to 50% have also been shown to benefit from surgical revascularization, such patients have been shown to have a prohibitively high mortality following PTCA, and should not be considered for PTCA unless surgery can not be performed (34).

The importance of complete revascularization may vary depending on the indication for coronary angioplasty. If angioplasty is performed principally for the relief of symptoms, it is increasingly clear that complete revascularization need not be obtained for complete symptom relief to be achieved (35). An example of this would be a patient who first developed angina several

years ago, following an inferior myocardial infarction, and in whom angiography reveals an occluded right coronary artery and subtotal occlusion of the left anterior descending artery (Fig. 5A). If the segments of the left ventricle supplied by the occluded right coronary artery are infarcted and akinetic, then dilation of the left anterior descending (LAD) artery lesion will in all likelihood produce complete resolution of symptoms. This can be defined as incomplete but adequate revascularization—adequate in that all ischemia-producing lesions had been dilated. It is not known whether there is any benefit in restoring coronary blood flow to occluded arteries sup-

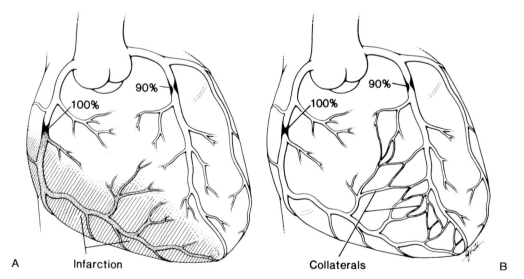

FIG. 5. A. Coronary diagram from a patient with an occluded right coronary artery and subtotal occlusion of the left anterior descending artery. If the segments of the left ventricle supplied by the occluded right coronary artery are infarcted and akinetic, then dilation of the left anterior descending artery lesion will in all likelihood produce complete resolution of symptoms. This has been termed incomplete but adequate revascularization; incomplete because an occluded vessel remains unrevascularized, but adequate since all ischemia-producing lesions will have been dilated. **B:** If the occluded right coronary artery was well collateralized and preserved motion in the inferior region of the left ventricle was present, dilation of the LAD would be termed incomplete and inadequate revascularization. Such a patient would continue to have inferior ischemia following dilation of the left anterior descending artery. In such a patient, if the occluded right coronary artery could not be dilated, surgical revascularization might be a better option.

TABLE 3. *Initial success and complication rates among patients with multivessel disease undergoing coronary angioplasty*

Series	Recruitment years	No. of Patients	Definition of clinical success	Clinical success	Study design	Death	Q-wave MI	Emergency CABG	Elective CABG	Any major complication	Complications	References
Bell et al.	1979 to 1988	1039	≥40% improvement in luminal diameter in ≥1 lesion, and no CABG during hospitalization	83%	Included emergency PTCA	2.5%	4.8%	4.9%	7.4%	NA	In-hospital mortality 1.7% when PTCA within 24 hr of MI excluded.	(6)
Cowley et al.	1979 to 1984	100	≥20% improvement in luminal diameter in ≥1 lesion, without Q-wave MI or emergent CABG	94%	Only pts with ≥2 vessels dilated, except for 12% with 1 vessel and a major branch dilated; 8 pts excluded because the 1st vessel attempted was unsuccessful	NA	2%	4%	NA	NA	Complications in the excluded 8 pts with unsuccessful PTCA of the 1st vessel attempted not reported	(11)
Doros et al.	1979 to 1986	428	≥20% improvement in luminal diameter with clinical improvement at 1 week ≥2 CHC classes	94%	Only pts with ≥2 vessels attempted, except for 10% of pts with 1 vessel and its major branch dilated; included emergency PTCA	1.4%	2.5%	2.1%	NA	4.0%	All 6 deaths resulted from abrupt closure ≥30 min following the procedure	(41)
Mata et al.	1980 to 1984	74	≥20% improvement in luminal diameter, or a residual stenosis ≤60%, in both vessels	85%	Only pts undergoing elective PTCA with ≥2 vessels attempted; 99% of pts had ≥1 lesion successfully dilated without complication	0	1.4%	0	NA	0	Emergency PTCA excluded.	(10)
O'Keefe et al.	1980 to 1989	3186	≤40% residual stenoses in ≥2 dilated lesions without Q wave MI, emergent CABG or death	92%	Only pts undergoing elective PTCA with ≥2 vessels attempted	1%	1.5%[a]	0.9%	NA	2.9%	Non-fatal Q-wave MI; excluded pts in whom the 1st vessel attempted was unsuccessful[a]	(3)

Study	Years	No. pts	Definition of success	Success	Comments						Notes	Ref
Myler et al.	1983 to 1986	494	≥35% stenosis reduction and residual stenosis < 50% in ≥1 vessel, clinical improvement at 1 week ≥1 CHC class	95%	Only pts in whom CR was anticipated with ≥2 vessel PTCA planned, except for 13% of pts with multivessel, not multilesion, dilation	0.4%	3%	2.8%	NA	3.8%	The 2 deaths were both due to multivessel abrupt closure	(40)
Vandormael et al.	1983 to 1988	637	≥30% reduction in luminal stenosis, residual stenosis < 50% in the most important vessel, without MI, CABG, or death	83%	Excluded pts with prior CABG or MI within 1 week	1.4[b]	0.9%[a]	6.9%	NA	NA	Pts with Q-wave MI undergoing CABG not included[a]. Procedural, not in-hospital death[b]	(9)
DiSciascio et al.	1982 to 1987	54	≥20% reduction in luminal stenosis, residual stenosis < 50% in the most important vessel, and clinical improvement ≥1 CHC class	93%	Included only pts with 3-vessel disease in whom 3-vessel dilation was planned; 12 patients had dilation of <3 vessels	0%	0%	1.8%	5.5%	7.3%	Non-Q MI occurred in an additional 11% of pts	(39)
Finci et al.	NA	100	<50% residual stenosis in the most important vessel without MI or CABG, and clinical improvement at 1 week ≥1 CHC class	85%	Included only pts in whom ≥2 vessel dilation was planned; 10% of pts had multilesion, not multivessel, disease	NA	5%[a]	5%	NA	8%	Included non-Q MI if CPK rose to >3 times normal value[a]	(38)
Ellis et al.	1986 to 1987	350	<50% residual stenosis in ≥1 lesion without MI, emergent CABG, or death	82%	Pts with acute MI excluded	1.1%	1.7%[a]	5.7[b]	NA	8.6%	Procedural, not in-hospital death.	(37)

CABG, coronary artery bypass surgery; MI, myocardial infarction; PTCA, percutaneous transluminal coronary angioplasty; NA, not available; Pts, patients; CHC, Canadian heart classification; CR, complete revascularization.

[a] Nonfatal MI without CABG.

[b] Nonfatal CABG.

plying akinetic areas of myocardium, but it is clearly not required to achieve complete resolution of angina, as in this case. However, if the occluded right coronary artery in this same patient was well collateralized and motion in the inferior region of the left ventricle was present, dilation of the LAD artery would be termed incomplete and inadequate revascularization, since there would likely be ischemia following even successful dilation of the left anterior descending artery (Fig. 5B). In such a patient, if the occluded right coronary artery could not be dilated, surgical revascularization might be a better option.

Among patients in whom angioplasty is performed with the goal of improving long-term survival, it is less clear whether incomplete but adequate revascularization is sufficient to achieve this goal. The severity of angina at the time of angioplasty may influence the need for complete revascularization, as has been found among surgery patients. A report from the CASS Registry indicates that, among patients with three-vessel disease and mild angina, there was no difference in the long-term outcome of patients receiving two or more bypass grafts, regardless of preoperative left ventricular function (27). However, among patients with severe angina and reduced left ventricular function, complete revascularization (placement of three or more grafts) was strongly associated with an improved survival on multivariate analysis. Recent data from the Mayo Clinic suggest that angioplasty patients with severe angina may also derive greater benefit from complete revascularization than patients with milder angina. Among 867 patients with multivessel disease in whom coronary angioplasty was successful, incomplete revascularization was not found to be independently associated with adverse outcome in the years following the procedure (6). However, among 937 patients undergoing coronary angioplasty for the treatment of severe rest angina, multivariate analysis revealed that incomplete revascularization *was* strongly associated with adverse outcome in the years following PTCA (36). It thus appears that the more severe the ischemic burden and left ventricular dysfunction, the more important it becomes to achieve complete revascularization.

INITIAL OUTCOME

Reported success rates following attempted dilation among patients with multivessel disease have varied, in part due to widely varying definitions of success, and whether success referred to clinical outcome among patients undergoing the procedure or to angiographic success as it related to a lesion or all lesions undergoing attempted dilation. Based on varying definitions, clinical success rates ranging from 83% to 96% have been reported (Table 3) (3,6,9–11,37–41). Several studies reporting initial success rates for coronary angioplasty in-

cluded patients undergoing angioplasty in the early 1980s. In recent years, success rates are higher, despite the fact that the complexity of cases has increased over the years (2). There are several patient series in which only patients with multivessel disease undergoing two- or three-vessel dilation are included (10,11,39), as well as series in which only patients in whom complete revascularization was thought to be achievable (11,39,40); however, such inclusion and exclusion criteria may introduce considerable bias.

The percentage of patients reported to suffer major complications during multivessel coronary angioplasty has varied as well, due in part to differences in the end points considered to represent major complications. Major complications, in which in-hospital death, emergency coronary artery bypass surgery, and Q-wave myocardial infarction were included as end points, have ranged from 1.3% to 8.6%. While virtually all patient series have included Q-wave myocardial infarction, emergency coronary artery bypass surgery, and procedural death as complications, the inclusion of elective bypass surgery and death in the days following the procedure as complications has been inconsistent. As many as 7.4% of patients may undergo elective coronary artery bypass surgery following coronary angioplasty, generally due to either unsatisfactory dilation results or the inability to dilate a lesion felt to be responsible for the patient's ischemia (6); such patients are often not included as having suffered a major complication. Occasionally, culprit vessel angioplasty is performed as a bridge to bypass surgery, and the goals of angioplasty may have been achieved despite the performance of elective bypass surgery. More commonly, however, angioplasty is performed with the goal of achieving sufficient revascularization to avoid surgery, and elective coronary artery bypass surgery during the same hospitalization usually represents a failure of the angioplasty strategy.

The use of procedural rather than in-hospital death as an end point is more controversial, however. It is often difficult to determine the exact cause of death, even among patients undergoing autopsy. Furthermore, cardiac death may occur days following coronary angioplasty. Therefore, the reporting of procedural rather than in-hospital death may be misleading, and death at any time during the hospitalization should be included as a complication of angioplasty. However, since the length of hospitalization varies from patient to patient, regionally and internationally, the reporting of 30-day mortality, as is the case following coronary artery bypass, should probably be encouraged.

The influence of the number of diseased vessels on complications during coronary angioplasty has been analyzed using data from 1,764 patients in the second NHLBI PTCA Registry undergoing coronary angioplasty between 1985 and 1986 (Table 4) (42). Major complications (death, nonfatal myocardial infarction, or emergency bypass surgery) occurred in 5.5% of patients

TABLE 4. *Influence of the number of diseased vessels on the occurrence of major complications during percutaneous transluminal coronary angioplasty[a]*

	Vessels diseased			
	Single (N = 838) n (%)	Double (N = 559) n (%)	Triple (N = 367) n (%)	p value
Death	2 (0.2)	5 (0.9)	8 (2.2)	<0.001
Nonfatal MI	29 (3.5)	29 (5.2)	19 (5.2)	NS
Emergency CABG	24 (2.9)	22 (3.9)	16 (4.4)	NS
Any of the above	46 (5.5)	45 (8.1)	34 (9.3)	<0.05

MI, myocardial infarction; CABG, coronary artery bypass surgery.

[a] From the National Heart, Lung, and Blood Institute Percutaneous Transluminal Coronary Angioplasty Registry.

with single-vessel disease, 8.1% of patients with double-vessel disease, and 9.3% of patients with triple-vessel disease.

Vascular complications following angioplasty have not generally been reported as major complications. However, vascular complications requiring vascular surgery or blood transfusion occur in approximately 2.2% of patients undergoing multivessel PTCA (3).

Lastly, it must be remembered that these major complications are not mutually exclusive, and generally occur within the same patient. For example, a patient with failed angioplasty may suffer myocardial infarction, require emergency bypass surgery, and subsequently die. Simply summing the percentage of patients with myocardial infarction, bypass surgery, and death may result in doubling or tripling the actual complication rate if an analysis of the total number of patients in whom a major complication occurred is not performed.

LESION ANALYSIS

There are several lesion characteristics which have been recognized as unfavorable for dilation, including the presence of a major branch originating from within the lesion (a bifurcation lesion) (43,44), long lesions (43,45,46), lesion eccentricity (43,45), apparent thrombus (43,46,47), and severely angulated lesions (46). Recently, an American College of Cardiology and American Heart Association (ACC/AHA) Joint Task Force developed a comprehensive lesion characterization scheme with anticipated angioplasty success rates (Table 5) (48). The scheme had not been validated, however, until Ellis et al. prospectively characterized 662 lesions among 350 patients undergoing attempted multivessel coronary angioplasty at four medical centers (37). These investigators, using a minor modification of the ACC/AHA schema, found lesion type to be a more powerful predictor of procedural outcome than any other variable included in multivariate analysis. The presence of

TABLE 5. *Schema for characterization of coronary lesions with anticipated angioplasty success rates[a]*

Type A Lesions[b]	Type B lesions[c]	Type C lesions[d]
Discrete (<10 mm) Concentric	Tubular (10–20 mm in length) Eccentric	Diffuse (>2 cm length) Excessive tortuosity of proximal segment
Readily accessible	Moderate tortuosity of proximal segment	Extremely angulated segments (>90 degrees)
Nonangulated segment	Moderately angulated segment	Total occlusion > 3 months old
Smooth contour	Irregular contour	Inability to protect major side branches
Little or no calcification	Moderate to heavy calcification	Degenerated vein grafts with friable lesions
Less than totally occlusive	Total occlusion < 3 months old	
Not ostial in location	Ostial in location	
No major branch involvement	Bifurcation lesions requiring double guide wires	
Absence of thrombus	Some thrombus present	

[a] Proposed by the American College of Cardiology/American Heart Association Task Force.
[b] High success rate (85%), low risk.
[c] Moderate success rate (60–85%), low risk.
[d] Low success rate (60%), high risk.

chronic total occlusion, stenosis bend of more than 60 degrees, and excessive tortuosity were found to be particularly predictive of failure.

The utility of this classification scheme is limited, in part, by the degree of interobserver variability associated with it. Ellis et al. found that 42% of lesions were assigned a different classification by a second angiographer; a subsequent study reported that 39% of lesions were classified differently by a second angiographer (49). Another limitation of this classification scheme is that it fails to adequately describe the modes of failure with the more difficult lesion characteristics, and the associated complication rates. It is important to identify lesions that have a low success rate with angioplasty and to distinguish between those associated with high and low complication rates. For example, angioplasty of angulated segments has been shown to be associated with a low success rate and a high complication rate. In an attempt to quantify the success and complication rates associated with angioplasty of angulated lesions, and identify factors associated with the increased risk and means of reducing that risk, Ellis et al. analyzed 27 clinical, anatomic, and procedural variables among 100 patients who underwent coronary angioplasty of lesions located at bends of 45 degrees or more and compared these results to 344 patients undergoing coronary angioplasty of nonangulated segments (37). These investigators found that the success rate associated with angioplasty of angulated lesions was significantly lower (70%), and the complication rate higher (13%), than the 89% success rate and 3.5% complication rate found among patients undergoing angioplasty of nonangulated lesions. On multivariate analysis, the use of noncompliant polyethylene terephthalate balloons and highly experienced angioplasty operators appeared to increase the likelihood of success and lower the complication rate. However, this was a retrospective analysis, and the confidence intervals indicating improved outcome with noncompliant balloons were very wide. Based on *in vitro* work with an acrylic arterial model, the investigators attributed the greater success with noncompliant balloons to the fact that such balloons may conform to angulated arterial segments at high inflation pressures to a greater extent than more compliant balloons, such as those made of polyethylene or polyolefin. In this study, deliberate balloon undersizing resulting in a balloon:artery ratio of 0.80 to 0.90 was associated with a complication rate of 7%, compared to a complication rate of 13% with normal balloon sizing (balloon:artery ratio of 0.91 to 1.00). However, the number of patients in whom this technique was employed was too small to permit any conclusion about its effectiveness.

Angioplasty of chronic totally occluded arteries, although associated with a lower success rate than angioplasty of subtotally occluded arteries, is associated with a low complication rate (37,50,51). A recent report by Bell et al., in which the long-term outcome of 354 patients undergoing attempted angioplasty of a chronic total occlusion was analyzed, revealed that patients in whom angioplasty was successful not only had a marked reduction in anginal symptoms but also a reduced need for coronary artery bypass surgery in the years following the procedure (51).

INTRACORONARY STENTS

Coronary dissection is a major factor limiting the wider application of coronary angioplasty. Occurring in approximately 5% of patients, coronary dissection resulting in acute closure is responsible for the majority of myocardial infarctions, emergency bypass surgery, and deaths occurring during coronary angioplasty (52). Although patients at the highest risk of suffering coronary dissection can be identified by the presence of specific lesion characteristics as described above, coronary dissection in most patients is unpredictable (46). Prolonged inflation with an autoperfusion catheter has been shown to restore patency to the majority of coronary arteries in which dissection and abrupt closure have occurred (53–55). However, patients with coronary dissection in whom treatment with an autoperfusion catheter is unsuccessful remain at high risk for suffering myocardial infarction or death (55).

Intracoronary stents show great promise in their ability to overcome acute closure due to coronary dissection. The impact of coronary stents is most dramatic when they are able to restore normal coronary blood flow beyond a collapsed lumen due to a coronary dissection, and when hemodynamic stability returns in a patient with ischemia and hemodynamic compromise due to abrupt closure. Although stent placement in the treatment of abrupt closure due to coronary dissection has been shown to be associated with lower success rates and higher complication rates than elective stent placement (56), the availability of intracoronary stents has allowed the angioplasty operator greater security in attempting complex multivessel dilation and has reduced the need for emergency bypass surgery in this setting. A preliminary analysis of the early clinical outcome of 33 consecutive patients at the Mayo Clinic in whom coronary dissection occurred that was refractory to treatment with an autoperfusion catheter revealed that myocardial infarction, emergency bypass surgery, or death occurred in 88% of patients (7 of 8) prior to the availability of intracoronary stents, compared to 12% of patients (3 of 25) in whom stent deployment was attempted (P. B. Berger, *unpublished report*).

Several intracoronary stents are currently under clinical investigation, including the Palmaz-Shatz, Gianturco-Roubin, Wiktor stents, and the Wallstent; among others. Direct comparisons of these stents in the clinical setting have just begun, as have prospective randomized studies of the stents in the setting of acute closure. It has been difficult to design prospective random-ized trials of stent placement in the setting of coronary dissection and abrupt closure, in view of the apparent beneficial effect of stent deployment compared to tradi-tional therapy in this clinical setting. Preliminary data suggest that some stents may reduce the occurrence of restenosis, especially when deployed within large arteries or vein grafts in the treatment of de novo atherosclerotic lesions, rather than restenotic lesions or coronary dissec-tions following balloon angioplasty. Definitive evidence of this will require prospective randomized trials.

Stent placement is most valuable in the treatment of abrupt closure due to coronary dissection, and is asso-ciated with a low incidence of myocardial infarction, emergency bypass surgery, and death among patients in whom these adverse cardiac events were common prior to the availability of stents. The incidence of early in-hospital closure following stent placement has not been fully studied with most stents, although it has been re-ported to occur in as many as 15% of patients with one stent design (57). Optimizing adjunctive therapy with anticoagulant and antiplatelet medications may reduce this.

FOLLOW-UP

Little is known about the long-term clinical outcome of patients with multivessel disease following angio-plasty, since angioplasty has only recently been applied to patients with multivessel disease. In examining re-ports in which patients have been followed for more than 6 months, by which time the vast majority of patients who will develop restenosis will have done so, it is impor-tant to carefully examine the different end points that have been included as adverse cardiac events during follow-up. If recurrent severe angina and repeat PTCA are included as cardiac events, the proportion of patients suffering an adverse outcome will be much higher than if only myocardial infarction, bypass surgery, and death are included, since more than one-third of patients un-dergoing PTCA will develop restenosis.

Ellis et al. analyzed the 2-year outcome of 350 patients undergoing coronary angioplasty (successful and unsuc-cessful) to identify determinants of event-free survival (7). After analyzing numerous clinical and angiographic variables, the presence of angina at rest, diabetes melli-tus, and stenosis of the proximal left anterior descending artery were found to be independently predictive of the combined adverse cardiac events of death, myocardial infarction, or coronary artery bypass surgery. Patients without these features had a 2-year event-free survival rate of 87%; there were no deaths during the follow-up period. In contrast, patients with two or more of these risk factors had a 2-year mortality rate greater than 25% and an event-free survival rate of less than 50%. Reduced left ventricular function was found to be the most power-ful predictor of survival; whether successful angioplasty influenced the survival among such patients cannot be determined from this study.

Vandormael et al. analyzed predictors of cardiac sur-vival among 637 consecutive patients with multivessel disease who underwent coronary angioplasty and who were followed for a period of 1 to 5 years (9). Advanced age, diabetes mellitus, and left ventricular dysfunction were all independently associated with adverse cardiac events during follow-up. When only patients with suc-cessful PTCA were considered, left ventricular dysfunc-tion was the only independent predictor of cardiac mortality.

RESTENOSIS

Analyses of restenosis following multilesion or multi-vessel angioplasty indicate that the risk of restenosis for each lesion dilated is not independent of the other le-sions dilated. Therefore, restenosis occurs less frequently than would have been predicted if the risk of restenosis for each dilation site was additive (10,11,58,59). How-ever, restenosis occurs with increasing frequency with each additional lesion dilated, and approximately half of the patients undergoing angioplasty of three or more le-sions will develop restenosis of at least one lesion (8,38,58–61). Therefore, patients being considered for multivessel angioplasty should be prepared to undergo two or more angioplasty procedures in order to achieve long-term clinical success. Although studies in which a high percentage of patients who underwent repeat angi-ography during the follow-up period reveal that angio-graphic restenosis of at least one lesion is not uncom-mon, many patients remain free of recurrent symptoms following multivessel angioplasty, despite angiographic evidence of restenosis (8,10,38,62).

There have been two patient series reported in which a high proportion of patients who had undergone multi-vessel dilation underwent follow-up coronary angiogra-phy. Mata et al. reported angiographic data from 61 of 63 consecutive patients (97%) in whom two-vessel angio-plasty had been successfully performed a mean of 5.5 months earlier (10). Restenosis, defined as either an in-crease in the postangioplasty diameter stenosis of 30% or more, or a luminal diameter stenosis of 70% or more at the angioplasty site, was present in 21 patients (34%) and in 30 of 132 (23%) successfully dilated segments. Reste-nosis had occurred in one of the dilated segments in 17 patients (28%), and in both of the dilated segments in 4 patients (6%). Four of the 21 patients with restenosis (19%) remained asymptomatic despite angiographic evi-dence of restenosis.

Finci et al. performed follow-up angiography on 77 of 85 consecutive patients (91%) in whom multivessel PTCA had been performed a mean of 12 months earlier (38). Restenosis, defined as 50% or more luminal diameter stenosis at the angioplasty site, was present in 39 of 77 patients (51%), and in 47 of 143 arteries dilated (33%). Restenosis was clinically silent in 14 of the patients (36%) with angiographic restenosis. The more frequent occurrence of restenosis and the greater proportion of clinically silent restenosis in the Finci series compared to the Mata series is undoubtedly due, in part, to the more inclusive definition of restenosis used by Finci et al.

PATIENT SUBGROUPS

There are a number of patient subgroups with multivessel disease in whom angioplasty is performed with increasing frequency and that warrant additional discussion.

The Elderly

The aged comprise a growing percentage of our population. Elderly patients are admitted to the hospital for unstable angina refractory to medical therapy in increasing numbers. Although recent reports have documented the growing use of coronary bypass surgery among the elderly, morbidity and mortality following bypass surgery among the elderly is markedly higher than that reported among younger patients (63,64). In view of these data, an increasing number of patients are being referred to angiography in hopes of finding anatomy suitable for coronary angioplasty. Multivessel disease is present in a majority of elderly patients undergoing coronary angiography. Often, however, the goal of angioplasty among such patients is not to dilate all lesions and render the patient asymptomatic, but rather to restore patients to their former level of activity without prolonged bed rest or inactivity. Angioplasty in the elderly has been reported to have similar success and complication rates to those seen among younger patients in most analyses (65–70), although success and complication rates were less favorable in an early analysis of the first NHLBI PTCA Registry (71) and in two studies of PTCA in octagenarians (72,73). The morbidity and mortality reported for angioplasty appears to be considerably lower than that reported for elderly patients undergoing bypass surgery (63,64). It appears that unfavorable lesion characteristics are more common among the elderly, including diffuse disease and coronary calcification (65); these are known to be associated with an increased risk of angioplasty (37). Therefore, high-risk elderly patients can be identified upon review of the coronary angiogram, and alternative treatment strategies considered in such patients.

Patients with Prior Bypass Surgery

Patients with prior bypass surgery are also increasingly referred for coronary angioplasty as the utilization of cor-

onary artery bypass surgery continues to grow. More than 300,000 coronary artery bypass grafting (CABG) procedures are performed annually in the United States (data from the National Center for Health Statistics). The majority of such patients have multivessel disease. Since more than 50% of vein grafts develop partial or complete occlusion within 10 years of bypass surgery (74,75), a growing number of patients are referred for angioplasty of vein grafts and, less commonly, internal mammary arteries. Patients with prior bypass surgery comprised 9% of patients in the NHLBI PTCA Registry from 1977 to 1981; the proportion of patients had risen to 13% in the Registry's second report which included the years 1985 to 1986 (2). Angioplasty of these conduits has been shown to have initial success rates nearly as high and complication rates similar to those associated with angioplasty of the native coronaries (76–78). However, restenosis occurs more frequently following angioplasty of vein grafts, occurring in approximately 50% of patients. Therefore, restenosis remains a significant limitation of the procedure. The reasons for the increased occurrence of restenosis following angioplasty of vein grafts are unclear; whatever the etiology, restenosis of vein grafts following PICA remains a major limitation of the procedure (77,79). Despite the increased risk of restenosis, many such patients are referred for angioplasty in order to avoid or postpone repeat bypass surgery. There are several reasons for this approach, including (i) morbidity and mortality rates following repeat bypass surgery are more than twice those for initial bypass surgery; (ii) advanced age or coexisting illness, which in and of themselves increase the risk of bypass surgery; and (iii) the reduction in angina is less significant following repeat CABG compared to initial CABG. In approximately half of patients undergoing coronary angioplasty following coronary bypass surgery, the native artery may be dilated instead of the vein graft, which will reduce the likelihood of restenosis. Several new interventional devices are believed to be highly effective in vein grafts and perhaps even more effective than balloon angioplasty, but a conclusion as to whether these devices truly result in a lower risk of restenosis awaits randomized trials.

The Young

Young patients with premature multivessel coronary artery disease are generally excellent surgical candidates, with preserved ventricular function and little comorbid illness. However, many physicians are reluctant to refer such patients for coronary artery bypass surgery because of their belief that such patients are likely to develop atherosclerotic disease within their grafts while they are still relatively young and require repeat coronary bypass surgery, with the increased risks associated with this procedure as outlined above. Follow-up studies of young patients undergoing coronary angioplasty reveal an excellent long-term prognosis (80). Reluctance to refer young patients, and the elderly, to bypass surgery if the coronary anatomy is suitable for angioplasty reflects a bias in favor of coronary angioplasty, the appropriateness of which will only be answered by subset analyses of the large ongoing randomized trials.

Patients with Reduced Ventricular Function

Patients with multivessel disease have, in general, lower left ventricular ejection fractions than patients with single-vessel disease, and a greater percentage have prior myocardial infarction as well. While increasing numbers of patients with reduced ventricular function are undergoing coronary angioplasty, little is known about the initial and long-term outcomes of such patients. A major concern has been that such patients will be less able to withstand abrupt closure, which may result in fatal myocardial infarction. However, abrupt closure occurs in approximately 5% of patients. Therefore, if the mortality among patients with reduced ventricular function who suffer these adverse outcomes was even two or three times higher than the mortality of patients with normal left ventricular function, a mortality difference of one or two patients per hundred patients undergoing angioplasty would be expected. Enthusiasm for the alternative option of coronary artery bypass surgery among such patients is dampened by the knowledge that reduced left ventricular function is the most powerful predictor of increased morbidity and mortality among patients undergoing the procedure, although suitable patients with multivessel disease with depressed left ventricular function derive the greatest survival benefit from bypass surgery (31).

In a recent report, Holmes et al. analyzed data from the second NHLBI PTCA Registry and compared the results of angioplasty among 126 consecutive patients with an ejection fraction of 40% or less (mean 35%), to 1,329 consecutive patients with an ejection fraction of over 40% (mean 61%) (81). Despite the fact that patients with reduced ventricular function had a higher incidence of prior myocardial infarction, prior coronary artery bypass surgery, congestive heart failure, multivessel disease, and chronic total occlusion than patients with preserved left ventricular function, initial clinical success (defined as ≥20% luminal diameter in one or more lesions dilated without major ischemic complications) was similar in the two groups (89% in the patients with an ejection fraction ≤ 40% versus 91% in those with an ejection fraction > 40%). The proportion of patients in whom every attempted lesion was successfully dilated was similar between the two groups as well (74% of patients with ejection fraction ≤ 40% versus 79% of patients with ejection fraction > 40%). The proportion of patients suffering death, nonfatal myocardial infarction, emergency, or elective coronary artery bypass surgery

was also similar between the two groups (10.0% versus 9.0%).

In a larger study from a single institution, Stevens compared the results of elective coronary angioplasty among 845 patients with ejection fractions of 40% or less to 8,117 patients with ejection fractions over 40% and found that clinical success was lower in the group with ejection fractions of 40% or less (81% versus 87% respectively, $p < 0.001$) (4). Although the incidence of nonfatal myocardial infarction and emergency bypass surgery was similar in the two groups, procedural mortality was markedly higher among patients with reduced ventricular function (4% versus 1% among patients with an ejection fraction > 40%, $p < 0.001$). Kohli reported the results of coronary angioplasty among a small group of patients (n = 61) with left ventricular ejection fractions of 35% or less; angioplasty was successful in 90% of the patients (82). Major complications occurred in 8.2% of the patients, with death occurring in 3.2% (two patients).

Because the majority of patients with reduced left ventricular function have one or more chronic total occlusions, they are less likely to be anatomically unsuitable for coronary angioplasty than patients with preserved ventricular function. However, it has been our approach to accept patients with reduced left ventricular function with suitable anatomy for angioplasty, and we do not regard the presence of reduced ventricular function per se as a strong contraindication. An exception to this is patients with a severe stenosis in their only remaining patent coronary artery. This is a strong relative contraindication to coronary angioplasty, and we generally refer such patients to bypass surgery unless their risk of surgery is felt to be prohibitively high. When performing angioplasty in such patients in whom abrupt closure is likely to result in major hemodynamic compromise, the use of a prophylactic intraaortic balloon pump (83) or placement of a cardiopulmonary support system (84) appears to be associated with improved safety.

DILATING STRATEGIES

Once the decision has been made to proceed with angioplasty in a patient with multivessel disease, a strategy should be planned prior to commencing the procedure. This should include identification of the lesion or lesions for dilation, the equipment to be used, and the order of dilation.

The Culprit Lesion Strategy

There are many instances in which, among patients with multivessel disease, a single lesion is responsible for most, or all, of a patient's ischemia. Such a lesion is termed a "culprit" lesion. Identification and dilation of a culprit lesion has become a popular strategy in patients with multivessel disease who undergo PTCA in the setting of unstable angina. Although it may be difficult to determine which of several lesions is the culprit lesion, coronary angiography, combined with knowledge of the location of electrocardiographic changes during chest pain and supplemented by the results of radionuclide imaging studies, can reliably identify the culprit lesion in over 80% of cases (35,85). The majority of patients undergoing culprit vessel angioplasty remain asymptomatic 1 year after the procedure, despite the fact that significant lesions in the coronary circulation were not dilated (35,85,86).

Little is known of the long-term consequences of culprit vessel angioplasty. In a preliminary report of the long-term outcome of 937 patients with multivessel disease and the recent onset of rest angina, the clinical outcome of patients who underwent either culprit lesion (n = 728) or multivessel (n = 209) coronary angioplasty was analyzed (36). Initial success and complication rates were similar between the two groups. Of course, fewer patients undergoing culprit vessel angioplasty achieved complete revascularization, defined as the dilation of all lesions by 70% or more. Patients were followed for a mean of 19 months following the procedure, and multivariate analysis revealed that incomplete revascularization was the strongest predictor of adverse cardiac events during the follow-up period. Therefore, as appears to be the case for patients with severe angina undergoing surgical revascularization in a CASS registry study (27), patients with unstable rest angina may derive greater long-term benefit from complete revascularization than from culprit vessel angioplasty resulting in incomplete revascularization.

Multivessel Dilation

Whether or not multivessel angioplasty is planned, angioplasty of the lesion that supplies the greatest amount of viable myocardium should generally be attempted first. The reason for this is twofold. First, when attempted dilation of this most important lesion is unsuccessful, hypotension or other hemodynamic consequences are most likely to occur. If less important lesions are initially dilated and hypotension occurs following the subsequent dilation of the more hemodynamically significant lesion, there is an increased risk that abrupt closure of all the recently dilated lesions may occur (87). If dilation of the most important lesion is performed initially and is unsuccessful, there is less chance that multivessel abrupt closure will occur. In addition, bypass surgery may be considered at that time, regardless of results that may be achieved following angioplasty of less significant lesions. If a suboptimal but acceptable result is achieved following dilation of the most hemodynamically significant lesion, a decision may be made to perform a staged procedure and dilate the remaining lesions 24 to 48 hr

later, at a time when abrupt closure of the first lesion is very unlikely to occur.

In certain cases, however, angioplasty of a less hemodynamically significant lesion should be performed initially, as in the case where an occluded vessel receives collateral blood flow from a subtotally occluded vessel of greater hemodynamic significance. If the occluded vessel is dilated initially, and normal blood flow is restored, collateral blood flow can reverse direction, making subsequent angioplasty of the more hemodynamically significant subtotally occluded artery less hazardous in the event that abrupt closure occurs.

If all the vessels being considered for dilation are roughly equivalent in terms of myocardium supplied, it is generally advisable to attempt the most difficult lesion first. If angioplasty of the most difficult lesion is unsuccessful, it may be advisable to consider alternative treatment strategies. In addition, should the dilation of the difficult lesion take longer and the amount of contrast administered be greater than anticipated, it may be advisable to complete the angioplasty procedure in a staged manner. This is difficult to do when less difficult lesions were initially dilated and it becomes advisable to stage the procedure while still in the middle of the longer, more difficult dilation.

Staged Procedure

There are certain patients in whom multivessel coronary angioplasty is planned and, while no single lesion constitutes a high risk lesion as described above, all of the vessels to be dilated provide blood flow to the majority and in some cases virtually all of the viable myocardium. The use of a staged procedure has been advocated in such patients (39). In a staged procedure, one or more lesions are generally dilated in a single setting, and the remaining lesions are dilated one or more days following the initial angioplasty procedure. Since abrupt closure is most likely to occur in the minutes or hours following dilation, it is believed that a staged multivessel angioplasty procedure is less likely to result in multivessel abrupt closure, which is associated with a high mortality. An additional benefit of a staged procedure is that patients are exposed to a lower amount of contrast over a brief time interval, which reduces the risk of acute renal failure from the nephrotoxic contrast agents. These benefits must be weighed against a greater duration of discomfort to the patient, and a longer hospital stay, with the greater expense that it entails. Such a staged procedure is particularly important in patients undergoing PTCA of an infarct-related artery. In the hours or days following myocardial infarction, only the infarct-related artery should be dilated; other vessels should, in most cases, be approached later.

It has generally been our practice to dilate all lesions in

a single setting, unless a suboptimal result occurs, in which case we will generally not dilate any additional lesions in the same procedure. This approach is based upon the knowledge that abrupt closure is unusual unless a significant coronary dissection or residual stenosis of more than 50% is present. Therefore, the likelihood that abrupt closure will occur in two lesions with adequate results is exceedingly small. The other setting in which we will perform a staged procedure is where the amount of contrast already used is large, usually greater than 400 cc. When contrast is increased above this amount, the likelihood of contrast-induced acute renal failure increases dramatically.

CONCLUSION

Percutaneous transluminal coronary angioplasty has evolved greatly since its initial description. As a result of improved equipment and, in particular, increased operator experience, the types of patients in whom angioplasty can be performed has expanded. At the current time, PTCA is most commonly performed among patients with multivessel disease and acute ischemic syndromes. Patient selection is of the utmost importance in optimizing the results of PTCA. For each patient, the risks and benefits of medical therapy, PTCA, and bypass surgery must be considered. For PTCA, particular consideration must be given to the need for complete revascularization, identification of a culprit lesion, analysis of the characteristics of the lesion or lesions to be dilated, and the potential for restenosis.

The future looks bright for angioplasty among patients with multivessel disease. Its eventual role will be dependent upon the outcome of the randomized trials of PTCA versus bypass surgery. In addition, therapies to prevent restenosis and the development of techniques to more successfully treat chronic total occlusions will have great importance.

REFERENCES

1. Gruentzig A. Transluminal dilation of coronary artery stenoses. *Lancet* 1978;1:263.
2. Detre K, Holubkov R, Kelsey S, Cowley M, Kent K, Williams D, Myler R, Faxon D, Holmes DJ, Bourassa M, Block P, Gosselin A, Bentivoglio L, Leatherman L, Dorros G, King S III, Galichia J, Al-Bassam M, Leon M, Robertson T, Passamani E and the coinvestigators of the National Heart, Lung, and Blood Institute's Percutaneous Transluminal Coronary Angioplasty Registry. Percutaneous transluminal coronary angioplasty in 1985–1986 and 1977–1981. The National Heart, Lung, and Blood Institute Registry. *N Engl J Med* 1988;318:265–270.
3. O'Keefe JH Jr., Rutherford BD, McConahay DR, Johnson WL Jr., Giorgi LV, Ligon RW, Shimshak TM, Hartzler GO. Multivessel coronary angioplasty from 1980 to 1989: procedural results and long-term outcome. *J Am Coll Cardiol* 1990;16:1097–1102.
4. Stevens T, Kahn JK, McCallister BD, Ligon RW, Spaude S, Rutherford BD, McConahay DR, Johnson WL, Giorgi LV, Shimshak TM, Hartzler GO. Safety and efficacy of percutaneous translu-

5. minal coronary angioplasty in patients with left ventricular dysfunction. *Am J Cardiol* 1991;68:313–319.
5. Reeder GS, Holmes DRJ, Detre K, Costigan T, Kelsey SF. Degree of revascularization in patients with multivessel coronary disease: a report from the National Heart, Lung, and Blood Institute Percutaneous Transluminal Coronary Angioplasty Registry. *Circulation* 1988;77:638–644.
6. Bell MR, Bailey KR, Reeder GS, Lapeyre ACIII, Holmes DRJ. Percutaneous transluminal angioplasty in patients with multivessel coronary disease: how important is complete revascularization for cardiac event-free survival? *J Am Coll Cardiol* 1990;16:553–562.
7. Ellis SG, Cowley MJ, DiSciascio G, Deligonul U, Topol EJ, Bulle TM, Vandormael MG. Determinants of 2-year outcome after coronary angioplasty in patients with multivessel disease on the basis of comprehensive preprocedural evaluation. Implications for patient selection. The Multivessel Angioplasty Prognosis Study Group. *Circulation* 1991;83:1905–1914.
8. Deligonul U, Vandormael MG, Kern MJ, Zelman R, Galan K, Chaitman BR. Coronary angioplasty: a therapeutic option for symptomatic patients with two and three vessel coronary disease. *J Am Coll Cardiol* 1988;11:1173–1179.
9. Vandormael M, Deligonul U, Taussig S, Kern MJ. Predictors of long-term cardiac survival in patients with multivessel coronary artery disease undergoing percutaneous transluminal coronary angioplasty. *Am J Cardiol* 1991;67:1–6.
10. Mata LA, Bosch X, David PR, Rapold HJ, Corcos T, Bourassa MG. Clinical and angiographic assessment 6 months after double vessel percutaneous coronary angioplasty. *J Am Coll Cardiol* 1985;6:1239–1244.
11. Cowley MJ, Vetrovec GW, DiSciascio G, Lewis SA, Hirsh PD, Wolfgang TC. Coronary angioplasty of multiple vessels: short-term outcome and long-term results. *Circulation* 1985;72:1314–1320.
12. CASS principal investigators and their associates. Coronary Artery Surgery Study (CASS): a randomized trial of coronary artery bypass surgery. Survival data. *Circulation* 1983;68:939–950.
13. Vandormael MG, Chaitman BR, Ischinger T, Aker UT, Harper M, Hernandez J, Deligonul U, Kennedy HL. Immediate and short-term benefit of multilesion coronary angioplasty: influence of degree of revascularization. *J Am Coll Cardiol* 1985;6:983–991.
14. Weintraub WS, Jones EL, King SB III, Craver J, Douglas JS, Guton R, Liberman H, Morris D. Changing use of coronary angioplasty and coronary bypass surgery in the treatment of chronic coronary artery disease. *Am J Cardiol* 1990;65:183–188.
15. Kennedy JW, Kaiser GC, Fisher L, Fritz JK, Myers W, Mudd JG, Ryan TJ. Clinical and angiographic predictors of operative mortality from the Collaborative Study in Coronary Artery Surgery (CASS). *Circulation* 1981;63:793–802.
16. Gersh BJ, Holmes DRJ. Coronary angioplasty as the preferred approach to treatment of multivessel disease: promising, appealing but unproved. *J Am Coll Cardiol* 1990;16:1104–1106.
17. RITA Trial Participants. Coronary angioplasty versus coronary artery bypass surgery: the Randomised Intervention Treatment of Angina (RITA) trial. *Lancet* 1993;341:573–580.
18. Tyras DH, Barner HB, Kaiser GC, Codd JE, Laks H, Pennington DG, Willman VL. Long-term results of myocardial revascularization. *Am J Cardiol* 1979;44:1290–1296.
19. Lawrie GM, Morris GC, Silvers A, Wagner WF, Baron AE, Beltangady SS, Glaeser DH, Chapman DW. The influence of residual disease after coronary bypass on the 5-year survival rate of 1274 men with coronary artery disease. *Circulation* 1982;66:717–723.
20. Samson M, Meester HJ, de Feyter PJ, Strauss B, Serruys PW. Successful multiple segment coronary angioplasty: effect of completeness of revascularization in single-vessel multilesions and multivessels. *Am Heart J* 1990;120:1–12.
21. Cukingnan RA, Carey JS, Wittig JH, Brown BG. Influence of complete coronary revascularization on relief of angina. *J Thorac Cardiovasc Surg* 1980;79:188–193.
22. Lavee J, Rath S, Tran-Quang-Hoa, Ra'anani P, Ruder A, Modan M, Neufeld HN, Goor DA. Does complete revascularization by the conventional method truly provide the best possible results? *J Thorac Cardiovasc Surg* 1986;92:279–290.
23. Schaff HV, Gersh BJ, Pluth JR, Danielson GK, Orszulak TA,

Puga FJ, Piehler JM, Frye RL. Survival and functional status after coronary artery bypass grafting: results 10 to 12 years after surgery in 500 patients. *Circulation* 1983;68[Suppl II]:II-200–II-204.

24. Gohlke H, Gohlke-Barwolf C, Samek L, Sturzenofecker P, Schumiger M, Roskamm H. Serial exercise testing up to 6 years after coronary bypass surgery: behavior of exercise parameters in groups with different degrees of revascularization determined by postoperative angiography. *Am J Cardiol* 1983;51:1301–1306.

25. Jones EL, Craver JM, Guyton RA, Bone DK, Hatcher CR, Riechwald N. Importance of complete revascularization in performance of the coronary bypass operation. *Am J Cardiol* 1983;51:7–12.

26. Holmes DRJ, Reeder GS, Vlietstra RE. Role of percutaneous transluminal coronary angioplasty in multivessel disease. *Am J Cardiol* 1988;61:9G–14G.

27. Bell MR, Gersh BJ, Schaff HV, Holmes DRJ, Fisher LD, Alderman EL, Myers WO, Parsons LS, Reeder GS and the investigators of the Coronary Artery Surgery Study. The effect of the completeness of revascularization on the long-term outcome of patients with three-vessel disease undergoing coronary artery bypass surgery: a report from the Coronary Artery Surgery (CASS) Study. *Circulation* 1992;86:446–457.

28. Ambrose JA, Tannenbaum MA, Alexopoulos D, Hjemdahl-Monsen CE, Leavy J, Weiss M, Borrico S, Gorlin R, Fuster V. Angiographic progression of coronary artery disease and the development of myocardial infarction. *J Am Coll Cardiol* 1988;12:56–62.

29. Little WC, Constantinescu M, Applegate RJ, Kutcher MA, Burrows MT, Kahl FR, Santamore WP. Can coronary angiography predict the site of a subsequent myocardial infarction in patients with mild to moderate coronary artery disease? *Circulation* 1988;78:1157–1166.

30. Mabin TA, Holmes DRJ, Bove AA, Hammes LN, Elveback LR, Orszulak TA. Follow-up clinical results in patients undergoing percutaneous transluminal coronary angioplasty. *Circulation* 1985; 71:754–760.

31. Alderman EL, Bourassa MG, Cohen LS, Davis KB, Kaiser GG, Killip T, Mock MB, Pettinger M, Robertson TL. Ten-year follow-up of survival and myocardial infarction in the Coronary Artery Surgery Study. *Circulation* 1990;82:1629–1646.

32. Mock MB, Fisher LD, Holmes DRJ, Gersh BJ, Schaff HV, Ryan TJ, Myers WO, Killip TKI. Comparison of effects of medical and surgical therapy on survival in severe angina pectoris and two-vessel coronary artery disease with and without left ventricular dysfunction: a Coronary Artery Surgery Study Registry study. *Am J Cardiol* 1988;61:1198–1203.

33. Weiner DA, Ryan TJ, McCabe CH, Chaitman BR, Sheffield T, Fisher LD, Tristani F. The role of exercise testing in identifying patients with improved survival after coronary artery bypass surgery. *J Am Coll Cardiol* 1986;8:741–748.

34. O'Keefe JR Jr, Hartzler GG, Rutherford BD, McConahay DR, Johnson WL, Giorgi RV, Ligon RW. Left main coronary angioplasty: early and late results of 127 acute and elective procedures. *Am J Cardiol* 1989;64:144–147.

35. Breisblatt WM, Barnes JV, Weiland F, Spaccavento LJ. Incomplete revascularization in multivessel percutaneous transluminal coronary angioplasty: the role for stress thallium-201 imaging. *J Am Coll Cardiol* 1988;11:1183–1190.

36. Berger PB, Bell MR, Garratt KN, Hammes L, Grill DE, Holmes DR Jr. Clinical outcome of patients with rest angina and multivessel disease undergoing culprit versus multivessel PTCA, and the influence of complete revascularization. *J Am Coll Cardiol* 1992;19(suppl A):138A.

37. Ellis SG, Vandormael MG, Cowley MJ, DiSciascio G, Deligonul U, Topol EJ, Bulle TM. Coronary morphologic and clinical determinants of procedural outcome with angioplasty for multivessel coronary disease. Implications for patient selection. Multivessel Angioplasty Prognosis Study Group. *Circulation* 1990;82: 1193–1202.

38. Finci L, Meier B, De Bruyne B, Steffenino G, Divernois J, Rutishauser W. Angiographic follow-up after multivessel percutaneous transluminal coronary angioplasty. *Am J Cardiol* 1987;60: 467–470.

39. DiSciascio G, Cowley MJ, Vetrovec GW, Kelly KM, Lewis SA.

Triple vessel coronary angioplasty: acute outcome and long-term results. *J Am Coll Cardiol* 1988;12:42–48.

40. Myler RK, Topol EJ, Shaw RE, Stertzer SH, Clark DA, Fishman J, Murphy MC. Multivessel coronary angioplasty: classification, results, and patterns of restenosis in 494 consecutive patients. *Cathet Cardiovasc Diagn* 1987;13:1–15.

41. Dorros G, Lewin RF, Janke L. Multiple lesion transluminal coronary angioplasty in single and multivessel coronary artery disease: acute outcome and long-term effect. *J Am Coll Cardiol* 1987;10:1007–1113.

42. Holmes DRJ, Holubkov R, Vlietstra RE, Kelsey SF, Reeder GS, Dorros G, Williams DO, Cowley MJ, Faxon DP, Kent KM, Bentivoglio LG, Detre K, and the coinvestigators of the National Heart, Lung, and Blood Institute Percutaneous Transluminal Coronary Angioplasty Registry. Comparison of complications during percutaneous transluminal coronary angioplasty from 1977 to 1981 and from 1985 to 1986: the National Heart, Lung, and Blood Institute Percutaneous Transluminal Coronary Angioplasty Registry. *J Am Coll Cardiol* 1988;12:1149–1155.

43. Cowley MJ, Dorros G, Kelsey SF, Van Raden M, Detre KM. Acute coronary events associated with percutaneous transluminal coronary angioplasty. *Am J Cardiol* 1983;53:12C–16C.

44. Meier B, Gruentzig AR, King SB III, Douglas JS, Hollman J, Ishinger T, Aueron F, Galan K. Risk of side branch occlusion during coronary angioplasty. *Am J Cardiol* 1984;53:10–14.

45. Meier B, Gruentzig AR, Hollman J, Ischinger T, Bradford JM. Does length or eccentricity of coronary stenoses influence the outcome of transluminal dilatation? *Circulation* 1983;67:497–499.

46. Ellis SG, Roubin GS, King SBI, Douglas JSJ, Weintraub WS, Thomas RG, Cox WR. Angiographic and clinical predictors of acute closure after native vessel coronary angioplasty. *Circulation* 1988;77:372–379.

47. Ischinger T, Gruentzig AR, Meier B, Galan K. Coronary dissection and total coronary occlusion associated with percutaneous transluminal coronary angioplasty: significance of initial angiographic morphology of coronary stenoses. *Circulation* 1986; 74:1371–1378.

48. Ryan TJ, Faxon DP, Gunnar RM, Kennedy JW, King SBI, Loop FD, Peterson KL, Reeves TJ, Williams DO, Winters WLJ. Guidelines for percutaneous transluminal coronary angioplasty: a report of the American College of Cardiology/American Heart Association Task Force on Assessment of Diagnostic and Therapeutic Cardiovascular Procedures (Subcommittee on Percutaneous Transluminal Coronary Angioplasty). *J Am Coll Cardiol* 1988;12:529–545.

49. Kleinman NS, Rodriguez AR, Raizner AE. Interobserver variability in grading of coronary arterial narrowings using the American College of Cardiology/American Heart Association grading criteria. *Am J Cardiol* 1992;69:413–415.

50. Stone GW, Rutherford BD, McConahay DR, Johnson WLJ, Giorgi LV, Ligon RW, Hartzler GO. Procedural outcome of angioplasty for total coronary artery occlusion: an analysis of 971 lesions in 905 patients. *J Am Coll Cardiol* 1990;15:849–856.

51. Bell MR, Berger PB, Bresnahan JF, Reeder GS, Bailey KR, Holmes DRJ. Initial and long-term outcome of 354 patients following coronary balloon angioplasty of total coronary artery occlusions. *Circulation* 1992;85:1003–1011.

52. Hollman J, Gruentzig AR, Douglas JRJ, King SB, Ischinger T, Meier B. Acute occlusion after percutaneous transluminal coronary angioplasty—a new approach. *Circulation* 1983;68:725–732.

53. Sinclair IN, McCabe GH, Sipperly ME, Baim DS. Abrupt reclosure: predictors, therapeutic options, and long-term outcome. *J Am Coll Cardiol* 1988;11:132A.

54. Palazzo AM, Gustafson GM, Santilli E, Kemp HG Jr,. Unusually long inflation times during percutaneous transluminal coronary angioplasty. *Cathet Cardiovasc Diagn* 1988;14:154–158.

55. Leitschuh ML, Mills RM, Jacobs AK, Ruocco NAJ, Larosa D, Faxon DP. Outcome after major dissection during coronary angioplasty using the perfusion balloon catheter. *Am J Cardiol* 1991;67:1056–1060.

56. Cannon AD, Roubin GS, Dean LS, Baxley SK, Agrawal SK. Acute and threatened closure complicating PTCA: treatment by intracoronary stenting. *Aust N Z J Med* 1991;21:506.

57. Strauss BH, Serruys PW, Bertrand ME, Puel J, Meier B, Goy JJ, Kappenberger L, Rickards AF, Sigwart U. Quantitative angiographic follow-up of the coronary Wallstent in native vessels and bypass grafts (European experience—March 1986 to March 1990). *Am J Cardiol* 1992;69:475–481.
58. Lambert M, Bonan R, Cote G, Crepeau J, de Guise P, Lesperance J, David PR, Waters DD. Early results, complications and restenosis rates after multilesion and multivessel percutaneous transluminal coronary angioplasty. *Am J Cardiol* 1987;60:788–791.
59. Vandormael MG, Deligonul U, Kern MJ, Kennedy H, Galan K, Chaitman B. Restenosis after multilesion percutaneous transluminal coronary angioplasty. *Am J Cardiol* 1987;60:44B–47B.
60. Roubin GS, King SBI. Restenosis after percutaneous transluminal coronary angioplasty: the Emory University Hospital experience. *Am J Cardiol* 1987;60:39B–43B.
61. DiSciascio G, Cowley MJ. Multivessel coronary artery disease. *Cardiovasc Clin* 1988;19:101–114.
62. Vandormael MG, Deligonul U, Kern MJ, Harper M, Presant S, Gibson P, Galan K, Chaitman B. Multilesion coronary angioplasty: clinical and angiographic follow-up. *J Am Coll Cardiol* 1987;10:246–252.
63. Edmunds LH, Stephenson LW, Edie RN, Ratcliffe MB. Openheart surgery in octogenarians. *N Engl J Med* 1988;319:131–136.
64. Weintraub WS, Jones EL, Craver J, Guyton R, Cohen CL. Determinants of prolonged length of hospital stay after coronary bypass surgery. *Circulation* 1989;80:276–284.
65. Macaya C, Alfonso F, Iniguez A, Zarco P. Long-term clinical and angiographic follow-up of percutaneous transluminal coronary angioplasty in patients ≥65 years of age. *Am J Cardiol* 1990;66:1513–1515.
66. Thompson RC, Holmes DRJ, Gersh BJ, Mock MB, Bailey KR. Percutaneous transluminal coronary angioplasty in the elderly: early and long-term results. *J Am Coll Cardiol* 1991;17:1245–1250.
67. Raizner AE, Hust RG, Lewis JM, Winters WLJ, Batty JW, Roberts R. Transluminal coronary angioplasty in the elderly. *Am J Cardiol* 1986;57:29–32.
68. Jones EL, Abi-Mansour P, Gruentzig AR. Coronary artery bypass surgery and percutaneous transluminal angioplasty in the elderly patient. *Cardiology* 1986;73:223–234.
69. Dorros G, Janke L. Percutaneous transluminal coronary angioplasty in patients over the age of 70 years. *Cathet Cardiovasc Diagn* 1986;12:223–229.
70. Zaidi AR, Hollman J, Frano I, Simpfendorfer C, Galan K. Percutaneous transluminal coronary angioplasty in patients over the age of 70 years. *Geriatrics* 1985;40:38–44.
71. Mock MB, Holmes DRJ, Vliestra RE, Gersh BJ, Detre KM, Kelsey SF, Orszulak TA, Schaff HV, Peihler JM, VanRaden MJ, Passamani ER, Kent JM, Gruentzig AR. Percutaneous transluminal coronary angioplasty (PTCA) in the elderly patient: experience in the National Heart, Lung, and Blood Institute PTCA Registry. *Am J Cardiol* 1984;53:89–91C.
72. Kern MJ, Deligonul U, Galan K, Zelman R, Gabliani G, Bell ST, Bodet J, Naunheim K, Vandormael M. Percutaneous transluminal coronary angioplasty in octagenarians. *Am J Cardiol* 1988;61:457–458.
73. Rich JJ, Crispino CM, Saporito JJ, Domat I, Cooper WM. Percutaneous transluminal coronary angioplasty in patients 80 years of age and older. *Am J Cardiol* 1990;65:675–676.
74. Campeau L, Enjalbert M, Lesperance J, Bourassa MG, Kwiterovich P, Wacholder S, Sniderman A. The relationship of risk factors to the development of atherosclerosis in saphenous vein grafts and the progression of disease in the native circulation: a study of 10 years after aortocoronary bypass surgery. *N Engl J Med* 1984;311:1329–1332.
75. Guthaner DF, Robert EW, Alderman EL, Wexler L. Long-term serial angiographic studies after coronary artery bypass surgery. *Circulation* 1979;60:250–259.
76. Plokker HWT, Meester BH, Serruys PW. The Dutch experience in percutaneous transluminal angioplasty of narrowed saphenous veins used for aortocoronary arterial bypass. *Am J Cardiol* 1991;67:361–366.
77. Douglas JS, Gruentzig AR, King SB III, Hollman J, Ischinger T, Meier B, Craver JM, Jones EL, Waller JL, Bone DK, Guyton R. Percutaneous transluminal coronary angioplasty in patients with prior coronary bypass surgery. *J Am Coll Cardiol* 1983;2:745–754.
78. Douglas JS, King S, Roubin G, Schlumpf M. Percutaneous angioplasty of venous aortocoronary graft stenoses: late angiographic and clinical outcome. *Circulation* 1986;74[Suppl II]:II–281.
79. Schwartz L, Bourassa MG, Lesperance J, Aldridge HE, Kazim F, Salvatori VA, Henderson M, Bonan R, David PR. Aspirin and dipyridamole in the prevention of restenosis after percutaneous transluminal coronary angioplasty: a randomized study. *N Engl J Med* 1988;318:1714–1719.
80. Stone GW, Ligon RW, Rutherford BD, McConahay DR, Hartzler GO. Short-term outcome and long-term follow-up following coronary angioplasty in the young patient: an 8-year experience. *Am Heart J* 1989;118:873–877.
81. Holmes DRJ, Detre KM, Williams DO, Kent KM, King SB III, Yea W, Steenkiste MS. Long-term outcome of patients with depressed left ventricular function undergoing percutaneous transluminal coronary angioplasty: the NHLBI PTCA Registry. *Circulation* 1992; (in press).
82. Kohli RS, DiSciascio G, Cowley MJ, Nath A, Goudreau E, Vetrovec GW. Coronary angioplasty in patients with severe left ventricular dysfunction. *J Am Coll Cardiol* 1990;16:807–811.
83. Kahn JK, Rutherford BD, McConahay DR, Johnson WL, Giorge LV, Hartzler GO. Supported "high risk" coronary angioplasty using intraaortic balloon pump counterpulsation. *J Am Coll Cardiol* 1990;15:1151–1155.
84. Lincoff AM, Popma JJ, Ellis SG, Vogel RA, Topol EJ. Percutaneous support devices for high risk or complicated coronary angioplasty. *J Am Coll Cardiol* 1991;17:770–780.
85. Wohlgelernter D, Cleman M, Highman HA, Zaret BL. Percutaneous transluminal coronary angioplasty of the "culprit lesion" for management of unstable angina pectoris in patients with multivessel coronary artery disease. *Am J Cardiol* 1986;58:460–464.
86. de Feyter PJ, Serruys PW, Arnold A, Simoons ML, Wijns W, Geuskens R, Soward A, van den Brand M, Hugenholtz PG. Coronary angioplasty of the unstable angina related vessel in patients with multivessel disease. *Eur Heart J* 1986;7:460–467.
87. Gaul G, Hollman J, Simpfendorfer C, Franco I. Acute occlusion in multiple lesion coronary angioplasty: frequency and management. *J Am Coll Cardiol* 1989;13:283–288.

Practical Angioplasty,
edited by David P. Faxon.
Raven Press, Ltd., New York © 1993.

CHAPTER 9

Coronary Angioplasty of Bifurcation Lesions

Geoffrey O. Hartzler

Bifurcation lesions present certain judgmental and technical challenges for coronary angioplasty (Fig. 1). Atheromatous plaque which is adjacent to, at, or involving the origin of a side branch has been associated with an increased incidence of side-branch closure during coronary angioplasty (1–3). Additionally, some practitioners have suggested that a relatively increased restenosis rate exists for successfully dilated bifurcation lesions (4). Consequently, and in the last decade, there have been numerous reports describing a variety of unique approaches to the management of bifurcation lesions (5–12).

THE PROBLEM

The immediate sequelae of balloon inflation within an atheromatous plaque are complex. In addition to trivial compression, gross splitting, cracking and localized dissection, some longitudinal shift of plaque within the arterial wall occurs, with potential for side-branch compromise or occlusion. In all likelihood, tiny tertiary branches are commonly occluded by balloon angioplasty, although they are not angiographically evident before or after the procedure, and are without clinical consequence. However, when plaque shift occludes a larger or major bifurcating side branch, myocardial ischemia and infarction can result. In an early report from Emory University (1), the risk of side-branch occlusion during coronary angioplasty was determined to be 5%. However, of the side branches judged to be at higher risk for occlusion, 14% became obstructed during coronary angioplasty.

In a survey of 50 major referral centers, bifurcation stenoses were estimated to occur with a frequency of approximately 9% in patients undergoing diagnostic coronary angiography (13). However, the overall frequency of bifurcation stenoses in any angioplasty population may differ from institution to institution, or operator to operator, depending upon referral patterns of more or less complex coronary disease and operator selection. In a recent 12-month laboratory experience by the author, 47 (9%) of 533 patients undergoing angioplasty had bifurcation lesions dilated; they represented approximately 3% of all stenoses.

HISTORY AND EVOLVING STRATEGIES FOR BIFURCATION ANGIOPLASTY

In the late 1970s and early 1980s, side-branch occlusion was more common as a direct result of the primitive and technically inadequate balloon catheters utilized. These first-generation, fixed-wire, highly compliant, and nonsteerable balloon catheters presented few management options. Further, the importance of careful analysis of each stenosis to include morphologic features and its location relative to side branches had not yet been appreciated. The subsequent development and use of high-resolution imaging systems for coronary angiography and angioplasty clearly allowed more optimal lesion assessment and selection. Still, operators were limited to the use of a single balloon without steerable guidewire. In the setting of acute side-branch occlusion, there was just one option to restore flow: emergency bypass surgery. Consequently, the presence of a bifurcation stenosis served as a relative contraindication to coronary angioplasty.

The introduction of the original over-the-wire angioplasty catheter (Simpson-Robert, Advanced Cardiovascular Systems, Inc.) offered no real improvement in the management of bifurcation lesions. Although shapeable, guidewires were stiff and nonsteerable. In 1983, the development of shapeable, yet flexible and steerable guidewires were pioneering accomplishments in coronary an-

G. O. Hartzler: University of Missouri at Kansas City, Kansas City, Missouri; and Mid-America Heart Institute, Kansas City, Missouri 64111

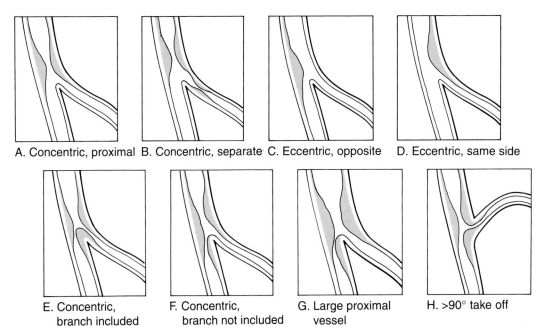

A. Concentric, proximal B. Concentric, separate C. Eccentric, opposite D. Eccentric, same side

E. Concentric, branch included F. Concentric, branch not included G. Large proximal vessel H. >90° take off

FIG. 1. The various anatomical situations that can occur with bifurcation lesions.

gioplasty, further increasing the applicability of the procedure to more patients and stenoses. These guidewires allowed the operator to probe, select, and reopen an occluded side-branch with improved control, success, and safety.

Kissing balloon angioplasty for peripheral vascular disease was first described in 1980 for treatment of the Leriche syndrome (14). Subsequently, two authors (1,9) attributed the introduction of kissing balloons for coronary angioplasty to Dr. Andreas Gruentzig. In 1984, Meier described the use of two over-the-wire balloon catheter systems for kissing balloon coronary angioplasty utilizing bifemoral arterial punctures and two guiding systems in 3 patients (5). Also in 1984, Zack and Ischinger described an essentially identical approach for treatment of 8 patients with bifurcation lesions (6). George et al. detailed a larger experience in 52 patients using kissing balloon techniques. They typically introduced one guide catheter via the femoral approach and the second via the brachial approach (9). In their series, two-thirds of balloon inflations were performed simultaneously, and one-third sequentially.

In 1984, McAuley et al. described a modified approach using a single guiding catheter through which two wires were placed, one a protective guidewire positioned in one of the bifurcating limbs and the second with dilating balloon positioned in the other bifurcating limb (7). In the face of side-branch closure as a sequel to dilatation of the primary vessel, the previously placed protective guidewire allowed access to the occluded side branch with an over-the-wire system. In 1985, Pinkerton et al. further described this two-wire, one-balloon approach to bifurcation lesions in 13 patients (8). They utilized dou-

ble arterial puncture and two guiding catheters for left coronary stenoses, but a single guide catheter for right coronary lesions, in concert with a single protective exchange wire plus a newly developed, fixed-wire, low-profile, yet steerable, balloon catheter (LPS, ACS). These authors concluded that the use of the kissing balloon technique was cumbersome and technically demanding, while noting excellent results with their approach of first dilating the major stenosis with the fixed-wire catheter, followed by its subsequent removal and passage of an over-the-wire balloon catheter for branch dilatation when required. Many subsequent technical variations on these approaches to bifurcation lesions have been reported, including crossing balloons (11), the double long-wire technique (12), the simultaneous use of two fixed-wire low-profile balloon catheters, the monorail variation of two-wire techniques, and even triple-wire usage for a trifurcation lesion (15).

Most practitioners and authors have observed that with two guidewires passed through a single guiding catheter, wrapping of guidewires can occur and complicate both wire manipulation and balloon advancement. Later, as guiding catheters appeared with larger internal diameters, and newer generation low-profile, fixed-wire balloon catheters came into existence (Probe, United States Cathater and Instrument Company), it became feasible to routinely introduce two balloon catheters through one guiding catheter for protection, and alternate or simultaneous balloon inflations. However, true steerability of these devices was compromised, and wrapping persisted as a problem within the catheter shaft and balloon segment. In the late 1980s, continued miniaturization of balloon catheters and guidewires came to allow the introduction of two complete, over-the-wire, steerable balloon catheter systems through a single guiding catheter and markedly facilitated the operator's ability to successfully dilate most bifurcation lesions.

Uncertainty continues regarding bifurcation lesion restenosis rates, with some authors suggesting a higher incidence of recurrence (4). The basis for any increase in restenosis rate remains unclear, although it has been postulated that there is a contribution from increased mechanical trauma to the bifurcating arterial segment due to the use of two intracoronary devices. Other possibilities include the relatively greater plaque burden shared by two branches, or the less satisfactory primary results obtained in earlier years of bifurcation angioplasty. The postulate that bifurcation restenosis rates are increased is not clearly supported by recent data which include analyses by Pinkerton et al. (16) and Renkin et al. (17). The definitive answer will remain elusive until large series of bifurcation lesions undergoing successful percutaneous transluminal coronary angioplasty are subject to a high degree of angiographic follow-up with patient populations controlled for other factors known to be associated with increased restenosis rates.

BIFURCATION CORONARY ANATOMY ASSOCIATED WITH SIDE-BRANCH CLOSURE

Regardless of the historical approach to bifurcation lesions and catheter systems utilized, the concern then and today remains the same: how to predict and prevent bifurcation or side-branch closure during balloon angioplasty. Obviously, optimal patient care and safety remain overriding considerations in coronary angioplasty. Secondary considerations include costs. If the operator chose to use a two-wire or two-balloon catheter system in all patients with bifurcation lesions, procedural costs would be excessively augmented in over 86% of patients with bifurcation stenoses, if the report from Emory University (1) is used as a branch occlusion model.

A strong argument can be made for minimizing the use of two-wire and two-balloon techniques. The approach itself is cumbersome and introduces some increased technical risk, largely due to additionally required intracoronary manipulations. Many side branches are not of large enough magnitude to justify the increased cost and effort of dual approaches. Many side branches originate by marked angulation from the parent vessel, therefore requiring excessive technical manipulation, which in itself may promote closure of the branch or parent vessel. Further, if the proximal stenosis is extremely severe, it may not be possible to easily pass two wires through both limbs of a bifurcation, due to wire-induced obstruction to the central lumen. Finally, as in other endeavors, angioplasty is generally best when kept simple.

Perhaps most bifurcation lesions have specific anatomic features which do not correlate with branch closure. If the origin or ostium of the side branch is free of significant occlusive disease, it is extremely unlikely that the branch will close despite placement of a balloon directly across the origin of the side branch for dilatation of discrete or diffuse lesions located immediately adjacent to the branch. This statement generally holds true, even in the presence of severe narrowings of the primary vessel that commence prior to and extend past the origin of the side branch.

By careful analysis of bifurcation morphology, the experienced operator may commonly identify a single wire/balloon strategy minimizing the chance of branch closure. For example, in the setting of bifurcation disease, multiple angiographic views may reveal that the bulk of the atheromatous plaque is, in fact, contralateral to the origin of the side branch, which itself is widely patient or only minimally narrowed. In these circumstances, it can be expected that the majority of plaque shift will be in the wall of the parent vessel contralateral to the side branch origin. Consequently, most bifurcation stenoses of this nature can be satisfactorily dilated with a single wire/balloon catheter system. Other bifurcation lesions may include substantial bulky plaque ipsilateral to the origin of the side branch which itself has some ostial disease. In this circumstance, it may be highly effective to place a single guidewire through the proximal portion of the bifurcation stenosis so as to select the side branch itself. A single balloon positioned in the proximal portion of the stenosis with distal aspect in the ostium effectively protects and dilates the ostium while preventing plaque shift into the branch ostium. Rarely, in well-selected bifurcation stenoses approached with single-balloon techniques, plaque may shift into an unprotected branch or parent vessel. If significant plaque shift continues to occur despite alternate single-balloon inflations in each branch of the bifurcation, it is appropriate to pass two balloons into the coronary artery and position them adjacent to each other, so as to encompass the parent vessel and the origin of the side branch for simultaneous inflations. Typically, and perhaps most safely, relatively low pressure inflations are utilized with attention focused upon the combined and additional dilating effect of the hugging portions of the balloons immediately proximal to the bifurcation. In the author's experience, it has been extremely uncommon to create adverse sequelae due to gross overexpansion in this segment, particularly when avoiding higher pressure simultaneous inflations, which are rarely required in the setting of predilatation at each site with a single balloon catheter system.

When using simultaneous balloon placement and inflation, the size of the balloon catheter selected for the parent vessel is based on the normal caliber of the artery immediately distal to the point of bifurcation. Similarly, the balloon size selected for the side branch would be that judged appropriate for the normal caliber of the side branch immediately past its origin. By using a strategy of initial low-pressure inflations followed by sequential increments in pressure within both balloons, it is possible to achieve wider patency in the larger segment immediately proximal to the bifurcation than that achievable with any single balloon catheter system, while effectively protecting and dilating both of the bifurcational limbs without overexpansion. Although this approach was technically cumbersome in earlier years and generally required the use of poorly steerable, fixed-wire balloon catheter systems, by the 1990s this could be easily accomplished with newer generation, extremely low profile, over-the-wire balloon catheter systems through one guiding catheter.

Obviously, there are anatomic circumstances where procedural safety is increased and outcome enhanced by alternate, sequential, or even simultaneous balloon inflations in a bifurcation stenosis as described above. The anatomy most typically correlating with, yet not clearly predicting branch closure, is the presence of severe, diffuse, and bulky atheromatous disease commencing prior to the branch and extending across the origin of the branch in the setting of additional, intrinsic, severe stenosis at the true ostium of the side branch. In this circumstance, even minor plaque shift during balloon inflation in the primary vessel may further narrow or occlude the side branch. When this anatomy is identified, it is appropriate to place two balloons simultaneously at the outset of the procedure for controlled, incremental inflations as described above. The author has observed that despite this particular anatomy and even with a single-wire balloon approach, branch occlusion occurs in less than 10% of cases. Still, this higher risk bifurcation anatomy should prompt strong consideration of a dual-wire/balloon approach and simultaneous inflations, particularly if the segment of parent artery immediately proximal to the bifurcation is larger than either of the bifurcating limbs.

CASE EXAMPLES

Case 1

Fig. 2A,B shows before and after cine frames in left anterior oblique (LAO) cranial projection. Figure 2A depicts a bifurcation stenosis with a high-grade tubular zone of narrowing in the distal right coronary artery at the bifurcation into the posterior descending branch and the posterolateral segment. The origin of the posterolateral segment is also approximately 60% narrowed, with minor tubular narrowing from the origin of the posterior descending branch. This type of bifurcation lesion can easily be dilated using a single-wire balloon strategy. By first placing the balloon in the distal right coronary, with the tip of the balloon catheter positioned in the postero-

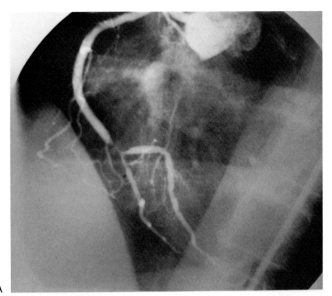

A

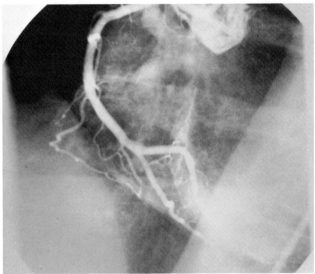

B

FIG. 2. Cine frames; left anterior oblique (LAO) cranial projection. **A:** Bifurcation stenosis with a high-grade tubular zone of narrowing in the distal right coronary artery at the posterior descending branch. **B:** Wide patency of the distal right coronary artery and the posterior descending branch achieved by angioplasty.

lateral segment, the bulk of the plaque was lifted away from the origin of the posterolateral segment. The balloon was then redirected across the distal right coronary lesion to encompass the origin of the posterior descending branch and achieved wide patency of both vessels as depicted in Fig. 2B.

Case 2

Fig. 3A illustrates a moderately complex bifurcation lesion involving the distal circumflex at the origin of a large obtuse marginal branch. There is marked proximal angulation with a high-grade tubular zone of narrowing extending to the bifurcation and significant intrinsic narrowing of both continuing limbs. Upon careful analysis of this projection [right anterior oblique (RAO) caudal], it is evident that the bulk of the plaque proximal to the bifurcation is ipsilateral to the origin of the obtuse marginal branch. The continuing distal circumflex past the obtuse marginal branch is approximately 60% narrowed at its origin, but the extent of plaque contralateral to the obtuse marginal is small. Dilatation was accomplished using a single-wire and balloon catheter system first positioned in the circumflex artery and extended into the obtuse marginal branch to effectively lift plaque away from the origin of the obtuse marginal. The balloon was then positioned across the origin of the obtuse marginal to better dilate the origin of the continuing distal circumflex. Fig. 3B illustrates the immediate postprocedural result.

Case 3

This case demonstrates the use of the classical two-wire technique for dilatation of a proximal left anterior descending (LAD) diagonal branch bifurcation stenosis. Fig. 4A illustrates the bifurcation stenosis, particularly as it involves the origin of the diagonal branch in an LAO cranial projection. Fig. 4B is an RAO cranial view depicting high-grade tubular narrowing of the proximal LAD artery immediately prior to the diagonal branch, which arises by a marked angle. This frame strongly suggests that a single balloon placed across the origin of the diagonal branch would shift much of the plaque located ipsilateral to the diagonal into the origin of that branch with further compromise. Fig. 4C and all subsequent frames are in the RAO cranial projection. Initially, a floppy-tipped guidewire was used to select the diagonal branch through a 2-mm balloon catheter. The balloon tip was advanced into the diagonal, followed by withdrawal of the guidewire and replacement with a 300-cm exchange wire. Fig. 4D illustrates the passage of a fixed-wire, steerable balloon catheter (LPS, ACS) alongside the previously placed exchange wire, for primary dilatation in the LAD artery itself. Fig. 4E demonstrates the achievement of wide angiographic patency in the LAD artery but significant compromise with filling defect at the origin of the diagonal branch due to plaque shift from the LAD artery proper. However, the exchange wire remains in place giving access to the vessel. Fig. 4F illustrates removal of the fixed-wire balloon catheter from the LAD artery and passage of an over-the-wire system into the diagonal branch by utilizing the previously placed exchange wire. Because the previous, successful dilatation of the LAD artery achieved wide patency, and because of the very localized nature of the increased obstruction at the origin of the diagonal branch, there is negligible chance for compromise to the

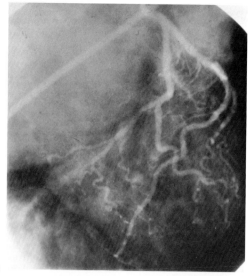

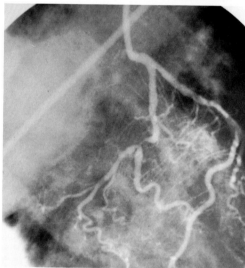

FIG. 3. Right anterior oblique (RAO) caudal projection. **A:** Moderately complex bifurcation lesion involving the distal circumflex artery at the origin of a large obtuse marginal branch. **B:** Vessels after dilatation.

previously dilated LAD artery by balloon inflation in this position. Fig. 4G illustrates the final result, with injection performed over the exchange wire. Wide patency has been restored to the ostium of the diagonal branch with no additional compromise of the LAD artery.

Case 4

This case illustrates the only quadrification lesion seen to date by the author in which a four-wire technique could reasonably be contemplated. Because of unusual vessel anatomy, angulations, and tortuosity, no single view adequately depicts the anatomy. Fig. 5A is an LAO, slightly cranial projection, demonstrating proximal LAD ectasia followed by a significant stenosis, which extends past the origin of the complex diagonal branch

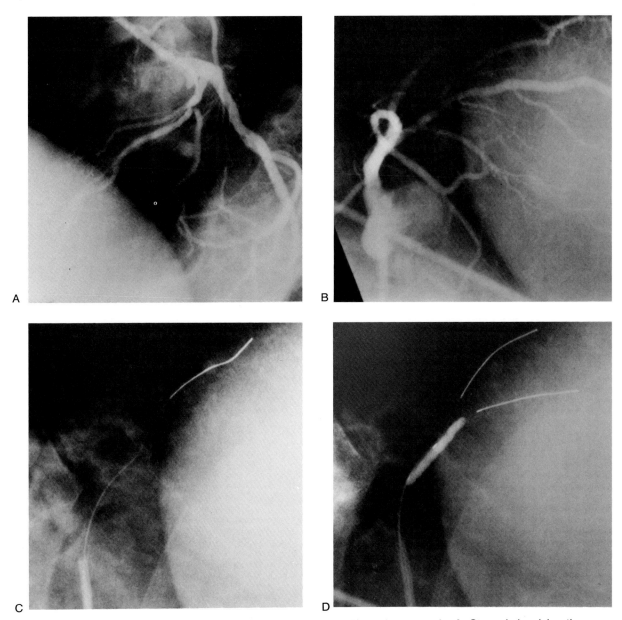

FIG. 4. Left anterior descending (LAD) diagonal branch bifurcation stenosis. **A:** Stenosis involving the origin of the diagonal branch; LAO cranial projection. **B:** Narrowing of the proximal LAD artery immediately prior to the diagonal branch; RAO cranial view. **C:** Exchange wire (300 cm) in place. **D:** Fixed-wire, steerable balloon catheter alongside the previously placed exchange wire; RAO projection. **E:** Angiographic patency in the LAD artery accompanied by plaque shift to the origin of the diagonal branch. The exchange wire remains in place. **F:** Removal of the fixed-wire balloon catheter, followed by passage of an over-the-wire system into the branch over the exchange wire. **G:** Wide patency restored to the ostium of the diagonal branch.

system. The first limb of the diagonal system contains an ostial stenosis, followed by an additional discrete lesion approximately 2 cm more distally. The second limb of the diagonal system (third vessel from left) is diseased and arises in an immediately adjacent location. The third limb of the diagonal system (fourth vessel from left) actually originates from the very origin of the preceding branch creating a marked right-angle entry from the proximal LAD artery. In this projection, due to vessel overlap, it appears that this final branch of the diagonal system may be a more proximally arising first diagonal branch with separate orifice from the LAD artery, an incorrect impression. Fig. 5B illustrates the first portions of this procedure performed with two guiding catheters containing a protective wire through each, and an over-the-wire balloon catheter through each guide. Simulta-

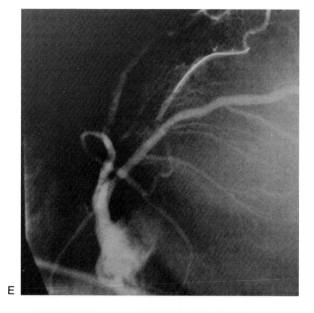

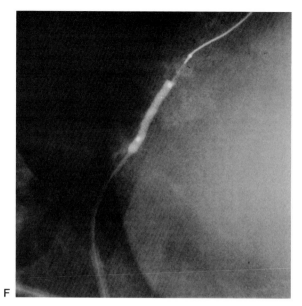

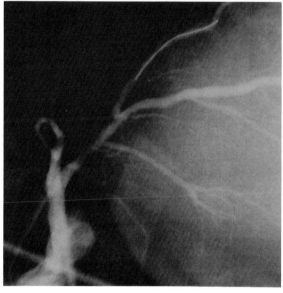

FIG. 4. *Continued.*

neous inflations were performed in pairs of arteries as initially depicted in Fig. 5B. Ultimately, inflations were performed in all vessels to include the more distal lesion in the most leftward of the three diagonal branches. Fig. 5C lacks precise detail but shows wide patency as achieved in the LAD, and the first two branches of the diagonal system. The most rightward branch of the diagonal system is also widely patent but required multiple complex angulated views to confirm that conclusion. The use of simultaneous balloon inflations in the LAD artery and first diagonal branch as seen in Fig. 5B proved necessary to obtain wide angiographic patency in the ectatic portion of the proximal LAD through the combined dilating diameters of the hugging portions of these balloons.

Case 5

Fig. 6A,B depicts a complex bifurcation lesion involving the proximal circumflex artery and origin of a large continuing first obtuse marginal branch. The LAO artery view illustrates bulky plaque immediately prior to the bifurcation, with much plaque upon the superior surface of the vessel and very high-grade narrowing of the obtuse marginal itself. Fig. 6B suggests additional, severe narrowing at the origin of the continuing distal circumflex. Consequently, and although use of a single balloon and wire system could be reasonably contemplated with balloon tip positioned in the first obtuse marginal branch, the chance of occlusion of the distal circumflex is increased. Fig. 6C demonstrates simulta-

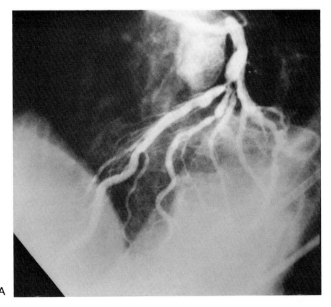

A

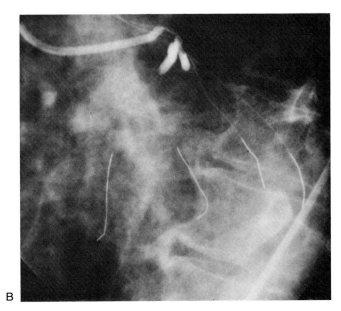

B

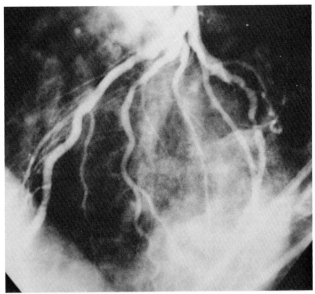

C

FIG. 5. A: Quadrification lesion; LAO, slightly cranial projection. Proximal LAD extasia followed by stenosis extending past the origin of the complex branch system. Ostial stenosis of the first limb of the diagonal system, with a discrete stenosis 2 cm more distal. Diseased second limb of the diagonal system. **B:** Simultaneous inflations of two over-the-wire balloon catheters. The two guiding catheters each contain a protective wire and a balloon catheter. **C:** Wide patency achieved in the LAD artery and the first two branches of the diagonal system.

neous balloon inflations using a 0.080-in diameter guiding catheter, a low-profile, fixed-wire balloon catheter (Slalom, ACS) positioned in the distal circumflex, and a second, very low profile, over-the-wire balloon catheter system (TEN, ACS) positioned in the first obtuse marginal branch. Fig. 6D,E depicts the final result, with achievement of wide angiographic patency at both branches and more effective dilatation of the larger, immediately proximal circumflex segment due to hugging.

Case 6

Fig. 7A,B demonstrates a complex, bifurcation lesion involving the proximal circumflex artery at the origin of

a large second obtuse marginal branch and continuing dominant distal circumflex artery. An ulcerating lesion is most definite in the LAO projection, with significant compromise at the origin of the distal circumflex. Again, a reasonable thought would be to use a single wire and balloon system positioning the balloon across the origin of the continuing distal circumflex. However, because of uncertainties about the ulceration and appreciation that the true proximal circumflex prior to the bifurcation was substantially larger than either of the distal branches, simultaneous balloon inflations were preferred. Fig. 7C,D depicts the use of a single 8 French 0.080-in internal diameter guiding catheter and two 3.5-mm ACS TEN balloon catheters passed over 0.010-in guidewires posi-

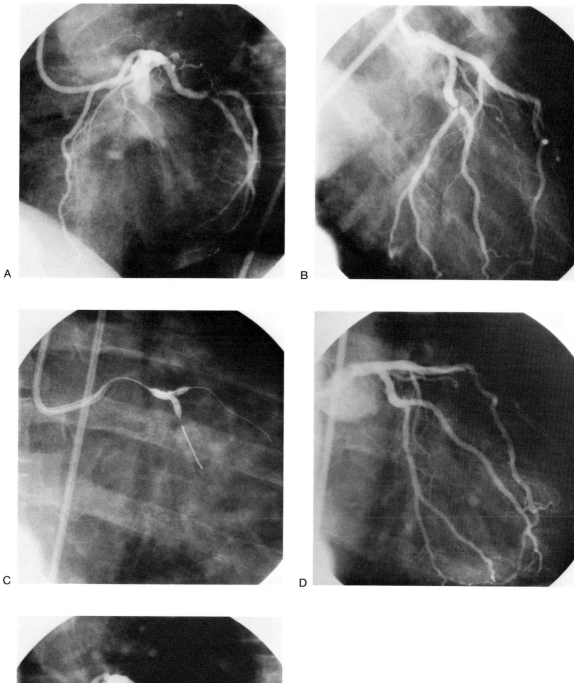

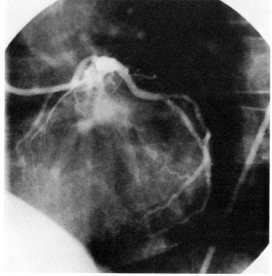

FIG. 6. A: Complex bifurcation lesion involving the proximal circumflex artery and a large continuing first obtuse marginal branch; LAO view. B: Severe narrowing at the origin of the continuing distal circumflex artery, RAO caudal view. C: Simultaneous balloon inflation using a 0.080-in diameter guiding catheter, a low-profile, fixed-wire balloon catheter at the distal circumflex artery, and a second, very low profile, over-the-wire balloon catheter system at the first obtuse marginal branch. D,E: Achievement of wide angiographic patency at both marginal branches and dilatation of the larger, immediately proximal, circumflex segment.

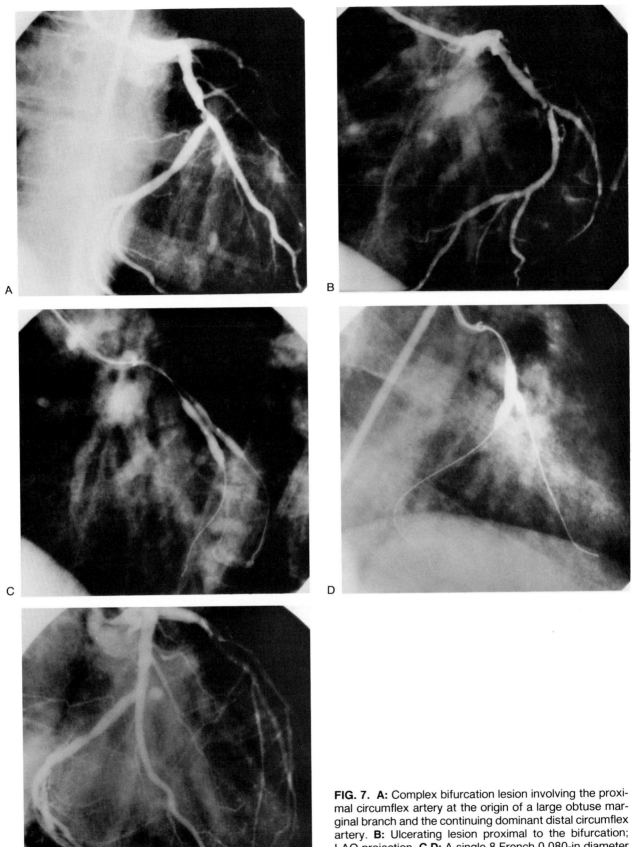

FIG. 7. A: Complex bifurcation lesion involving the proximal circumflex artery at the origin of a large obtuse marginal branch and the continuing dominant distal circumflex artery. **B:** Ulcerating lesion proximal to the bifurcation; LAO projection. **C,D:** A single 8 French 0.080-in diameter guiding catheter and two 3.5-mm balloon catheters passed over one 0.010-in guidewires positioned directly in the bifurcation. **E,F:** Vessels after angioplasty.

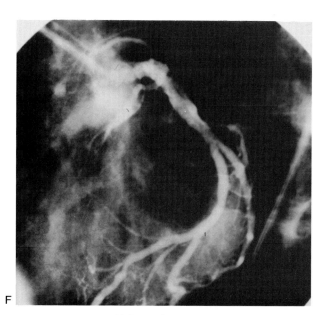

FIG. 7. *Continued.*

tioned directly in the bifurcation. Fig. 7E,F depicts the final result.

ROLE OF ALTERNATIVE TECHNOLOGIES

To date, no clear role for alternative technologies has been identified for the treatment of bifurcation lesions. Individual operators have anecdotally described the use of directional coronary atherectomy, suggesting that decreasing the bulk of the bifurcation stenosis may yield improved primary results. This hypothesis is far from established. Directional atherectomy remains limited to large vessels without tortuosity or significant angulation, and if applied to bifurcation lesions would require minimal angulation between the two branches. Additionally, there is some theoretic if not real chance of vessel perforation by inappropriate atherectomy at the summit of tissue located between the bifurcating limbs. Presently, it is impractical to consider a kissing atherectomy strategy and placement of a protective guidewire could potentially lead to an adverse primary atherectomy outcome. The author has utilized atherectomy following initial simultaneous balloon inflations to further reduce residual plaque bulk at the origin of inadequately dilated bifurcating branches. However, as a primary strategy for the treatment of most bifurcation lesions, atherectomy has a limited role.

Similarly, the excimer laser has a very limited role for primary treatment of bifurcation lesions, in part because of safety issues. Although an effective debulking modality, the coaxial approach required by current excimer laser systems can expose the summit of tissue between the bifurcating branches to laser pulses with increased potential for arterial perforation, a complication experienced by the author. A newer, directional laser catheter may have greater safety and utility for this anatomy.

CONTEMPORARY APPROACH TO BIFURCATION LESIONS

At the present time, the author's approach to bifurcation lesions is influenced by available technologies, personal observation, and experience. First, the vast majority of stenoses involving, at, or near the origin of a side branch do not lead to occlusion of the side branch during coronary angioplasty with a single balloon. Since a high likelihood of branch occlusion can be reasonably accurately predicted by careful analysis of quality angiograms obtained in multiple angulated views, the author's bias is to utilize a single wire and balloon system whenever possible. For example, of the 47 bifurcation lesions previously described, only 4 were subject to two-wire, double, or kissing balloon techniques. No side branches were lost in any of the procedures.

Presently, when it is concluded that two-wire and two-balloon systems are required, the author's favored approach is to use a single 8 French, large lumen (0.080 in) internal diameter guiding catheter, a double access hemostatic valve, and two completely over-the-wire balloon catheter systems (ACS TEN or omega catheters with 0.010 in guidewires). Each balloon catheter with guidewire introduced, yet contained within the catheter shaft, is introduced into the hemostatic valve and advanced to the end of the guiding catheter prior to sequential selection of each bifurcating limb. This approach allows the simultaneous passage of two 3.5-mm balloons through a single guide, while preserving excellent distal guide injections. Using an incremental balloon inflation strategy, assessment of interim results can be easily obtained without loss of access to either branch. Problems of guidewire, balloon, and catheter shaft wrapping are minimized. When necessary, balloons of different sizes can be passed back into the bifurcation lesion by use of exchange wires or attachable wire segments.

CONCLUSION

Most bifurcation lesions can be safely and effectively dilated using a single guidewire and single over-the-wire balloon catheter. More complex bifurcation lesions create greater technical challenge because of the need for dual access, with or without simultaneous balloon inflations. Regardless, contemporary catheter technology now allows primary success rates which are equivalent to those achieved during routine angioplasty.

REFERENCES

1. Meier B, Gruentzig AR, King SB, Douglas JS, Hollman J, Ischinger T, Aueron F, Galan K. Risk of side branch occlusion during coronary angioplasty. *Am J Cardiol* 1984;53:10–14.
2. Vetrovec GW, Cowley MJ, Wolfgang TC, Ducey KC. Effects of percutaneous transluminal coronary angioplasty on lesion associated branches. *Am Heart J* 1985;109:921–925.
3. Arora RR, Raymond RE, Dimas AP, Bhadwar K, Simpendorfer C. Side branch occlusion during coronary angioplasty: incidence, angiographic characteristics and outcome. *Cathet Cardiovasc Diagn* 1989;18:210–212.
4. Weinstein JS, Baim DS, Sipperly ME, McCabe CH, Lorell BH. Salvage of branch vessels during bifurcation lesion angioplasty: acute and long-term follow-up. *Cathet Cardiovasc Diagn* 1991;22:1–6.
5. Meier B. Kissing balloon coronary angioplasty. *Am J Cardiol* 1984;54:918–920.
6. Zack PM, Ischinger T. Experience with a technique for coronary angioplasty of bifurcational lesions. *Cathet Cardiovasc Diagn* 1984;10:433–443.
7. McAuley BJ, Sheehan DJ, Simpson JB. Coronary angioplasty of stenoses at major bifurcations: simultaneous use of multiple guidewires and dilatation catheters. *Circulation* 1984;70:II–108 (abst).
8. Pinkerton CA, Slack JD, Van Tassel JW, Orr CM. Angioplasty for dilatation of complex coronary artery bifurcation stenoses. *Am J Cardiol* 1985;55:1626–1628.
9. George BS, Myler RK, Stertzer SH, Clark DA, Cote G, Shaw RE, Fishman-Rosen J, Murphy M. Balloon angioplasty of coronary bifurcation lesions: the kissing balloon technique. *Cathet Cardiovasc Diagn* 1986;12:124–138.
10. Oesterle SN, McAuley BJ, Buchbinder M, Simpson JB. Angioplasty at coronary bifurcations: single-guide, two-wire technique. *Cathet Cardiovasc Diagn* 1986;12:57–63.
11. Nakhjavan FK, Wertheimer JH, Goldman A. "Crossing balloons": a new technique for complex angioplasty. *J Am Coll Cardiol* 1986;8:980–981.
12. Vallbracht C, Kober G, Kaltenbach M. Double long-wire technique for percutaneous transluminal coronary angioplasty for narrowings at major bifurcations. *Am J Cardiol* 1987;60:907–909.
13. Baim DS, Ignatuim EJ. Use of percutaneous coronary angioplasty: results of a current survey. *Am J Cardiol* 1988;61:36–86.
14. Velasquez G, Castaneda-Zuniga W, Formanek A, Zollikoter C, Barreto A, Nikoloff D, Amphatz K, Sullivan A. Nonsurgical aortoplasty in leriche syndrome. *Radiology* 1980;134:359–360.
15. Hartzler GO. Three-wire technique: a unique approach to percutaneous coronary angioplasty of a trifurcation lesion. *Cathet Cardiovasc Diagn* 1987;13:174–177.
16. Pinkerton CA, Slack JD, Nasser WK, Pinto RD, Center D, Orr CM, VanTassel J, Waller B. Pattern of restenosis after percutaneous transluminal coronary angioplasty of bifurcation stenoses. *J Interven Cardiol* 1989;2:147–148.
17. Renkin J, Sijns W, Hanet C, Michel X, Cosyns J, Col J. Angioplasty of coronary bifurcation stenoses: immediate and long-term results of the protecting branch technique. *Cathet Cardiovasc Diagn* 1991;22:167–173.

Practical Angioplasty,
edited by David P. Faxon.
Raven Press, Ltd., New York © 1993.

CHAPTER 10

Total Occlusion

Bernhard Meier

Although the chapter focuses on coronary angioplasty for chronic total occlusions without antegrade flow, specific aspects of spontaneously recanalized occlusions, occlusions with bridging collaterals, and subtotal stenoses, as well as their special approach and results, are discussed when appropriate.

PATHOPHYSIOLOGY

The main components of a chronic total coronary occlusion are an atherosclerotic plaque and a thrombus or several thrombi. Multiple thrombi testify to prior plaque fissures and nonocclusive blood clots or occlusive clots that were partially recanalized. The texture of the most recent thrombus is a determinant of success. The older and the more fibrosed it is, the smaller the chance to cross it with the recanalization device.

A coronary wedge pressure of 45 mmHg or more indicates sufficient collateralization to prevent chest pain or ischemia (1). Collaterals, that are preexisting or immediately recruited at the time of acute occlusion, prevent necrosis altogether, or at least confine the damage to the subendocardium (2–8). Young patients with insignificant coronary disease and an acute thrombotic coronary occlusion rarely possess collaterals, in contradistinction to patients with longstanding disease and a subtotal stenosis of the vessel in question. The latter stand a greater chance of preserving their myocardium yet a smaller chance of spontaneous recanalization. This makes them typical candidates for coronary balloon recanalization. Unfortunately, their lesions are likely to have been tight prior to occlusion. In addition, they may have been eccentric which further increases the intricacy of a percutaneous recanalization attempt.

SELECTION CRITERIA

Although the interventional cardiologist faces only a negligible risk of a periinterventional infarction when dealing with chronic total occlusions, he is hampered by technical problems. The technique of bypass surgery is the same whether the vessel in question is totally occluded or only stenosed. The cardiac surgeon does not distinguish in his indications between a chronic total occlusion and a stenosis. He takes into account only size and state of the distal vessel and viability of the dependent myocardium. Like the cardiologist, the surgeon relishes the low-risk aspect of a total occlusion. An acute or late postoperative occlusion of a graft implanted into a chronically occluded vessel should not cause a myocardial infarction. It merely reestablishes the preoperative status.

Thus, chronically occluded coronary vessels continue to play a major role in favor of selecting bypass surgery over angioplasty, particularly at advanced age where longstanding disease with a high percentage of collateralized occlusions is prevalent. On the other hand, coronary recanalization by angioplasty is not infrequently attempted in patients in whom surgery is not seriously considered because of small vessel size, low symptom level, and excellent spontaneous prognosis.

Indications for coronary recanalization by angioplasty weigh the technical difficulties expected and the clinical risks projected on the one side and the likely subjective benefit on the other side. The degree of limitation by symptoms and the amount of viable myocardium at stake are the key parameters in predicting the improvement of the patient. The indication threshold is low for a recanalization attempt that is part of the diagnostic coronary angiogram since it means little additional inconvenience and cost. The threshold is intermediate if the patient is still hospitalized, but it should be high if the patient is at home.

B. Meier: Cardiology, University Hospital, 3010 Bern, Switzerland

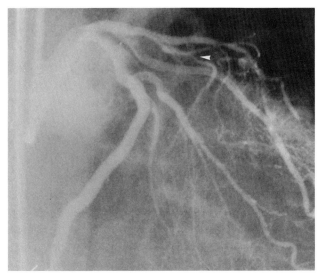

FIG. 1. Contraindication to a recanalization attempt of a chronic total coronary occlusion because of the absence of a stump. The vessel tapers smoothly into a small septal and diagonal branch (*arrowhead*). There is no nipple to probe.

Clinical Findings

Typical candidates for coronary recanalization have effort angina but no rest angina. A well-collateralized total occlusion functionally imitates a 90% stenosis (9). It keeps the myocardium alive but cannot prevent clinically apparent ischemia during phases with increased oxygen demand. Such episodes are not strictly confined to

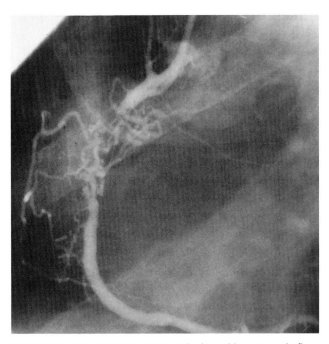

FIG. 2. Chronic total coronary occlusion with antegrade flow through bridging collaterals (vasa vasorum and local side-branches). The well-developed local collaterals testify to the chronicity of the occlusion, which constitutes a contraindication to a recanalization attempt.

physical exercise but may exceptionally occur in the context of transient hypertension or tachycardia, for instance during mental stress. This may mimic unstable angina and unnecessarily prompt coronary care surveillance or emergency revascularization.

Ventricular Function

Noncontracting myocardium appears to be a logical contraindication to a revascularization attempt of the occluded culprit vessel. However, noncontracting myocardium may be stunned (10) or hibernating (11) rather than irreversibly damaged. Stunning (delayed resumption of function after reflow) plays a minor role in the indication for a recanalization attempt of a chronically occluded vessel, although reflow can be present in the form of collaterals. Hibernation (stalled function to pre-

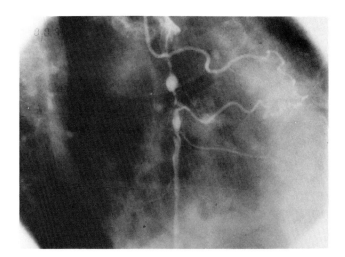

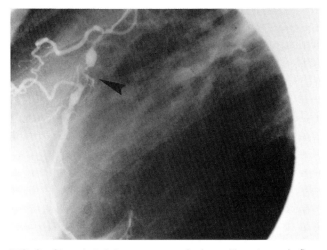

FIG. 3. Chronic total coronary occlusion with antegrade flow through internuncial collaterals not readily detected as such. The right anterior oblique view (*top*) gives the impression of a tight stenosis with a preserved lumen. Only the lateral view (*bottom*) unveils the total occlusion with local collaterals (*arrowhead*) and thus the contraindication to angioplasty.

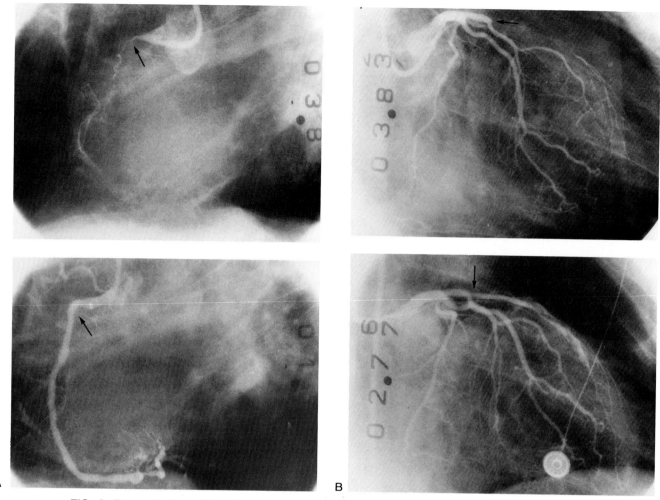

FIG. 4. Recanalization of two chronic total occlusions in a single session. The sites are indicated by arrows. **A:** The right coronary artery receives collaterals from the left coronary artery and is recanalized first. **B:** The left anterior descending coronary artery has ipsilateral collaterals and is recanalized second. Both arteries are treated with a Judkins 7 French guiding catheter and a Magnum wire and 3.0-mm Magnarail balloon. The sites of occlusion are indicated by arrowheads.

serve life during marginal oxygen supply) is a more obvious reason for noncontracting myocardium that supports a recanalization attempt. To date, a reliable practical method is lacking to identify hibernating myocardium with potential for recovery after normalization of coronary blood flow. Positron emission tomography holds some promise (12) but it is extremely costly, time-consuming, and restricted to the few equipped centers. Thallium scintigraphy with reinjection is more practical but less specific (13). A way to tell is to recanalize and see what happens. Obviously, such an approach needs to be scrutinized by a randomized study for its risk–benefit and/or cost–benefit profile.

Left ventricular function at rest is not improved immediately after recanalization of a chronically occluded coronary artery, but pacing can document instant amelioration of regional and global left ventricular function and left ventricular end-diastolic pressure (14,15). Left ven-

tricular function at rest tends to improve, albeit late, and only with sustained recanalization of chronic coronary occlusions (16,17).

Overall, left ventricular recuperation is at best a secondary goal for recanalization of chronic total coronary occlusions because it is inconsistent, slow, and hard to document by crude assessment of global left ventricular ejection fraction (17,18).

Angiography

The projection of success is based primarily on duration, length, and aspect of the occlusion. An occlusion flush at the orifice of the vessel or tapering into a small sidebranch is a contraindication for angioplasty (Fig. 1). So is an old occlusion recanalized by bridging collaterals that may consist of vasa vasorum and/or internuncial

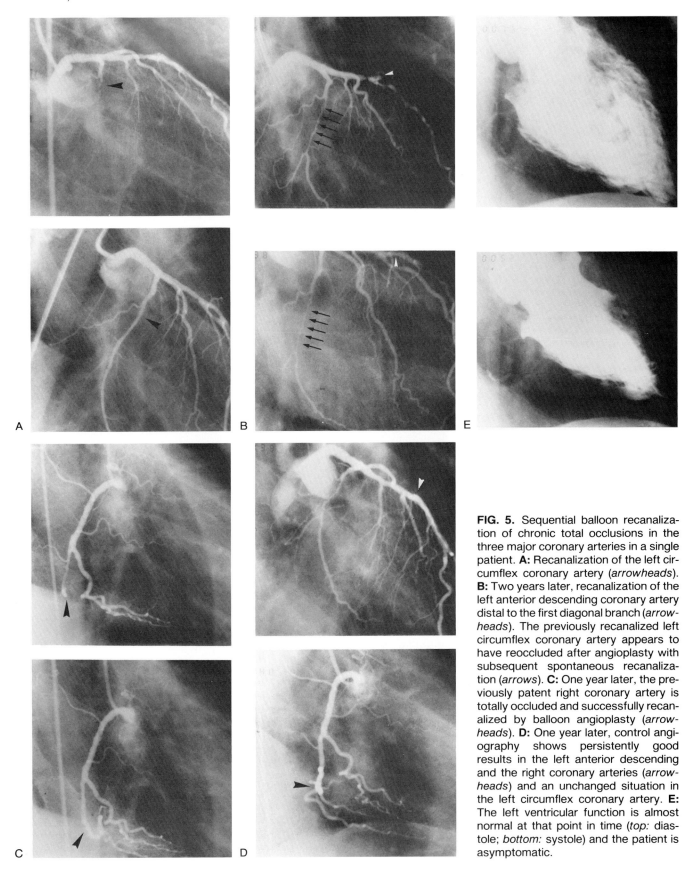

FIG. 5. Sequential balloon recanalization of chronic total occlusions in the three major coronary arteries in a single patient. **A:** Recanalization of the left circumflex coronary artery (*arrowheads*). **B:** Two years later, recanalization of the left anterior descending coronary artery distal to the first diagonal branch (*arrowheads*). The previously recanalized left circumflex coronary artery appears to have reoccluded after angioplasty with subsequent spontaneous recanalization (*arrows*). **C:** One year later, the previously patent right coronary artery is totally occluded and successfully recanalized by balloon angioplasty (*arrowheads*). **D:** One year later, control angiography shows persistently good results in the left anterior descending and the right coronary arteries (*arrowheads*) and an unchanged situation in the left circumflex coronary artery. **E:** The left ventricular function is almost normal at that point in time (*top:* diastole; *bottom:* systole) and the patient is asymptomatic.

TABLE 1. *Conventional angioplasty of chronic total coronary occlusion*

	Pool	Boston	Rotterdam/Ghent	Redwood City	Richmond	Geneva	Boston	A.A./Atl. S Fran.	Kansas City	Atlanta	Rochester
Year of Report		1983	1985	1985	1986	1987	1988	1989	1990	1992	1992
Reference		(24)	(18)	(25)	(26)	(27)	(28)	(29)	(30)	(31)	(32)
Number of Patients	2676[a]	13[a]	49	76	46[a]	100	169	484[a]	905[a]	480[a]	354[a]
Age of occlusion (months)											
mean	8	1	2	7	2	4		8	12		2
range		0.03–?	0.03–10	0.13–120	0.1–17	0.25–48		0.06–108			0–>3
Collaterals visible	67%	100%	76%		100	100%		74%			40%
Prior infarction	58%	38%	19%	39%	50%	76%	66%			55%	63%
Primary success	67%	54%	57%	53%	63%	56%	63%		72%	69%	66%
Emergency surgery	2%	0%	2%	1%	4%	0%	2%		1%		3%
Infarction	2%	0%	18%	11%	0%	2%	0%		1%	2%	4%
In-hospital death	1%	0%	0%	0%	0%	0%	0%		1%	1%	2%
Mean follow-up (months)	26	6	7	7	8	8		24		36	32
Recurrence[b]	62%	43%	65%	75%		55%		77%		54%	59%
restenosis	45%	39%				35%		56%		38%	45%
reocclusion	17%	4%				20%		21%		16%	14%
Long-term clinical improvement[c]	69%[d]	86%[d]	64%	75%	100%	82%[d]				69%	60%

[a] Including functional occlusions.
[b] Of patients with primary success and follow-up angiograhy.
[c] Of patients with primary success.
[d] Including repeat angioplasty.
A.A., Ann Arbor; Atl., Atlanta; S Fran., San Francisco.

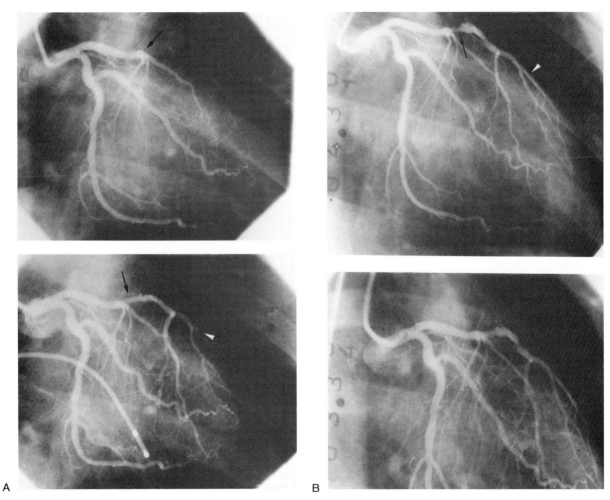

FIG. 6. Distal embolization during coronary balloon recanalization. **A:** During recanalization of the left anterior descending coronary artery (*arrows*), a fragment of the occluding material has been embolized into the diagonal branch blocking it (*arrowhead*). **B:** A control angiogram 15 months later (*top*) reveals a mild restenosis in the left anterior descending coronary artery (*arrow*) and spontaneous recanalization of the diagonal branch (*arrowhead*). The left anterior descending coronary artery is treated with repeat angioplasty (*bottom*).

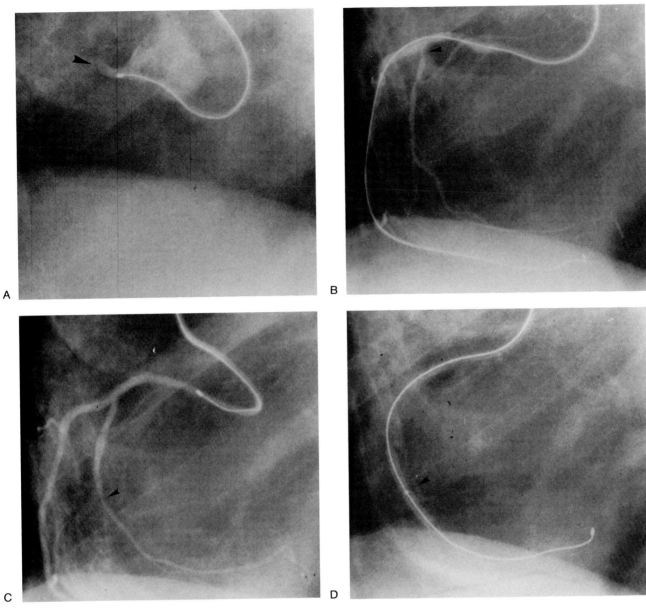

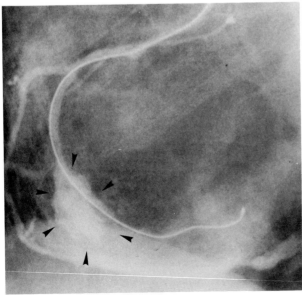

FIG. 7. Rupture of a branch of the right coronary artery during balloon inflation distal to a segment recanalized by balloon angioplasty. **A:** Chronically occluded right coronary artery (*arrowhead*) with a Magnum wire ready for the recanalization attempt. **B:** Successful recanalization with a 3-mm balloon unexpectedly reveals a stenosed early takeoff (*arrowhead*) of the left ventricular branch of the right coronary artery. **C:** After dilatation of the takeoff with the same 3-mm balloon, a segment more distal appears stenosed (*arrowhead*). **D:** The same 3-mm balloon is inflated in this segment (*arrowhead*). **E:** After deflation, a rupture of the artery (*arrowheads*) with drainage into the right ventricle is seen; this is not felt by the patient and has no clinical sequelae. Oversizing of the balloon is to be held responsible for this complication. Had the artery been visible on the preangioplasty film, it would probably not have been dilated at all because the assumed stenosis was just a variation in caliber of the genuinely small vessel. Certainly, a smaller balloon would have been selected for a premeditated angioplasty of such a vessel. Thus, the total occlusion is indirectly responsible for the mismanagement of the patient.

collaterals (Fig. 2). Such lesions may be difficult to tell from tight stenoses (Fig. 3) and account for most of the rare failures to pass a modern coronary guidewire through an assumedly nontotal lesion.

It appears unwise to attempt recanalization of chronic total coronary occlusions in patients with more than one additional lesion. The average amount of time, fluoroscopy, and contrast medium to be invested into recanalization of an occlusion corresponds to that of at least two nontotal lesions. Notwithstanding, even two total occlusions can occasionally be successfully treated in a single session if they are properly selected (Fig. 4). Figure 5 illustrates a case of total occlusions of the three major coronary arteries that occurred sequentially over three years and were recanalized individually as they happened, with satisfactory follow-up.

Adequate visualization of the distal part of the occluded artery via collaterals is an absolute prerequisite. First, there is little hope of reconstructing a vessel that is obliterated over its entire length. Second, myocardial areas of occluded vessels completely devoid of collateral blood flow are always akinetic and never hibernating.

Bypass Grafts

The literature on balloon recanalization of chronically occluded saphenous vein bypass grafts is scarce (19–23). A considerable quantity of thrombus has to be expected in an occluded bypass graft. Even when using urokinase during balloon recanalization as advocated by some (20–22), the acute reocclusion and actual recurrence rates must be exorbitant. For these reasons, one report strongly advocates against this indication (23).

RESULTS

The literature frequently confounds functional occlusions with total occlusions, although the respective success and complication rates are disparate. Hence, comparison of data has to be done with caution.

Primary Success

Success rates vary from 53% to 72%, with a mean of 67%, in 2,192 pooled patients and are presented in Table 1 (18,24–32). The highest success rates derive from series which included technically less challenging functional occlusions (30,31).

The key factor for success is the age of the occlusion (18,24–28,33,34). The primary decline in chance of success occurs during the first 4 weeks after the occlusion (26). The length of the occlusion is also important (25). Only angiographically ideal occlusions (short, straight segment in large vessel) with a sound clinical indication should be tackled if they are more than a few months old.

Complications

Reocclusion after balloon recanalization cannot cause an acute infarction. It merely reinstitutes the preintervention status. Thus, the risk of complications during attempts to recanalize chronic total coronary occlusions is lower than that of angioplasty of nonoccluded coronary arteries albeit still higher than that of diagnostic coronary angiography.

Only the largest series report in-hospital deaths (30–32). They occurred largely secondary to problems with dilated sites other than the total occlusions. There is a recent report of intractable fatal ventricular fibrillation in a patient with acute reocclusion of a recanalized left anterior descending coronary artery. The patient had unstable angina to begin with, which suggests a subtotal occlusion rather than a total occlusion, and there is no discussion of the possible mechanism of the problem that led to the demise of the patient (35). Subtotal occlusions may also have been the explanation for the complications attributed to the angioplasty site reported in a paper on patients with unstable angina and balloon recanalization (36). This series included a patient who died from a thrombus inadvertently retracted from the occluded site in the left anterior descending coronary artery into the left main stem, from where it embolized, occluding the proximal left circumflex coronary artery.

Distal embolizations occur with some regularity but they are usually benign events (Fig. 6). The only coronary rupture reported with recanalization of chronic occlusions, involved a diagonal branch. It had a benign course (37). Figure 7 shows another example of coronary rupture during a recanalization attempt which, however, happened at a location distant from the recanalized segment. Perforations with the guidewire are perhaps more common but should not cause clinical problems provided they are recognized before the balloon is advanced. Extracardiac complications, such as stroke and bleeding from the arterial entry site, are an additional hazard as with all cardiac catheterizations.

In the literature, the need for emergency bypass surgery varies between 0% and 4%, with an average below

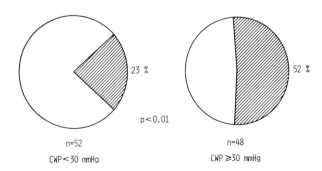

FIG. 8. Boosting influence of a high coronary wedge pressure (CWP) on subsequent restenosis after coronary angioplasty (40) ▨. The recurrence rate is twice as high in arteries with a coronary wedge pressure ≥ 30 mmHg.

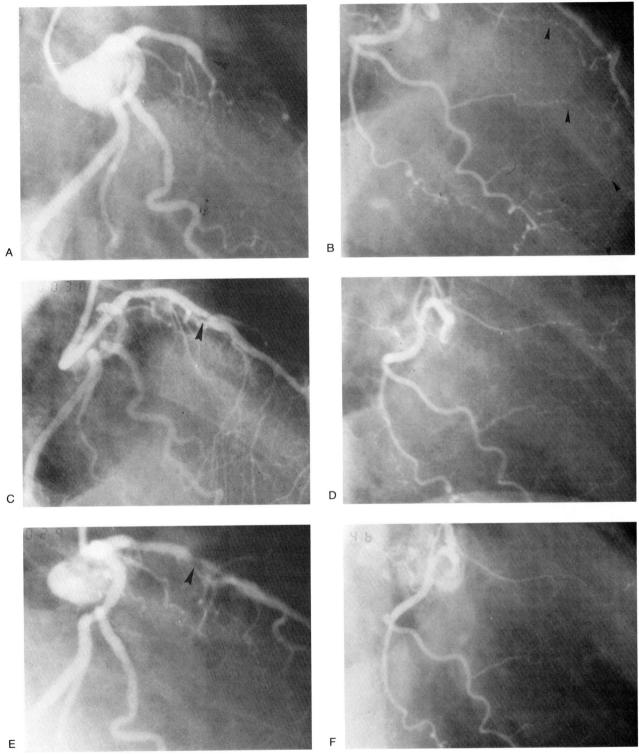

FIG. 9. Instantly recruited collaterals 3 months after their disappearance with successful recanalization of the recipient vessel. **A:** Totally occluded left anterior descending coronary artery (*arrowhead*). **B:** Copious collateralization (*arrowheads*) of the left anterior descending coronary artery from the nondominant right coronary artery. **C:** Result after successful recanalization of the left anterior descending coronary artery (*arrowhead*). **D:** Immediate disappearance of the collaterals documenting a good hemodynamic result. **E:** Restenosis (*arrowhead*) 3 months later with maintained patency. **F:** The collaterals from the right coronary artery are still absent because the lesion is not tight enough. **G:** Balloon occlusion of the left anterior descending coronary artery (*arrow*) and simultaneous contrast medium injection into the right coronary artery via a separate arterial catheter proves instant recruitment of the collaterals (*arrowheads*) having remained dormant (on standby) since the recanalization. **H:** Result of repeat angioplasty (*arrowhead*). **I:** Normal left ventricular function at the time of repeat angioplasty (*top:* diastole; *bottom:* systole).

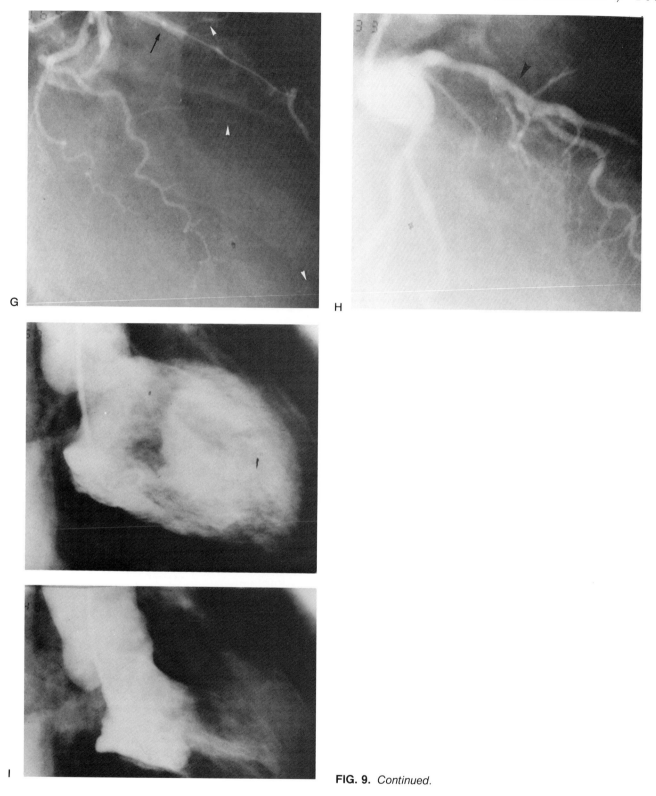

FIG. 9. Continued.

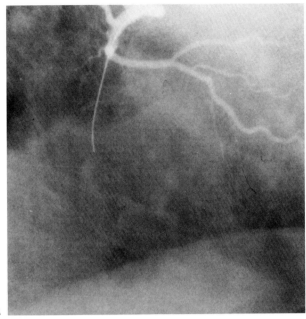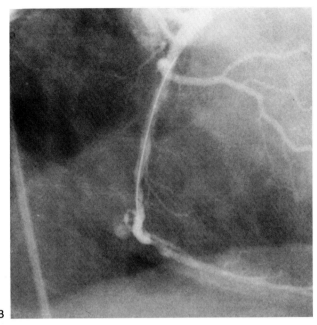

FIG. 10. Successful recanalization of a chronic total occlusion of the right coronary artery with a 3.5-mm Omniflex fixed-wire balloon catheter. **A:** The balloon gets stuck halfway through the occlusion. A contrast medium injection through the guiding catheter fails to inform about the correct or incorrect placement of the balloon, even after partial withdrawal of the balloon catheter. **B:** An inflation is made without ascertaining the correct position. In this case, it yields a good recanalization. Had the passage been subintimal or into a small sidebranch, such a blind balloon inflation could have had detrimental consequences.

2% (Table 1). Abrupt vessel reclosure is frequent but it constitutes no reason for emergency surgery. Neither does the failure to pass the occlusion. These events do not impair the situation of the patient compared to the beginning of the procedure, with the rare exception of exclusive local collaterals that were damaged during an unsuccessful recanalization attempt. A more conceivable reason for immediate surgery is a closure of an important vessel proximal to the occlusion.

Q-wave infarctions in this setting are possible in the case of an occlusion of a significant proximal sidebranch or impairment of collaterals by dissection or embolization. Events of the kind have been reported only once, however, and have not been unequivocally linked to the recanalization attempt (30). Similar mechanisms account for the 0% to 18% (mean 2%) reported rates of subendocardial infarctions documented by creatine kinase elevations (Table 1).

Recurrence

In the major reports on chronic total coronary occlusion angioplasty, recurrence rates per patient with initial success and control angiography average 62%, and range from 43% to 77% (Table 1). The global recurrence rate encompasses only 17% complete reocclusions, the remainder being restenoses which are easier to deal with by angioplasty. For comparison, the average restenosis rate reported in a compiled cohort of almost 10,000 patients

with coronary angioplasty for mixed indications is only 28% (38). Less than ideal results that are more commonly encountered with recanalization have been documented to boost recurrence (39), but collaterals are likely to account for most of this difference (Fig. 8). They are a prerequisite for angioplasty of chronic total coronary occlusions and lead to a high recurrence rate by exerting competitive pressure even after being no longer visibly functional (40).

It is safe to assume that some of the reocclusions subsumed under recurrences are silent acute occlusions. They probably occur in at least 10% of patients during the first hours after angioplasty. They may be picked up by a final injection into the contralateral artery showing persistence or reappearance of collaterals, or by a positive stress test the day after the intervention.

True restenoses may be partial or may progress to complete reocclusion. They exhibit the histologic features common to all restenoses after angioplasty, namely smooth muscle cell proliferation. Consequently, their time of appearance is expected to be identical to that of the recurrence of stenoses after angioplasty, that is, several weeks to a few months after the intervention.

Clinical Follow-up

Medium term clinical improvement after successful recanalization of chronic coronary occlusions has been documented be it in the form of fewer cardiac symptoms

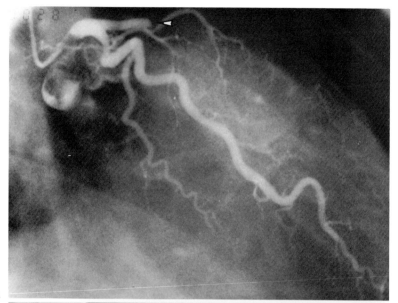

A

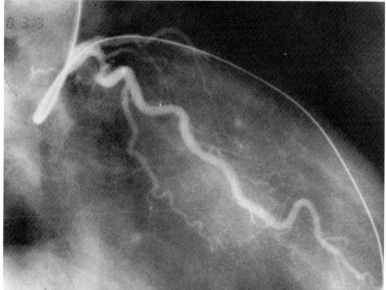

B

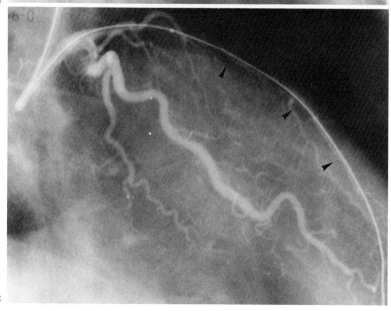

C

FIG. 11. Distal contrast medium injection through a Magnarail (monorail-type) balloon catheter to ascertain correct balloon placement before inflation. **A:** Chronic total occlusion of the proximal left anterior descending coronary artery (*arrowhead*). **B:** A Magnum wire is advanced across the occlusion. A contrast medium injection through the guiding catheter does not provide opacification of the distal vessel to assure a correct intraluminal path of the wire. **C:** After advancement of the Magnarail balloon catheter across the occlusion, injection of the same amount of contrast medium opacifies the distal left anterior descending coronary artery (*arrowheads*). The contrast medium passes through the short wire lumen of the Magnarail catheter feigning a distal injection. The balloon can now be safely inflated. **D:** Result of the recanalization (*arrowhead*).

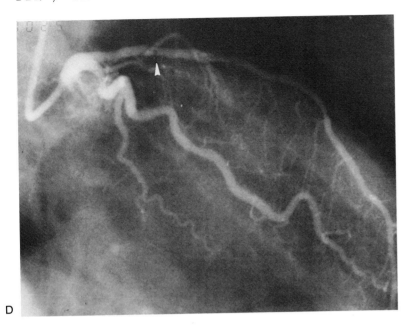

D

FIG. 11. *Continued.*

or events (41,42) or improved exercise tests (17). Acute infarctions occur in about 1% of patients per year of follow-up, but their incidence is identical in patients with successful and those with failed recanalization (32). This marks these infarctions as a result of disease progression rather than vessel reocclusion. To reiterate: not a single myocardial infarction has been reported that was indubitably attributable to such a reocclusion. Figure 9 illustrates that collaterals that had promptly disappeared with successful recanalization are immediately recruitable in case of need, even several months later. Whether there is a time limit for their standby availability remains unknown.

About 30% of patients undergo repeat angioplasty and bypass surgery after successful coronary angioplasty for complete chronic occlusion compared to only about

20% of patients with stenoses (28); however, a reduced need for coronary bypass surgery is the primary benefit that separates patients with a successful balloon recanalization attempt from those with a failed one (31,32,41,42).

CONVENTIONAL TECHNIQUES

Floppy coronary guidewires may easily negotiate tight and eccentric nontotal lesions but they tend to buckle and curl when used for chronic total occlusions. Stiffer wires succeed where floppy wires fail (25). Since even the most rigid conventional coronary guidewires are still quite flexible, bracing of the guidewire by advancement of the balloon catheter close to the tip is needed to pro-

FIG. 12. Incomplete disappearance of collaterals after balloon recanalization of a chronic total occlusion (left anterior descending coronary artery) documenting an incomplete hemodynamic result and heralding a restenosis in a patient with a stenosis of the donor vessel (right coronary artery). Repeat angioplasty yields a better result and the donor vessel subsequently progresses to a total occlusion protected by the formerly recipient vessel. **A:** Total occlusion (*arrowhead*) of the left anterior descending coronary artery (*top*) with a generous collateral vessel (*arrows*) from the posterior descending branch of the right coronary artery which has a significant stenosis (*large arrowhead*) itself (*bottom*). **B:** Angiographically successful recanalization (*arrowhead*) of the left anterior descending coronary artery (*top*). However, the watershed in the collateral vessel (*large arrows*) from the right coronary artery is still located at the distal third of the left anterior descending coronary artery (*bottom*) reflecting an inadequate hemodynamic result of the recanalization, a harbinger of the subsequent restenosis. **C:** After repeat angioplasty 3 months later for recurrent stenosis and symptoms, the angiographic result (*top; arrowhead*) is not superior to that in (B), achieved with the first intervention. The watershed in the collateral vessel (*large arrows*), however, is now appreciated at its desired site between the two arteries (*bottom*). The lesion in the right coronary artery has progressed (*large arrowheads*). **D:** Nine months later, a routine control angiogram while the patient is asymptomatic shows normal patency (*arrowhead*) of the left anterior descending coronary artery (*top*) with reversed collateral flow to the distal posterior descending branch of the right coronary artery (*arrows*) which is now occluded (*large arrowhead*) at the site of the former stenosis (*bottom*). No further intervention is considered necessary.

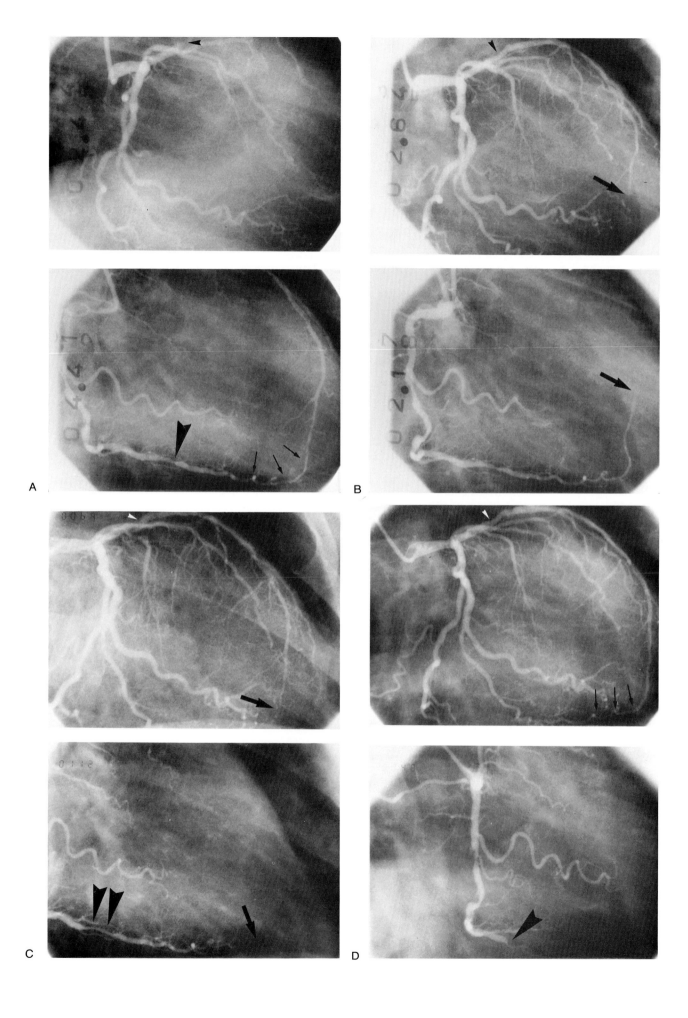

A

B

C

D

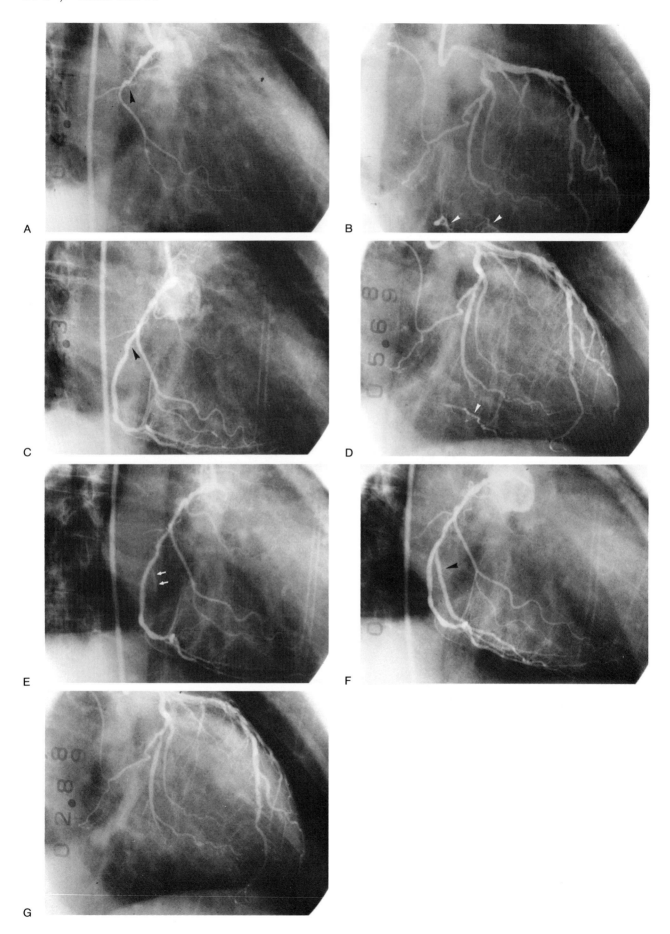

vide adequate stiffness. The use of single-lumen bracing catheters, in the form of perfusion catheters (43) and hollow wires (44), has been proposed to avoid wasting a balloon catheter in case of failure to pass. This implies a potentially tedious exchange maneuver to a balloon catheter if the occlusion can be crossed which, after all, is the rule rather than the exception with reasonable indications. Although the exchange maneuver can be significantly simplified using a monorail-type bracing catheter (45), the price of the balloon catheter added to the bracing device wastes a good part of the savings achieved with the cheaper bracing catheter in failed cases. Fixed-wire balloons have also been recommended for chronic occlusions, the sturdy Omniflex (Medtronic) as single instrument (46) and the sleek Probe (USCI) in conjunction with a probing catheter (47).

In case a preocclusion film exists, it should be consulted before and, if need arises, during the recanalization attempt. It gives information about the length of the occlusion and the course of the distal vessel. A late freeze-frame of a contrast medium injection into the artery providing the collaterals shows the distal part of the occluded vessel. It may be used simultaneously or alternately with a freeze-frame showing the stub of the proximal part of the occluded vessel. Repeat injections of contrast medium into the donor vessel during the recanalization attempt are helpful and practical in case of ipsilateral collaterals, but cumbersome in case of contralaterals (48,49).

It cannot be overemphasized how essential it is to inject contrast medium through the tip of the balloon catheter (or bracing catheter) whenever progression stops, or doubt about the correct path arises. Such injections should be repeated after crossing the occlusion. This assures that the correct lumen is being recanalized and prevents inadvertent placement of the balloon in a small branch originating from the area of the occlusion and running in the assumed direction of the vessel to be recanalized. Conventional over-the-wire systems lend themselves perfectly to distal injections. Fixed-wire balloons (50–53), such as Omniflex (Medtronic), Probe (USCI), Ace (SciMed), Orion Lightning (Cordis), Integra (Datascope) or One to One (Sorin) do not allow distal

contrast medium injections (Fig. 10); neither do monorail balloon catheters (Schneider) (54,55) or other rapid exchange systems such as RX (Advanced Cardiovascular Systems) or Express (SciMed). When injecting contrast medium through the guiding catheter with a monorail-type system, however, dye will enter the central lumen together with the guidewire proximal to the balloon, and will emerge from the tip of the catheter. This perfectly substitutes for a gentle distal injection (Fig. 11).

Advice applicable to all angioplasties involving collateralized arteries is to document the integral disappearance of collaterals at the end of the procedure. This demonstrates a good hemodynamic result. This is particularly important if the donor artery is stenosed as well (Fig. 12). It may also uncover an otherwise unrecognized incomplete revascularization (Fig. 13).

NEW DEVICES

Modified Guidewires

The Magnum wire (Schneider) features a Tefloncoated solid-steel shaft with a diameter of 0.021 in (0.53 mm), a flexible, shapeable distal part, and an olive-shaped ball tip 1 mm in diameter (56). It is compatible with the Magnum, Magnarail, and Mega Balloons of Schneider and some balloon models of other manufacturers. It has been particularly designed for angioplasty of chronic total occlusions in coronary arteries, yet it can be used for routine coronary angioplasty of nontotal lesions as well as for peripheral angioplasty (57). A randomized study on patients with total coronary occlusions, unassociated with acute infarction and devoid of antegrade flow, compared the performance of the Magnum system with that of a variety of conventional systems (58). The primary success rate of 67% was in the Magnum group versus 45% in the conventional group. Crossover successes were also more frequent in the Magnum group (39% versus 12%). Overall, the Magnum system needs minor adjustments from conventional technique but facilitates several basic maneuvers such a wire steering, guiding catheter placement and stabilization for

FIG. 13. Incomplete revascularization during recanalization of a right coronary artery detected by incomplete disappearance of collaterals and immediately remedied. **A:** Total occlusion (*arrowhead*) before recanalization. **B:** Collaterals (*arrowheads*) from the left coronary artery to several branches of the distal right coronary artery. **C:** Apparently successful recanalization of the right coronary artery (*arrowhead*). **D:** A contralateral contrast medium injection shows disappearance of the collaterals to the left ventricular branch but persistence of the collaterals (*arrowhead*) to the posterior descending branch of the right coronary artery. **E:** A repeat contrast medium injection into the right coronary artery reveals a so far unrecognized early bifurcation and the stump (*small arrows*) of the still totally occluded posterior descending branch. **F:** Result after additional recanalization of the posterior descending branch of the right coronary artery (*arrowhead*). **G:** A contralateral contrast medium injection shows complete disappearance of all collaterals to the right coronary artery.

backup, and balloon advancement. The 1-mm size of the current ball tip represents a compromise. It serves as an important safety feature, without overly increasing the resistance encountered when crossing the occluded segment. It reduces the risk of subintimal passage and practically eliminates the possibility of vessel perforation.

The Omniflex balloon (Medtronic), a sturdy fixed-wire balloon, added 24% to the 53% (total 77%) success rate achieved with conventional systems in 97 patients with occlusions deemed less than 3 months old, and 28% to 21% (total 49%) in 57 patients with occlusions older than 3 months (46). This study was not randomized but still suggests an advantage of the Omniflex system over conventional systems. Surprisingly, the disadvantage of the fixed leading wire and the impossibility of distal contrast medium injections (Fig. 10) seemed not to hamper the performance of the Omniflex balloon catheter in the hands of the authors.

Drills

The Rotacs system (Osypka), introduced at first for the peripheral circulation (59) and more recently for coronary arteries (60), is the only drilling device used routinely and unguided by a previously placed wire for chronic total occlusions. It features a smooth metallic tip rotating at or below 200 revolutions per minute. A central lumen allows distal dye injections and the use of an exchange wire to insert a conventional balloon for the actual angioplasty once the occlusion has been crossed. Success rates reported are comparable to those with conventional systems, a result which is considered progress by the authors, in light of the complexity of the occlusions attempted and the fact that the system was generally used after failure to pass with a conventional coronary guidewire.

The Kensey high speed drill (Cordis), rotating with up to 100,000 revolutions per minute, seems to be somewhat stuck in the investigational stage it entered in 1987 (61), at least as far as the coronary arteries are concerned. Endeavors to effect technical improvements are ongoing (62).

Atherectomy

None of the various atherectomy devices tested in coronary arteries (63–66) has been used to approach chronic occlusions without passing a guidewire first. They have, therefore, no value concerning the principal aspect of occlusion angioplasty, that is, the actual recanalization.

A slow rotational atherectomy device has been tested in vitro for recanalization of occluded human peripheral arteries without prior guidewire passage. It proved successful but resulted in extensive wall damage (67).

Laser

Two laser devices have clinically been used for initial passage through chronic total occlusions. In 4 of 10 cases with failure of conventional systems, an Argon laser heated ball tip guidewire called Hot Tip (Trimedyne) successfully crossed the chronic occlusion (68). There was one perforation without clinical consequences. Nevertheless, the enthusiasm for Hot Tip recanalization has cooled rapidly and the technique has practically been abandoned.

The results of the bare Argon laser instrument Lastac (GV Medical) are again comparable to those achieved with less costly mechanical means, but they are claimed to be superior because of the highly intricate cases attempted (69). A mere mechanical component is undoubtedly present with these catheters, which unite many of the pertinent features of mechanical devices for chronic occlusions (e.g., sturdiness, bluntness). The importance of this component could be easily assessed by a randomized study with and without turning on the laser. Yet, nobody seems anxious to undertake such a study.

Over-the-wire Excimer laser catheters have been used to treat chronic total occlusions (70). Since the laser power was only used to replace or complement balloon dilatation once an ordinary guidewire had crossed the occlusion, these methods will not be further discussed in this chapter.

Computer-assisted lasers may be triggered on-line by spectral analysis of the target tissue to avoid perforation of the normal vessel wall (71,72). Such concepts are fascinating but unlikely to ever reach routine use in catheterization laboratories. The smartest laser might be a laser guided by a human eye collaborating with a cunning and experienced human brain. However, angioscopic visibility in coronary arteries is still insufficient to reliably differentiate tissues, even through angioscopes free of laser channels which further impair resolution and flushing capabilities.

Ultrasound

Ultrasound breaks down solid materials like tartar, kidney stones, or calcified plaques while being relatively atraumatic to soft tissues. A 20-kHz ultrasonic catheter successfully ablated human calcified atherosclerotic plaques in vitro and recanalized vessel occlusions in an animal model (73). Again, there will be a long and rocky road to clinical application of this concept. It is seriously jeopardized by the fact that chronic occlusions rarely consist of chunks of calcium to be broken up or of poorly attached thrombi that might be removed by the shock wave. The elastic fibrous tissue they are predominantly made of is not a suitable target for ultrasound.

High-frequency Waves

Coronary angioplasty using high-frequency electricity (600 Hz) has been reported but total occlusions have not been tackled (74). This method might have some potential unless the local heat development proves prohibitive.

PERSPECTIVE

The clinical yield of chronic total coronary occlusion angioplasty will never match that of coronary angioplasty of stenoses, even if technical success can be improved. Recanalization angioplasty, a low-yield procedure, has to remain low-risk, and should also be low-cost. This sets limits to new tools and techniques. Laser technology holds the highest potential for passing old occlusions; yet it has to be disqualified for risk and cost reasons. Mechanical drills hold a lower potential for recanalization but they are more simple to handle, less costly, and less risky. Blunt and sturdy wires are even simpler and the closest relatives of conventional coronary guidewires in terms of user-friendliness and price. Hence, genuinely mechanical tools are likely to remain the mainstay of revascularization equipment, starting with the simplest. However, even these devices will have to prove their superiority to conventional means in randomized studies, which so far have been done only for one (58).

Although chronic total coronary occlusions, in contrast to stenoses, are no clinical menace, they frequently solicit revascularization and are the reason for selecting bypass surgery over angioplasty. Both the reduction of the need for bypass surgery and the salutary clinical follow-up results justify investments to improve recanalization techniques. As a side product, we will enjoy refinement of gear for coronary angioplasty of nontotal lesions.

REFERENCES

1. Meier B, Luethy P, Finci L, Steffenino GD, Rutishauser W. Coronary wedge pressure in relation to spontaneously visible and recruitable collaterals. *Circulation* 1987;75:906–913.
2. Schwartz F, Flameng W, Ensslen R, Sesto M, Thorman J. Effect of coronary collaterals on left ventricular function at rest and during stress. *Am Heart J* 1978;95:570–577.
3. Hamby RI, Antablian A, Schwartz A. Reappraisal of the functional significance of the coronary circulation. *Am J Cardiol* 1976;38:305–309.
4. Rogers WJ, Hood WP, Mantle JA, Baxley WA, Kirklin JK, Zorn GL, Nath HP. Return of left ventricular function after reperfusion in patients with myocardial infarction: importance of subtotal stenoses or intact collaterals. *Circulation* 1984;69:338–349.
5. Saito Y, Yasuno M, Ishida M, Suzuki K, Matoba Y, Emura M, Takahashi M. Importance of collaterals for restoration of left ventricular function after intracoronary thrombolysis. *Am J Cardiol* 1985;55:1259–1263.
6. Nitzberg WD, Nath HP, Rogers WJ, Hood WP, Whitlow PL, Reeves R, Baxley WA. Collateral flow in patients with acute myocardial infarction. *Am J Cardiol* 1985;56:729–736.
7. Schwartz H, Leiboff RH, Bren GB, Wasserman AG, Katz RJ, Varghese PJ, Sokil AB, Ross AM. Temporal evolution of the human coronary circulation after myocardial infarction. *J Am Coll Cardiol* 1984;4:1088–1093.
8. Cohen M, Rentrop KP. Limitation of myocardial ischemia by collateral circulation during sudden controlled coronary artery occlusion in human subjects: a prospective study. *Circulation* 1986;74:469–476.
9. Flameng W, Schwartz F, Hehrlein FW. Intraoperative evaluation of the functional significance of coronary collateral vessels in patients with coronary artery disease. *Am J Cardiol* 1978;42:187–192.
10. Braunwald E, Kloner RA. The stunned myocardium: prolonged, postischemic ventricular dysfunction. *Circulation* 1982;66:1146–1149.
11. Rahimtoola SH. The hibernating myocardium. *Am Heart J* 1989;117:211–221.
12. Tillisch J, Brunken R, Marshal R, Schwaiger M, Mandelkern M, Phelps M, Schelbert H. Reversibility of cardiac wallmotion abnormalities predicted by positron tomography. *N Engl J Med* 1986;314:884–888.
13. Dilsizian V, Rocco TP, Freedman NM, Leon MB, Bonow RO. Enhanced detection of ischemic but viable myocardium by the reinjection of thallium after stress-redistribution imaging. *N Engl J Med* 1990;323:141–146.
14. Meier B. Coronary angioplasty for chronic total occlusion. In: Meier B, ed. *Interventional Cardiology.* Toronto: Hogrefe & Huber, 1990:145–174.
15. Meier B. Chronic total occlusion. In: Topol EJ, ed. *Textbook of Interventional Cardiology.* Philadelphia: WB Saunders, 1990:300–326.
16. Singh A, Murray RG, Chandler S, Shiu MF. Myocardial salvage following elective angioplasty for total coronary occlusion. *Cardiology* 1987;74:474–478.
17. Melchior JP, Doriot PA, Chatelain P, Meier B, Urban P, Finci L, Rutishauser W. Improvement of left ventricular contraction and relaxation synchronism after recanalization of chronic total coronary occlusion by angioplasty. *J Am Coll Cardiol* 1987;4:763–768.
18. Serruys PW, Umans V, Heyndrickx GR, van den Brand M, de Feyter PJ, Wijns W, Jaski B, Hugenholtz PG. Elective PTCA of totally occluded coronary arteries not associated with acute myocardial infarction: short-term and long-term results. *Eur Heart J* 1985;6:2–12.
19. Finci L, Meier B, Steffenino GD. Percutaneous angioplasty of totally occluded saphenous aortocoronary bypass graft. *Int J Cardiol* 1986;10:76–79.
20. Sievert H, Köhler KP, Kaltenbach M, Kober G. Re-opening long-segment occlusions of aorto-coronary vein bypasses: short and long-term results. *Dtsch Med Wochenschr* 1988;113:637–640.
21. Hartmann J, McKeever L, Teran J, Bufalino V, Marek J, Brown A, Goodwin M, Amirparviz F, Motarjeme A. Prolonged infusion of urokinase for recanalization of chronically occluded aortocoronary bypass grafts. *Am J Cardiol* 1988;61:189–191.
22. Marx M, Armstrong WP, Wack JP, Bernstein RM, Brent B, Francoz R, Gregoratos G. Short-duration, high-dose urokinase for recanalization of occluded saphenous aortocoronary bypass grafts. *Am J Roentgenol* 1989;153:167–171.
23. De Feyter PJ, Serruys P, van den Brand M, Meester H, Beatt K, Suryaprananta H. Percutaneous transluminal angioplasty of a totally occluded venous bypass graft: a challenge that should be resisted. *Am J Cardiol* 1989;64:88–90.
24. Dervan JP, Baim DS, Cherniles J, Grossman W. Transluminal angioplasty of occluded coronary arteries: use of a movable guide wire system. *Circulation* 1983;68:776–784.

25. Kereiakes DJ, Selmon MR, McAuley BJ, McAuley DB, Sheehan DJ, Simpson JB. Angioplasty in total coronary artery occlusion: experience in 76 consecutive patients. *J Am Coll Cardiol* 1985;6:526–533.

26. DiSciascio G, Vetrovec GW, Cowley MJ, Wolfgang TC. Early and late outcome of percutaneous transluminal coronary angioplasty of subacute and chronic total coronary occlusion. *Am Heart J* 1986;111:833–839.

27. Melchior JP, Meier B, Urban P, Finci L, Steffenino G, Noble J, Rutishauser W. Percutaneous transluminal coronary angioplasty for chronic total coronary arterial occlusions. *Am J Cardiol* 1987;59:535–538.

28. Safian RD, McCabe CH, Sipperly ME, McKay RG, Baim DS. Initial success and long-term follow-up of percutaneous transluminal coronary angioplasty in chronic total occlusions versus conventional stenoses. *Am J Cardiol* 1988;61:23G–28G.

29. Ellis SG, Shaw RE, Gershony G, Thomas R, Roubin GS, Douglas JS, Topol EJ, Stertzer SH, Myler RK, King SB III. Risk factors, time course and treatment effect for restenosis after successful percutaneous transluminal coronary angioplasty of chronic total occlusion. *Am J Cardiol* 1989;63:897–901.

30. Stone GW, Rutherford BD, McConahay DR, Johnson WL Jr, Giorgi LV, Ligon RW, Harzler GO. Procedural outcome of angioplasty for total coronary artery occlusion: an analysis of 971 lesions in 905 patients. *J Am Coll Cardiol* 1990;15:849–856.

31. Ivanhoe RJ, Weintraub WS, Douglas JS Jr, Lembo NJ, Furman M, Gershony G, Cohen CL, King SB III. Percutaneous transluminal coronary angioplasty of chronic total occlusions: primary success, restenosis, and long-term clinical follow-up. *Circulation* 1992;85:106–115.

32. Bell MR, Berger PB, Bresnahan JF, Reeder GS, Bailey KR, Holmes DR. Initial and long term outcome of 354 patients following coronary balloon angioplasty of total coronary artery occlusions. *Circulation* 1992;85:1003–1011.

33. Holmes DR Jr, Vlietstra RE, Reeder GS, Breshnahan JF, Smith HC, Bove AA, Schaff HV. Angioplasty in total coronary artery occlusion. *J Am Coll Cardiol* 1984;3:845–849.

34. La Veau PJ, Remetz MS, Cabin HS, Hennecken JF, McConnell SH, Rosen RE, Cleman MW. Predictors of success in percutaneous transluminal coronary angioplasty of chronic total occlusions. *Am J Cardiol* 1989;64:1264–1269.

35. Rupprecht HJ, Brennecke R, Roth T, Erbel R, Meyer J. Recanalization of chronic coronary occlusion in patients with stable and unstable angina. *Cor Vasa* 1990;6:256–261.

36. Plante S, Laarman GJ, de Feyter PJ, Samson M, Rensing BJ, Umans V, Suryapranata H, van den Brand M, Serruys PW. Acute complications of percutaneous transluminal coronary angioplasty for total occlusion. *Am Heart J* 1991;121:417–426.

37. Meier B. Benign coronary perforation during percutaneous transluminal coronary angioplasty. *Br Heart J* 1985;54:33–35.

38. Meier B. Restenosis after coronary angioplasty: review of the literature. *Eur Heart J* 1988;9[Suppl C]:1–6.

39. Ellis SG, Shaw RE, King SB III, Myler RK, Topol EJ. Restenosis after excellent angiographic result for chronic total coronary artery occlusion—implications for newer percutaneous revascularization devices. *Am J Cardiol* 1989;64:667–668.

40. Urban P, Meier B, Finci L, DeBruyne B, Steffenino G, Rutishauser W. Coronary wedge pressure: a predictor of restenosis after coronary balloon angioplasty. *J Am Coll Cardiol* 1987;10:504–509.

41. Finci L, Meier B, Righetti A, Rutishauser W. Long-term results of successful and failed angioplasty for chronic total coronary arterial occlusion. *Am J Cardiol* 1990;66:660–662.

42. Warren RJ, Black AJ, Valentine PA, Manolas EG, Hunt D. Coronary angioplasty for chronic total occlusion reduces the need for subsequent coronary bypass surgery. *Am Heart J* 1990;120:270–274.

43. De Swart JBRM, Van Gelder LM, Van der Krieken AM, El Gamal MIH. A new technique for angioplasty of occluded coronary arteries and bypass grafts, not associated with acute myocardial infarction. *Cathet Cardiovasc Diagn* 1987;13:419–423.

44. Smith LDR, Katritsis D, Webb-Peploe MM. Use of a hollow wire to facilitate angioplasty of occluded vessels. *Br Heart J* 1989;61:326–330.

45. Meier B. Magnarail probing catheter: new tool for balloon recanalization of chronic total coronary occlusions. *J Invas Cardiol* 1990;2:227–229.

46. Hamm CW, Kupper W, Kuck KH, Hofmann D, Bleifeld W. Recanalization of chronic, totally occluded coronary arteries by new angioplasty systems. *Am J Cardiol* 1990;66:1459–1463.

47. Little T, Rosenberg J, Seides S, Lee B, Lindsay J Jr, Pichard AD. Probe angioplasty of total coronary occlusion using the probing catheter technique. *Cathet Cardiovasc Diagn* 1990;21:124–127.

48. Grollier G, Commeau P, Foucault JP, Potier JC. Angioplasty of chronic totally occluded coronary arteries: usefulness of retrograde opacification of the distal part of the occluded vessel via the contralateral coronary artery. *Am Heart J* 1987;114:1324–1328.

49. Sherman CT, Sheehan D, Simpson JB. Simultaneous cannulation: a technique for percutaneous transluminal coronary angioplasty of chronic total occlusions. *Cathet Cardiovasc Diagn* 1987;13:333–336.

50. Myler, RK, Mooney MR, Stertzer SH, Clark DA, Hidalgo BO, Fishman J. The balloon on a wire device: a new ultra-low-profile coronary angioplasty system/concept. *Cathet Cardiovasc Diagn* 1988;14:135–140.

51. Thomas ES, Williams DO, Neiderman AL, Douglas JS, King SB III. Efficacy of a new angioplasty catheter for severely narrowed coronary lesions. *J Am Coll Cardiol* 1988;12:694–702.

52. Rizzo TF, Ciccone J, Werres R. Dilating guide wire: use of a new ultra-low-profile percutaneous transluminal coronary angioplasty system. *Cathet Cardiovasc Diagn* 1989;16:258–262.

53. Feldman RL, Hennemann WW III. New steerable, ultra-low-profile, fixed-wire angioplasty catheter: initial experience with the Cordis Orion steerable PTCA balloon catheter. *Cathet Cardiovasc Diagn* 1990;19:142–145.

54. Finci L, Meier B, Roy P, Steffenino G, Rutishauser W. Clinical experience with the Monorail balloon catheter for coronary angioplasty. *Cathet Cardiovasc Diagn* 1988;14:206–212.

55. Mooney MR, Douglas JS Jr, Mooney JF, Madison JD, Brandenburg RO, Fernald R, Van Tassel RA. Monorail Piccolino catheter: a new rapid exchange/ultralow profile coronary angioplasty system. *Cathet Cardiovasc Diagn* 1990;20:114–119.

56. Meier B, Carlier M, Finci L, Nukta E, Urban P, Niederhauser W, Favre J. Magnum wire for balloon recanalization of chronic total coronary occlusions. *Am J Cardiol* 1989;64:148–154.

57. Villavicencio R, Meier B. Left axillary approach for balloon recanalization of an occlusion of the right common femoral artery. *Vasa* 1991;20:186–187.

58. Pande AK, Meier B, Urban P, de la Serna F, Villavicencio R, Dorsaz PA, Favre J. Magnum/Magnarail versus conventional systems for recanalization of chronic total coronary occlusions: a randomized comparison. *Am Heart J* 1992;123:1182–1186.

59. Vallbracht C, Liermann D, Prignitz I, Beinborn W, Landgraf H, Paasch C, Roth FJ, Kollath J, Schoop W, Bamberg W, Kaltenbach M. Results of low speed rotational angioplasty for chronic peripheral occlusions. *Am J Cardiol* 1988;62:935–940.

60. Kaltenbach M, Vallbracht C. Reopening of chronic coronary artery occlusions by low speed rotational angioplasty. *J Interven Cardiol* 1989;2:137–145.

61. Kensey KR, Nash JE, Abrahams C, Zarins CK. Recanalization of obstructed arteries with a flexible, rotating tip catheter. *Radiology* 1987;165:387–389.

62. Kensey KR. The Kensey catheter: what have we learned to date? *J Invas Cardiol* 1991;3:25–31.

63. Hinohara T, Selmon MR, Robertson GC, Braden L, Simpson JS. Directional atherectomy. New approaches for treatment of obstructive coronary and peripheral vascular disease. *Circulation* 1990;81[Suppl IV]:79–91.

64. Dick RJL, Haudenschild CC, Popma JJ, Ellis SG, Muller DW, Topol EJ. Directional atherectomy for total coronary occlusions. *Cor Art Dis* 1991;2:189–199.

65. Sketch MH, Phillips HR, Lee MM, Stack RS. Coronary transluminal extraction endarterectomy. *J Invas Cardiol* 1991;3:13–18.

66. Meany TB, Friedman HZ, O'Neill WW. Coronary rotational atherectomy: clinical application. *J Invas Cardiol* 1991;3:19–24.

67. Franzen D, Höpp HW, Hilger HH. Limitations of low speed rotational angioplasty—an angioscopic and histological study. *Cor Vasa* 1991;4:186–191.

68. Bowes RJ, Oakley GD, Fleming JS, Myler RK, Stertzer SH, Shaw RE, Cumberland DC. Early clinical experience with a hot tip laser wire in patients with chronic coronary artery occlusion. *J Invas Cardiol* 1990;2:241–245.

69. Mast EG, Plokker HWM, Ernst JMPG, Bal ET, Tjon Joe Gin RM, Ascoop CAPL. Percutaneous recanalization of chronic total coronary occlusions: experience with the direct Argon laser assisted angioplasty system (LASTAC). *Herz* 1990;15:241–244.

70. Werner GS, Buchwald A, Unterberg C, Voth E, Kreuzer H, Wiegand V. Recanalization of chronic total coronary arterial occlusions by percutaneous Excimer-laser and laser-assisted angioplasty. *Am J Cardiol* 1990;66:1445–1450.

71. Deckelbaum LI, Lam JK, Cabin HS, Clubb KS, Long MB. Discrimination of normal and atherosclerotic aorta by laser-induced fluorescence. *Lasers Surg Med* 1987;7:330–335.

72. Laufer G, Wollenek G, Hohla K, Horvat R, Henke KH, Buchelt M, Wutzl G, Wolner E. Excimer laser-induced simultaneous ablation and spectral identification of normal and atherosclerotic arterial tissue layers. *Circulation* 1988;78:1031–1039.

73. Siegel RJ, Fishbein MC, Forrester J, Moore K, DeCastro E, Daykhosky L, DonMichael TA. Ultrasonic plaque ablation. A new method of recanalization of partially or totally occluded arteries. *Circulation* 1988;78:1443–1448.

74. Höher M, Hombach V, Kochs M, Eggeling T, Haerer W. Angioplastie mittels Hochfrequenz bei Koronararterienstenosen. *Herz* 1990;15:245–252.

Practical Angioplasty,
edited by David P. Faxon.
Raven Press, Ltd., New York © 1993.

CHAPTER 11

Interventional Approaches in the Postbypass Patient

John S. Douglas, Jr.

Aortocoronary bypass surgery is an effective procedure which has resulted in initial relief of symptoms in a majority of patients treated during the 25 years since its initial application (1,2). However, subsequent long-term follow-up of patients revealed that angina pectoris recurred in a significant proportion of patients due to progression of native coronary artery disease, or development of new stenoses, or occlusions in graft conduits (3–8). Significant new native coronary artery disease has been documented to occur in approximately 5% of postoperative patients annually in the first five years postoperatively (6–9), and progression in venous conduits is even more common (10–15). Only about 80% of saphenous veins are patent and free of significant narrowing at 1 year following surgery, and at 5 and 10 years about 70%, and 45% to 50%, respectively, are widely patent. Although long-term patency of internal mammary artery grafts was shown to be more favorable by Loop and colleagues in the mid 1980s, thousands of patients were initially treated without arterial grafts, and hundreds of thousands continue to receive venous grafts annually. It is uncertain whether an increasing recognition of internal mammary artery anastomotic problems is related to the more frequent use of this conduit, to increasing recognition of the importance of early recatheterization of patients who have recurrent symptoms, or to reduced technical expertise as a result of the proliferation of low-volume surgical programs is uncertain. The progressive deterioration of native vessel and graft conduit lumina following surgery results in recurrent ischemic symptoms in 4% to 8% of patients annually (3,4,5,16), as well as an increasing need for repeat revascularization

procedures. At Emory University Hospital, reoperative coronary artery bypass grafts (CABG) constituted 5.4% of coronary surgical procedures in 1982 to 1984, but 9.8% of total volume in 1985 to 1987 and 12.9% in 1988 to 1990. Similarly, reoperations at the Cleveland Clinic increased by 230% in 1985 to 1987 compared to 1979 to 1981 (17), in spite of the advent and increasing utilization of percutaneous transluminal coronary angioplasty (PTCA) in this patient group. An increasing need for repeat revascularization procedures will be observed in the next decade as the enormous pool of postoperative patients continues to grow and age. Unfortunately, reoperative coronary surgery is associated with a substantially increased risk of in-hospital death and nonfatal Q-wave myocardial infarction. In the most experienced hands, the risk of these important complications is three times that of the initial operation (17). At Emory University Hospital the operative mortality in 1,406 patients undergoing coronary artery reoperation between 1980 and 1990 was 7.2%. In New York State in 1989, the operative risk for first reoperation was 10.6% and 24.5% for second reoperations (18). Unfortunately, in addition to the increased operative risk, reoperative surgery is associated with less complete angina relief (19,20) and a reduced graft patency at 5 years of 65% for saphenous vein grafts (SVG), and 88% for internal mammary artery (IMA) grafts in patients undergoing recatheterization (17). These factors have fostered a conservative approach to reoperation in symptomatic patients (21) and encouraged the use of percutaneous angioplasty strategies whenever possible (22–51b).

INDICATIONS

Patients who experience a recurrence of symptoms following coronary bypass surgery are a very heterogenous

J. S. Douglas, Jr.: Emory University School of Medicine, and Cardiovascular Laboratory, Emory University Hospital, Atlanta, Georgia

group, and selection for PTCA must be based on a careful weighing of multiple factors, including the likelihood of a successful procedure, risk of complications, and probability of long-term symptomatic benefit compared to other viable options (21,23,51,52). Since the ability to effectively relieve ischemia with PTCA in the post-CABG patient is as much influenced by the time since operation as by the type of conduit (SVG vs. native coronary artery vs. IMA graft) and location of the stenotic lesion, indications for intervention will be discussed relative to postoperative interval.

Ischemia Within Days or Weeks of CABG

Patients who present with recurrent ischemia within days or weeks of operation usually have acute graft thrombosis. However, an isolated technical problem may exist at proximal or distal anastomotic sites (see Fig. 1), the wrong vessel may have been bypassed, or the culprit vessel may have been unsuitable due to diffuse disease, or inaccessible due to intramyocardial position. Data from Canada indicate that 8% to 15% of vein grafts close by 1 month after surgery (11,53–55) and, even with aspirin therapy, 7% of vein grafts may close by as early as 9 days postoperatively, with up to 17% of patients having at least one closed graft at that time (54,55). When symptoms recur early after surgery, coronary arteriography is

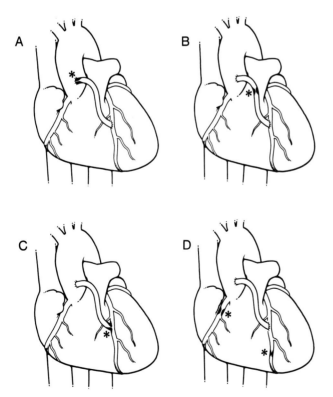

FIG. 1. Sites of saphenous vein graft and native coronary stenoses: proximal anastomosis (**A**), mid-vein graft (**B**), distal anastomosis (**C**), and native vessel sites (**D**) in ungrafted vessel and distal to graft insertion.

indicated to pinpoint the problem. If a focal stenosis is present at a graft anastomosis, PTCA across suture lines has been safe, in our experience and that of others (56), even a few days postoperatively, as long as balloon sizing is conservative. If the vein or internal mammary artery graft is thrombosed, or if the culprit vessel was not bypassed, the target should be the native vessel stenosis if at all possible. If the native vessel is not a reasonable target (e.g., a very old occlusion) and the graft is thrombosed, it may be reasonable to pass a guidewire or perhaps a balloon catheter across the occlusion to test the length of the thrombosed segment. Extensive thrombosis within a graft is not a very reasonable target for the balloon alone, and thrombolytic therapy a few days postoperatively has been anecdotally reported to cause cardiac tamponade. Novel methods of thrombectomy are in developmental stages. Thrombectomy with routine PTCA equipment is sometimes feasible, but frequently of limited efficacy. In a small number of patients, short segment occlusions of internal mammary artery grafts have been recanalized using guidewires and balloon catheters without thrombolytic therapy.

Ischemia 1 to 12 Months Post-CABG

In our experience, the majority of patients presenting at this time have conduit stenosis (see Figs. 1–4) although conduit thrombosis or even new native coronary disease may be present. Stenoses in internal mammary artery grafts may occur proximally (35,36), but are much more frequent at the coronary implantation site (see Fig. 4), where the success of PTCA is extremely high and restenosis rates are low. Short-segment total occlusions of internal mammary artery grafts are rarely seen and, in a limited experience, successful dilatation has frequently been possible. These short-segment occlusions can be visualized only by meticulous attention to late filming in order to demonstrate passage of contrast well down the graft, and almost to the implantation site. Saphenous vein grafts with distal anastomosis lesions can be dilated quite safely, and recurrence rates are less than 25% for lesions occurring at this time (see Fig. 2). Lesions in the mid saphenous vein graft occurring less than 1 year postoperatively are due to intimal hyperplasia, and these lesions can be safely dilated (see Table 1) or removed with directional atherectomy. The risk of distal embolization is quite low. Recurrence rates for mid graft lesions are rather high with conventional balloon angioplasty, but long-term success is sometimes achieved. When both the native vessel and the surgical conduit to a myocardial segment have lesions suitable for PTCA, we frequently dilate both the conduit and the native vessel in that order. Although the proximal anastomotic site (aortosaphenous vein graft junction) has a higher restenosis rate with conventional angioplasty, long-term success for up to a decade has been obtained in some patients. We and

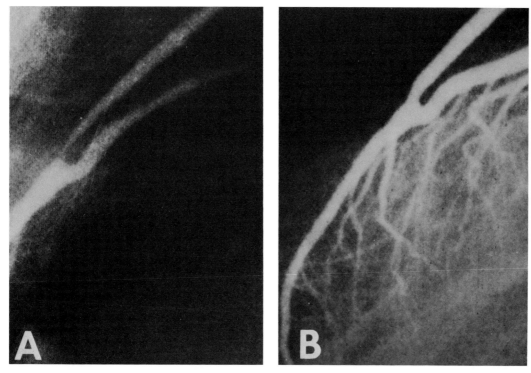

FIG. 2. A 57-year-old male underwent saphenous vein bypass grafting to the distal left anterior descending (LAD) artery in January, 1981 and developed disabling angina a few months later. Coronary arteriography in July, 1981 (**A**) revealed high-grade stenosis at the junction of the saphenous vein graft to the LAD artery (left lateral view). Percutaneous transluminal coronary angioplasty was successful (residual stenosis 13%) and recatheterization 9 months later showed a widely patent anastomosis (**B**). The patient subsequently remained completely asymptomatic and at last follow-up over 10 years later (November, 1991), had a negative stress electrocardiogram. From Douglas et al. (23), with permission from the American College of Cardiology.

others have applied directional atherectomy for aortosaphenous vein graft junction (see Fig. 5) stenoses with good initial results (57,57a). The effectiveness of this strategy will be clearer when long-term restenosis rates are available. Technically, excimer laser use seems partic-

ularly attractive for this site; however, long-term results are not yet known (57b). Stenting is problematic. One would prefer to avoid having the stent wires protruding into the aorta, but this may be necessary to conclusively stent an ostial site (57c).

Ischemia 1 to 3 Years After CABG

Patients who are seen 1 to 3 years following coronary bypass surgery frequently have new stenotic lesions in grafts and native coronary arteries, and palliation is often possible at low risk. Whenever possible, dilatation of native coronary arteries is preferable, due to lower restenosis rates. New internal mammary artery graft lesions are rare in this time frame. Occasionally, patients are seen with distal implantation site stenoses, and a history of angina persisting ever since surgery. Lesions in proximal and mid saphenous vein graft sites can be dilated with little risk of distal embolization, except in patients with diabetes or hyperlipidemia, where atherosclerosis is sometimes observed in vein grafts that have been implanted for less than 3 years.

Ischemia Developing More Than 3 Years Post-CABG

The symptomatic patient seen several years following coronary bypass surgery is frequently a candidate for

FIG. 3. Results of follow-up vein graft angiography in patients who underwent angioplasty of stenoses at the distal anastomosis (junction of saphenous vein graft and coronary artery) showing excellent patency. Dashed lines denote repeat angioplasty in three of four patients who developed restenosis. From Douglas et al. (23), with permission from the American College of Cardiology.

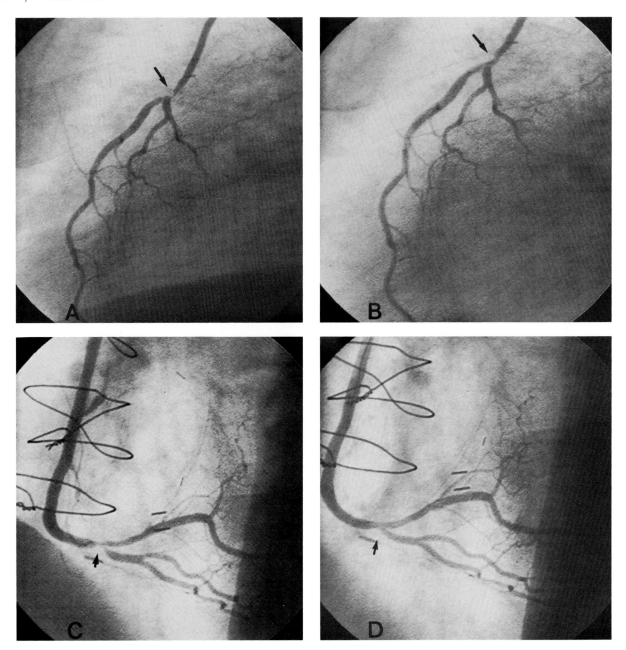

FIG. 4. A 58-year-old developed recurrent angina pectoris 3 months after triple coronary bypass surgery. Coronary arteriography revealed severe stenosis at the anastomosis of the left internal mammary artery (LIMA) graft to the LAD (**A**) and significant unbypassed coronary disease distal to the insertion of the saphenous vein graft (SVG) to the right coronary artery (**C**). A saphenous vein graft to the circumflex coronary artery was patent. Angioplasty of the LIMA anastomosis was successful (**B**) using a 2.5-mm diameter over-the-wire balloon device, and the distal right coronary artery bifurcation was successfully dilated (**D**) via the SVG using a double-balloon approach in which a 2.5-mm over-the-wire balloon was placed in the PDA and a 3-mm over-the-wire balloon was placed in the continuation of the distal right coronary artery. The low complication rate with PTCA of LIMA insertion sites made it possible for the operator to move ahead and dilate the right coronary artery once a good initial result was obtained with the LIMA-LAD junction dilatation. Repeat angiography at 4 months revealed no restenosis. The patient remained asymptomatic 14 months after PTCA. This patient illustrates use of angioplasty to correct both a graft problem and unbypassed native coronary disease.

TABLE 1. *Results of vein graft PTCA*

Author (Date)	Reference	Number of patients	Success (%)	AMI	CABG	Death
Gruentzig et al. (1979)	22	5	60	–	–	0
Ford et al. (1980)	22a	7	86			0
Douglas et al. (1983)	23	62	94	0	0	0
El Gamal et al. (1984)	24	44	93	1	1	0
Block et al. (1984)	25	40	78	2	0	0
Dorros et al. (1984)	26	33	79	0	1	0
Corbelli et al. (1985)	27	47	92	–	–	0
Reeder et al. (1986)	28	19	84	–	–	0
Douglas et al. (1986)	29	235	92	1	0	1
Cote et al. (1987)	30	101	85	16 (7%)[a]	3 (1.3%)	0
Ernst et al. (1987)	30a	33	97	1	1	0
Pinkerton et al. (1988)	31	100	93	–	–	–
Dorros et al. (1988)	32	53	83	–	–	–
Reed et al. (1989)	32a	52	90	1	–	1
Cooper et al. (1989)	33	24	75	0	–	0
Platko et al. (1989)	49	101	92	–	0	1
Plokker et al. (1991)	50	454	90	12	4	4
Douglas et al. (1991)	50a	599	90	13 (2.8%)	6 (1.3%)	3 (0.7%)
TOTAL		2009	89	14 (2.3%)[b]	21 (3.5%)	7 (1.2%)

AMI, acute myocardial infarction; CABG, coronary artery bypass graft.
[a] Q-wave + non–Q-wave AMI.
[b] Q-Wave AMI.

multisite PTCA (see Fig. 6). Vein graft lesions more than 3 years after surgery frequently have atheromatous elements, and embolization documented by creative kinase (CPK) elevation is seen in 10% to 20% of cases, but lower or higher rates may be encountered depending on case selection. Predictors of vein graft embolization include the presence of lesion-associated thrombus, eccentricity (see Fig. 7), irregular surfaces or lesion ulceration, and diffuse disease in the vein graft (58). Fortunately, small distal emboli are well tolerated. Extensive thrombus formation in saphenous vein grafts is not easily managed with direct PTCA (59). Prolonged intracoronary admin-

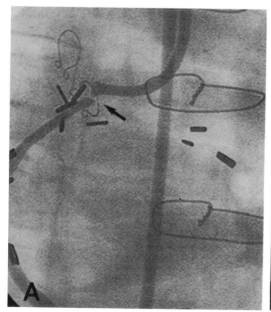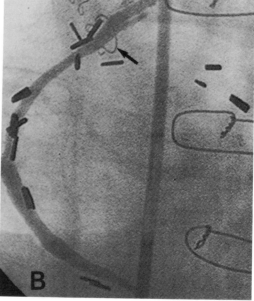

FIG. 5. High-grade stenosis was present at the most proximal portion of the saphenous vein graft (SVG) to right coronary artery (RCA) in a 65-year-old male with disabling symptoms, a patent left internal mammary artery (LIMA) to left anterior descending (LAD) artery and patent SVGs to two obtuse marginal coronary arteries. Lesions at this site have a high restenosis rate, although we have documented 9-year patency in a patient dilated 5 months postoperatively. This lesion (**A**) was discovered 7 years after bypass surgery and responded well to directional atherectomy (**B**).

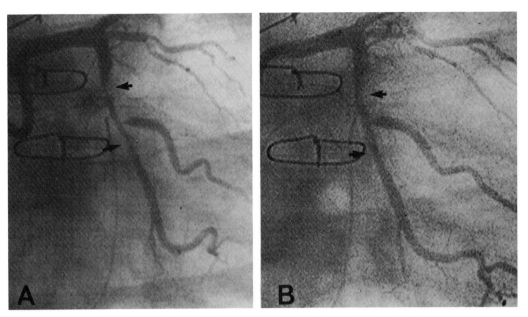

FIG. 6. Complex disease in the circumflex coronary artery of a 51-year-old male who developed disabling angina 4 years after bypass surgery. Saphenous vein grafts to the LAD, RCA, and two diagonal coronary arteries were widely patent. The new native coronary disease in the circumflex system (**A**) was dilated using a left Amplatz 2 guide catheter to obtain good support. A guide catheter with side holes was used due to mild ostial left main disease. A 2.5-mm diameter, 3 cm long over-the-wire compliant balloon was used to dilate the circumflex artery and a 2.5-mm balloon-on-a-wire was placed in the obtuse marginal. In spite of the excellent angiographic appearance (**B**), abrupt closure occurred within an hour of angioplasty and rePTCA with 3-mm diameter balloons yielded a result identical with (**B**). No postangioplasty complications were noted and the patient remains asymptomatic.

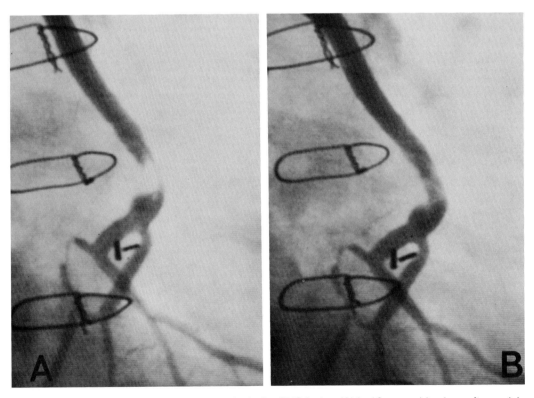

FIG. 7. This is an example of a very eccentric, bulky SVG lesion (**A**) in 10-year-old vein graft supplying two smaller circumflex branches. This type of vein graft problem in a symptomatic patient who has no other ischemia-producing lesions can be approached with angioplasty, although the risk of distal embolization is significantly increased. The site is not favorable for directional atherectomy because the larger, more posterior limb of the SVG is not long enough to accommodate the nose cone of the atherectomy device, and the more anterior branch is rather small. Stenting with a Palmaz-Schatz stent would be a reasonable option. Balloon angioplasty was carried out with a good result and only minimal evidence of distal embolization. (**B**) Three years later symptoms recurred and reoperation was recommended to bypass multiple new obstructive lesions and this graft, which was occluded.

istration of thrombolytic agents has been performed, and initial results have been somewhat favorable when the angiographic evidence of thrombus has been lessened and successful dilatation can be accomplished (60–63). In our early experience with this strategy several years ago, the amount of patient discomfort associated with a prolonged intracoronary infusion was quite significant and reocclusion rates were high, engendering a conservative approach. In addition, complications of thrombolytic therapy, including infarction (64–65) and significant bleeding, have been reported. When we see intracoronary thrombus at a potential PTCA site, we frequently give 5 to 7 days of intravenous heparin followed by PTCA, with or without intracoronary thrombolytic therapy, at the time of the dilatation.

Percutaneous transluminal coronary angioplasty of old native coronary artery stenoses in previously operated patients can present some unique challenges, due to the fibrocalcific nature of the lesions. Commonly, PTCA can be performed in spite of these factors; however, ostial lesions of the right coronary artery may require excimer laser use, old left main coronary lesions frequently require PTCA plus atherectomy, and stenoses in distal sites may require balloon-on-a-wire devices with high-pressure capability. In our experience, saphenous vein

graft lesions more than 5 years after surgery have evidence of distal embolization in over 20% of patients, and the restenosis rate is relatively high, particularly for lesions that are greater than 1 cm in length. In spite of these limitations, angioplasty is frequently helpful in patients who have high-grade stenoses in grafts to arteries of moderate size, or in patients in whom reoperation is not a viable option due to multiple previous coronary bypass operations (see Fig. 8), severe pulmonary disease, cancer, or other extenuating circumstances. When a lesion in a graft conduit can be successfully dilated and the patient benefitted, even for less than a year, this strategy may be reasonable as long as the risk to the patient is small. In certain cases the long-term patency of the dilated graft is surprisingly good. Even when restenosis occurs, the amount of time bought may allow development of collateral flow sufficient to avoid infarction and/or disabling symptoms.

Management of Acute Myocardial Infarction in the Post-CABG Patient

Although approximately 3% of post-CABG patients experience acute myocardial infarction (AMI) annually

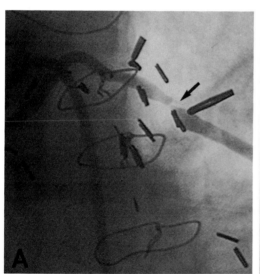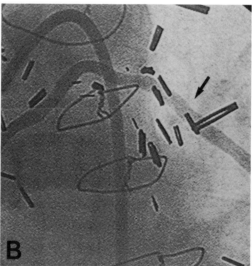

FIG. 8. Severe disabling angina pectoris recurred in a 65-year-old male who had previously had three coronary bypass operations, the last 6 years ago. **A:** Severe focal stenosis was present in the mid portion of the SVG to LAD. The SVG to the circumflex coronary artery was patent and the right coronary artery was occluded. Left ventricular function was normal. The abrupt angle in the proximal SVG ruled out directional atherectomy. After premedication with aspirin, Persantine, and dextran, a 3.5-mm diameter Palmaz-Schatz stent was placed and overexpanded with a 4-mm balloon inflated to 16 atm to yield an excellent result (**B**) with no evidence of distal embolization. The patient received anticoagulation treatment with Coumadin and is currently asymptomatic. Use of an Amplatz guide catheter was helpful in obtaining adequate support to advance the stent around the sharp bend in the saphenous vein graft. Results of conventional balloon angioplasty at Emory University Hospital suggest that dilatation of a mid SVG lesion 6 years post-CABG would be associated with a 20% to 25% incidence of CPK elevation greater than 340, and a restenosis rate of roughly 30% at 6 months, but continued attrition subsequently (45,50a). Results of the multicenter experience with placement of the Palmaz-Schatz stent in mid SVG sites suggest a restenosis rate at 6 months of about 25% when de novo lesions are stented (77a). It remains to be determined whether progressive restenosis would be noted in the stented vein grafts.

(66), optimal therapy in this group is controversial. There are no randomized trials to guide therapy. Data from the myocardial infarction triage and intervention (MITI) registry indicate that reperfusion strategies in patients with prior CABG are associated with increased risk (67), undoubtedly related to the higher prevalence of prior infarction and multivessel disease in these patients (68). In approximately two-thirds of cases, the infarct-related vessel is an occluded graft, and extensive thrombus formation is common (69–71). Although intravenous thrombolytic therapy has been applied in small groups of post-CABG patients (72) and is a reasonable strategy, many investigators favor emergency coronary angiography and thoughtful intervention based on the anatomic findings (69–71,73). Kahn et al. reported 90% survival in 72 patients undergoing direct PTCA without antecedent thrombolytic therapy and achieved success in 85% of SVGs and 100% of native coronary arteries, at 5.1 ± 4.0 hr from onset of symptoms (73). The ACC/AHA Task Force Report on Early Management of Acute Myocardial Infarction considered primary PTCA for vein graft recanalization to be a Class IIa intervention (acceptable, of uncertain efficacy, and may be controversial; weight of evidence in favor of usefulness/efficacy) (74).

TECHNICAL APPROACHES

Preparation of Patient

Optimal conditions for the performance of interventional procedures and routine measures to prepare patients for these procedures have been described in detail (52,75,76). In our experience, patients with prior surgery are handled in standard fashion, unless poor left ventricular function or an increased potential for ischemic hemodynamic compromise exist. In such patients, intraaortic balloon pumping or standby may be indicated, and advance consultation with surgical colleagues is of increased importance. We have not found cardiopulmonary support with in-lab cardiopulmonary bypass to be necessary in a broad spectrum of patients presenting with native vessel and conduit problems following coronary bypass surgery.

Native Vessel Intervention

Approaches to native coronary artery sites in the post-CABG patient may present unique challenges. In treatment of the protected left main coronary artery lesion, the interventionalist commonly encounters a very old fibrocalcific lesion which responds poorly to conventional balloon angioplasty. We have found directional atherectomy to be helpful (see Fig. 9) even in the presence of moderate calcification, but predilatation with a high pressure balloon is usually required. The excimer

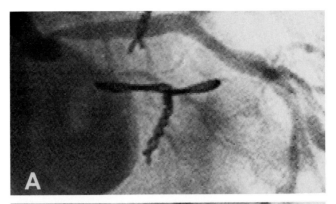
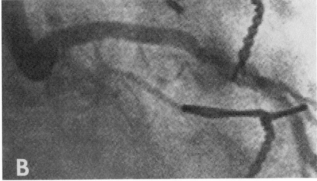

FIG. 9. Ostial left main coronary artery stenosis in a 66-year-old patient 2 years following bypass surgery (**A**). This type of lesion responds poorly to balloon angioplasty and, in this case, directional atherectomy was quite successful in achieving an excellent improvement in lumen diameter without complications (**B**).

laser and rotational atherectomy have also been used, and follow-up angioplasty or atherectomy is usually required. Recanalization of chronic occlusions may be required when conduits are thrombosed or too diffusely diseased for rehabilitation. A need for more aggressive strategies with stiffer guidewires and high-pressure balloons may be expected in this patient subset. Passage of dilatation catheters or other interventional devices via graft conduits into distal native sites is frequently required. When very long venous grafts have been implanted which wrap the heart (snake grafts), an extra long balloon catheter shaft (or shortened guide catheter) may be required to reach the lesion. Extra catheter length may also be needed when the right internal mammary is inserted quite distally in the right coronary artery or circumflex system and when a very redundant arterial graft is present. If retrograde passage is required from graft insertion into more proximal segments of the native coronary arteries, special guidewire strategies, high-performance balloon catheters, and optimal guide catheter backup become important (77). (See left IMA and SVG interventions below for a discussion of guide catheter selection.) When ischemia may be relieved by either a graft or native vessel intervention, a decision should be based on safety factors and durability of the interventional result.

Saphenous Vein Graft Intervention

In our practice an 8 French guide catheter is routinely used for SVG procedures. A multipurpose shape is chosen for most vein grafts to the right coronary artery, a multipurpose or right Judkins shape for a horizontal or inferiorly directed SVG to the left anterior descending (LAD) artery, and a left Amplatz 1.5 or 2 for superiorly oriented SVGs to the LAD artery and for virtually all diagonal and circumflex vein grafts. Guide catheters with side holes are frequently used and are especially helpful with smaller vein grafts or ostial SVG lesions. For ostial stenoses where guide catheter seating is difficult or impossible, a diagnostic catheter and balloon-on-a-wire may be required to achieve success. For rigid ostial lesions, initial dilatation with a small balloon-on-a-wire may be required simply to permit entrance of a definitive over-the-wire balloon when backup support is poor. Because of higher restenosis rates with balloon dilatation of ostial graft lesions, directional atherectomy (DCA) is frequently used (see Fig. 5), either after PTCA with a 2-mm balloon or as a primary approach. Lesions in the mid portion of SVGs occurring within 3 years of CABG frequently respond to less than 10 atm and rarely cause distal embolization. Slight balloon oversizing is safe in this time frame, but as vein grafts age, the risk of vein graft rupture increases, and balloon oversizing has an increased risk for that reason. In general, we size the balloon 1:1 for the vein graft and reserve oversizing for suboptimal results. Eccentric or ledgelike SVG lesions respond well to atherectomy, and results with the Palmaz-Schatz stent have been favorable in focal lesions. Because of obligatory Coumadin anticoagulation with stents, we commonly use directional atherectomy for de novo mid SVG lesions with favorable angiographic features, and stenting for restenotic lesions where DCA has a very high restenosis rate. When a suboptimal result has been obtained in vein graft lesions with balloon angioplasty or other strategies, a prolonged inflation with a perfusion balloon may yield significant improvement. In our experience, the presence of obvious intragraft thrombus is associated with an increased risk of distal embolization with infarction and also acute closure. Direct infusion of thrombolytic agents into the vein graft has a limited effect unless the infusion is prolonged, and results with these prolonged infusions have been less favorable in our experience than the literature suggests (61–63). Whereas placement of Palmaz-Schatz stents in the presence of obvious thrombus should be avoided, placement of these stents in bulky eccentric atheromatous lesions seems, in our experience and in the multicenter experience, to minimize or in some cases prevent

distal atheroembolization (77a). Angioplasty of distal anastomotic site lesions in vein grafts is associated with a very low immediate complication rate (23) and a favorable long-term outlook. These lesions occurring within a year of bypass surgery usually are easy to cross and respond to a low balloon inflation pressure; however, occasionally an inexplicably rigid lesion may be present, perhaps related to a tight suture line. When vein grafts enter native vessels at a right angle, there may be a tendency for any device to pass retrograde or in the case of the LAD artery, to pass directly into the septal perforating branches and an over-the-wire system may be desirable to enhance steerability. Whereas distal anastomotic lesions appearing within a year or so of surgery have a favorable outlook, lesions occurring many years following surgery have a much higher rate of atheroembolism and restenosis more in keeping with lesions observed in mid-vein graft sites.

Internal Mammary Artery Graft Intervention

Although stenotic lesions may be encountered throughout internal mammary grafts, the most common (and the most favorable site for PTCA) is at the anastomosis of the mammary artery with the native coronary artery. Virtually all lesions in either the left internal mammary artery (LIMA) or right internal mammary artery (RIMA) can be successfully approached from the leg; however, an arm approach may be easier if there is a problem seating the 7 or 8 French guide catheter, and especially if poor guide support is noted in the presence of severe graft tortuosity or very distal lesion location. In general, we use an 8 French IMA guide catheter for both RIMA and LIMA when good backup support is required (or 7 French, if vessels are small) and favor a balloon-on-a-wire for most dilatations. An over-the-wire dilatation system is used when maximal steerability is required, in the presence of a total occlusion requiring recanalization, or if retrograde passage into proximal native coronary artery sites is necessary. Perfusion balloons and stents may be useful when PTCA fails (78,79). Use of novel brachial guide catheter shapes has been reported to produce success when PTCA is unsuccessful from a femoral approach (79a). In patients with significant subclavian artery stenosis (or even occlusion), dilatation may be performed before CABG with a high success rate so that the surgeon can use the LIMA for coronary bypass or to improve symptoms in a patient with a LIMA graft already in place (80,81). To enhance patient comfort during internal mammary artery graft interventions, a recent blind study indicates that ioxaglate, a low osmolar ionic dimer was much better tolerated than the nonionic monomer, iopamidol. The improved tolerance may be related to a lower osmolality, 320 mOsm/kg of water versus 370 mOsm/kg of water (82).

MANAGEMENT OF COMPLICATIONS

Coronary Embolism

Coronary embolization is a rare complication of native vessel PTCA and is seen most often in patients with intracoronary thrombus (acute infarction, unstable angina, total occlusions) (83). Iatrogenic air embolism is usually recognized by transient chest pain and ST elevation following contrast injection, whereas atheroembolism is suspected when ischemia unaccountably develops and persists immediately after dilatation of a chronic lesion. In general, the clinical consequences of coronary embolization are proportional to the volume of embolic material. In native coronary interventions, minimal or no myocardial necrosis is the rule. The same is not necessarily true in vein grafts where atheromas are larger and friable, and thrombus formation is common. We observed seven coronary emboli during 235 vein graft angioplasty procedures, a 3% occurrence rate (29). One patient had Q-wave infarction, four had non–Q-wave infarction, and two had prolonged ischemic pain without infarction. All embolic events occurred in grafts in place for over 3 years. Cote reported two Q-wave infarctions during 101 vein graft PTCA procedures and both occurred over 5 years post-CABG (30). Dorros noted three coronary emboli in 53 vein graft procedures; one patient died of extensive myocardial infarction (32). Saber et al. reported postmortem findings in a patient who died of cardiogenic shock related to extensive atheroembolism of the coronary microcirculation following vein graft PTCA (84). This potential for coronary emboli is a major factor limiting intervention in older vein grafts. The frequency of this complication can be minimized by careful selection of patients, and avoiding large and eccentric vein graft lesions or thrombus-laden grafts. Once embolization has occurred, treatment is generally of a supportive nature (heparin, intravenous nitroglycerin, morphine, intraaortic balloon pumping if needed), but intragraft thrombolytic therapy may be successful in selected patients (32).

VESSEL PERFORATION

Perforation of a coronary artery or graft is a potential complication of all coronary interventions. Perforation during native vessel angioplasty has been related to guide wire penetration, inflation of a balloon catheter in a subintimal location and excessive expansion of a coronary artery during balloon inflation (85–89). This complication fortunately is exceedingly rare and in postoperative patients, the mediastinal fibrosis that is present offers some protection against free perforation. Saphenous vein graft rupture was first reported to occur during 235 vein graft procedures at Emory University Hospital (29). Prolonged balloon inflation at the site of perforation and

reversal of anticoagulation therapy was usually effective in stabilizing the limited perforation in our experience and that of others (90–92). A perfusion balloon catheter is best if technically feasible. In spite of the mediastinal scarring that is present, however, extensive hemorrhage and cardiac tamponade requiring emergency surgery and/or vein graft occlusion may occur. A fatal outcome has been reported secondary to vein graft rupture (92). Although use of oversized balloons has been encouraged with vein graft dilatation, older vein grafts may rupture with only slight balloon oversizing. In one patient, rupture occurred with a balloon:artery ratio of 1.12:1 (92). As with native vessel angioplasty, it has been our practice to size the balloon to the normal adjacent vessel and to reserve oversizing for situations where a suboptimal result occurs.

Abrupt Closure

In native vessel PTCA, abrupt closure is the most common serious complication. It occurs in 3% to 5% of patients and accounts for most of the morbidity and mortality related to the procedure. Abrupt closure is less common in saphenous vein graft angioplasty and occurred in 1.5% of 448 procedures in five reported series (24,25,27,29,30). Vein graft closure may be related to embolic phenomena, localized occlusive thrombus, or tissue flaps. Prolonged balloon inflations and thrombolytic therapy are frequently successful in restoring flow when localized occlusive thrombus formation is present. Abrupt closure related to dissection and tissue flaps may respond to prolonged inflation with a perfusion balloon or stent placement and, in the case of a very localized dissection, may be treated with directional atherectomy. If satisfactory reinstitution of flow cannot be accomplished or if an acceptable angiographic result cannot be obtained, surgical revascularization may warrant consideration. In our experience with 1,263 post-CABG patients undergoing PTCA over a 9-year period, 46 (3.6%) required reoperation during the same hospitalization (92a). Three (6.5%) died and 11 (24%) experienced nonfatal Q-wave myocardial infarction. Fifteen of the 46 patients (33%) had vein graft PTCA with or without concomitant native vessel dilatation. The survival rate at 3 years for this group of 46 patients was 91% ± 4%.

Restenosis

Recurrence of stenosis after PTCA limits application of the technique and increases morbidity and expense. The restenosis rate reported following native vessel PTCA has been in the 25% to 35% range. Overall restenosis rates reported following vein graft angioplasty are higher, but are dependent both on location of the lesion and the length of time since surgery. In our experience with 672 vein graft lesions, restenosis was noted to occur in 32% of patients dilated within 6 months of surgery, in 43% after 6 months to 1 year, in 61% after 1 to 5 years, and in 64% more than 5 years following surgery ($p <$ 0.02) (50a). Restenosis occurred in 68% of lesions at the aortosaphenous vein graft junction, 61% of mid-vein graft lesions, and 45% of lesions at the distal anastomosis. Stents, atherectomy, and excimer angioplasty have been used for treatment of vein graft lesions with reasonably good success. Restenosis rates following directional atherectomy for de novo lesions appear similar to those for balloon angioplasty, whereas directional atherectomy in restenotic lesions is associated with an even higher restenosis rate than balloon angioplasty (93). In a recent multicenter experience with excimer laser angioplasty, restenosis rates for vein graft lesions was 61% (94). More favorable results have been reported recently from the multicenter use of the Palmaz-Schatz stent in mid saphenous lesions. In 230 stents, the implantation procedural efficacy was 98%, and patient major complications were observed in 2.6% of the patients (77a). Early complications consisted of subacute thrombotic closure (1%), embolic episodes (2.1%), urgent CABG (1.6%), Q-wave myocardial infarction (1%), and in-hospital death (1.6%). On late follow-up, 1.6% of patients died suddenly (all with patent stents at autopsy) and the per site angiographic restenosis rate was 26% (n = 99). Restenosis rates were lower for de novo vein grafts (19%), compared to restenotic lesions (33%). This experience led the authors to conclude that stenting may be preferable to conventional angioplasty; however, significant complications were observed and a determination of efficacy will depend on carrying out randomized trials comparing balloon angioplasty with stents.

Restenosis following internal mammary graft PTCA is uncommon, but recatheterization has not been performed routinely in any series. Of 71 successful procedures from 14 reports in the literature, restenosis was documented in only 5 patients. This is consistent with our experience at Emory. The majority of reported patients had PTCA of the anastomosis of graft with native coronary. Very little is known about restenosis following PTCA at other IMA sites. In the largest reported series of IMA dilatations, actuarial survival at 1 and 5 years was 95% and 93%, respectively.

CONCLUSION

The growing arsenal of coronary artery interventional strategies has its broadest application in the heterogenous group of patients who have had prior bypass surgery. Many problems remain in the treatment of conduit and native vessel disease, but progress has been rapid and the future of interventional cardiology has never been brighter.

REFERENCES

1. Kolessov VI. Mammary artery-coronary artery anastomosis as method of treatment for angina pectoris. *J Thorac Cardiovasc Surg* 1967;54:535–544.
2. Favaloro RG. Saphenous vein auto graft replacement of severe segmental coronary artery occlusion: operative technique. *Ann Thorac Surg* 1968;5:334–339.
3. Campeau L, Lesperance J, Hermann J, Corbara F, Grondin CM, Bourassa MG. Loss of the improvement of angina between 1 and 7 years after aortocoronary bypass surgery. *Circulation* 1979;60 [Suppl I]:I-1–I-5.
4. Cameron A, Kemp HG, Shimomura S, Santilli E, Green GE, Hutchinson JE, et al. Aortocoronary bypass surgery, a 7-year follow-up. *Circulation* 1979;60[Suppl I]:I-9–I-13.
5. Johnson WD, Kayser KL, Pedraza PM. Angina pectoris and coronary bypass surgery. *Am Heart J* 1984;108:1190–1197.
6. Bourassa MG, Enjalbert M, Campeau L, Lesperance J. Progression of coronary artery disease between 10 and 12 years after coronary artery bypass graft surgery. In: Roskamm H, ed. *Prognosis of Coronary Heart Disease. Progression of Coronary Arteriosclerosis.* Berlin: Springer Verlag; 1983:150.
7. Frick MH, Valle M, Harjola PT. Progression of coronary artery disease in randomized medical and surgical patients over a 5-year angiographic follow-up. *Am J Cardiol* 1983;52:681.
8. Palac RT, Hwang MH, Meadows WR, Croke RP, Pifarre R, Loeb HS, Gunnar RM. Progression of coronary artery disease in medically and surgically treated patients 5 years after randomization. *Circulation* 1981;64[Suppl II]:II-17.
9. Hwang MH, Meadows WR, Palac RT, Piao ZE, Pifarre R, Loeb HS, et al. Progression of native coronary artery disease at 10 years: insights from a randomized study of medical versus surgical therapy for angina. *J Am Coll Cardiol* 1990;16:1066–1070.
10. Lawrie GM, Lie JT, Morris GC, Beazley HL. Vein graft patency and intimal proliferation after aortocoronary bypass; early and long-term angiopathologic correlations. *Am J Cardiol* 1976; 38:856.
11. Fitzgibbon GM, Burton JR, Leach AJ. Coronary bypass graft fate. Angiographic grading of 1400 consecutive grafts early after operation and of 1132 after one year. *Circulation* 1978;57:1070.
12. Hamby RI, Aintablian A, Handler M, Voleti C, Weisz D, Garvey JW, et al. Aortocoronary saphenous vein bypass grafts. Long-term patency, morphology and blood flow in patients with patent grafts early after surgery. *Circulation* 1979;60:901.
13. Bourassa MG, Enjalbert M, Campeau L, Lesperance J. Progression of atherosclerosis in coronary arteries and bypass grafts: ten years later. *Am J Cardiol* 1984;53:102C.
14. Bourassa MG, Fisher LD, Campeau L, Gillespie MJ, McConney M, Lesperance J. Long-term fate of bypass grafts: The Coronary Artery Surgery Study (CASS) and Montreal Heart Institute experiences. *Circulation* 1985;72[Suppl V]:V-71–V-78.
15. Fitzgibbon GM, Leach AJ, Kafka HP, Keon WJ. Coronary bypass graft fate: long-term angiographic study. *J Am Coll Cardiol* 1991;17:1075–1080.
16. Kirklin JW, Akins CW, Blackstone EH, Booth DC, Califf RM, Cohen LS, et al. ACC/AHA guidelines and indications for coronary artery bypass graft surgery. *Circulation* 1991;83:1125–1173.
17. Loop FD, Lytle BW, Cosgrove DM, Woods EL, Stewart RW, Golding LAR, et al. Reoperation for coronary atherosclerosis. *Ann Surg* 1990;212:378–386.
18. Hannan EL, Kilburn H, O'Donnell JF, Lukacik G, Shields EP. Adult open heart surgery in New York State. *JAMA* 1990;264:2768–2774.
19. Lytle BW, Loop FD, Cosgrove DM. Fifteen hundred coronary reoperations: results and determinants of early and late survival. *J Thorac Cardiovasc Surg* 1987;93:847–859.
20. Cameron A, Kemp HG Jr, Green GE. Reoperation for coronary artery disease: 10 years of clinical follow-up. *Circulation* 1988;78[Suppl I]:I-158–I-162.
21. Mills RM, Kalan JM. Developing a rational management strategy for angina pectoris after coronary bypass surgery: a clinical decision analysis. *Clin Cardiol* 1991;14:191–197.
22. Gruentzig AR, Senning A, Siegenthaler WE. Nonoperative dilatation of coronary-artery stenosis. Percutaneous transluminal coronary angioplasty. *N Engl J Med* 1979;301:61–68.

22a. Ford WB, Wholey MH, Zikria EA, Miller WH, Samadani SR, Koimattur AG, et al. Percutaneous transluminal angioplasty in the management of occlusive disease involving the coronary arteries and saphenous vein bypass grafts. *J Thorac Cardiovasc Surg* 1980;79:1–11.

23. Douglas JS Jr, Gruentzig AR, King SB III, Hollman J, Ischinger T, Meier B, et al. Percutaneous transluminal coronary angioplasty in patients with prior coronary bypass surgery. *J Am Coll Cardiol* 1983;2:745–754.

24. El Gamal M, Bonnier H, Michels R, Heijman J, Stassen E. Percutaneous transluminal angioplasty of stenosed aortocoronary bypass grafts. *Br Heart J* 1984;52:617–620.

25. Block PC, Cowley MJ, Kaltenback M, Kent KM, Simpson J. Percutaneous angioplasty of stenoses of bypass grafts or of bypass graft anastomotic sites. *Am J Cardiol* 1984;53:666–668.

26. Dorros G, Johnson WD, Tector AJ, Schmahl TM, Kalush S, Janke L. Percutaneous transluminal coronary angioplasty in patients with prior coronary artery bypass surgery. *J Thorac Cardiovasc Surg* 1984;87:17–26.

27. Corbelli J, Franco I, Hollman J, Simpfendorfer C, Galan K. Percutaneous transluminal coronary angioplasty after previous coronary artery bypass surgery. *Am J Cardiol* 1985;56:398–403.

28. Reeder GS, Bresnahan JF, Holmes DR Jr, Mock MB, Orszulak TA, Smith HC, Vlietstra RE. Angioplasty for aortocoronary bypass graft stenosis. *Mayo Clin Proc* 1986;61:14–19.

29. Douglas J, Robinson K, Schlumpf M. Percutaneous transluminal angioplasty in aortocoronary venous graft stenoses: immediate results and complications. *Circulation* 1986;74[Suppl II]:II-281.

30. Cote G, Myler RK, Stertzer SH, Clark DA, Fishman-Rosen J, Murphy M, Shaw RE. Percutaneous transluminal angioplasty of stenotic coronary artery bypass grafts: 5 years' experience. *J Am Coll Cardiol* 1987;9:8–17.

30a. Ernst JMPG, van der Feltz TA, Ascoop CAPL, Bal ET, Vermeulen FEE, Knaepen PJ, et al. Percutaneous transluminal coronary angioplasty in patients with prior coronary artery bypass grafting. *J Thorac Cardiovasc Surg* 1987;93:268–275.

30b. Douglas JS Jr, King SB III, Roubin GS. Percutaneous transluminal coronary angioplasty in patients with prior coronary artery bypass grafting. *J Am Coll Cardiol* 1987;93:272–275.

31. Pinkerton CA, Slack JD, Orr CM, Vantassel JW, Smith ML. Percutaneous transluminal angioplasty in patients with prior myocardial revascularization surgery. *Am J Cardiol* 1988;61:15G–22G.

32. Dorros G, Lewin RF, Mathiak LM, Johnson WD, Brenowitz J, Schmahl T, Tector A. Percutaneous transluminal coronary angioplasty in patients with two or more previous coronary artery bypass grafting operations. *Am J Cardiol* 1988;61:1243–1247.

32a. Reed DC, Beller GA, Nygaard TW, Tedesco C, Watson DD, Burwell LR. The clinical efficacy and scintigraphic evaluation of postcoronary bypass patients undergoing percutaneous transluminal coronary angioplasty for recurrent angina pectoris. *Am Heart J* 1989;117:60.

33. Cooper I, Ineson N, Demirtas E, Coltart J, Jenkins S, Webb-Peploe M. Role of angioplasty in patients with previous coronary artery bypass surgery. *Cathet Cardiovasc Diagn* 1989;16:81–86.

34. Sketch MH Jr, Perez JA, Quigley PJ, Herndon J, O'Connor CM, Tcheng JE, et al. Internal mammary artery graft angioplasty: clinical and angiographic follow-up. *J Am Coll Cardiol* 1989;13:221.

35. Stullman WS, Hilliard K. Unrecognized internal mammary artery stenosis treated by percutaneous angioplasty after coronary bypass surgery. *Am Heart J* 1987;113:393–395.

36. Vivekaphirat V, Yellen SF, Foschi A. Percutaneous transluminal angioplasty of a stenosis at the origin of the left internal mammary artery graft: a case report. *Cathet Cardiovasc Diagn* 1988;15:176–178.

37. Zaidi AR, Hollman JL. Percutaneous angioplasty of internal mammary artery graft stenosis: case report and discussion. *Cathet Cardiovasc Diagn* 1985;11:603–608.

38. Crean PA, Mathieson PW, Richards AF. Transluminal angioplasty of a stenosis of an internal mammary artery graft. *Br Heart J* 1986;56:473–475.

39. Dorros G, Lewin RF. The brachial artery method to transluminal internal mammary artery angioplasty. *Cathet Cardiovasc Diagn* 1986;12:341–346.

40. Steffenino G, Meier B, Finci L, von Segesser L, Velebit V. Percutaneous transluminal angioplasty of right and left internal mammary artery grafts. *Chest* 1986;90:849–851.

41. Salinger M, Drummer E, Furey K, Bott-Silverman C, Franco I. Percutaneous angioplasty of internal mammary artery graft stenosis using the brachial approach: a case report. *Cathet Cardiovasc Diagn* 1986;12:261–265.

42. Singh S. Coronary angioplasty of internal mammary artery graft. *Am J Med* 1987;82:361–362.

43. Hill DM, McAuley BJ, Sheehan DJ, Simpson JB, Selmon MR, Anderson ET. Percutaneous transluminal angioplasty of internal mammary artery bypass grafts. *J Am Coll Cardiol* 1989;13:221A.

44. Pinkerton CA, Slack JD, Orr CM, VanTassel JW. Percutaneous transluminal angioplasty involving internal mammary artery bypass grafts: a femoral approach. *Cathet Cardiovasc Diagn* 1987;13:414–418.

45. Douglas J, King S, Roubin G, Schlumpf M. Percutaneous angioplasty of venous aortocoronary graft stenosis: late angiographic and clinical outcome. *Circulation* 1986;74[Suppl II]:II-281.

46. Kereiakes DJ, George B, Stertzer SH, Myler RK. Percutaneous transluminal angioplasty of left internal mammary artery grafts. *Am J Cardiol* 1984;55:1215–1216.

47. Shimshak TM, Giorgi LV, Johnson WL, McConahay DR, Rutherford BD, Ligon R, et al. Application of percutaneous transluminal coronary angioplasty to the internal mammary artery graft. *J Am Coll Cardiol* 1988;12:1205–1214.

48. Kussmaul WG. Percutaneous angioplasty of coronary bypass grafts: an emerging consensus. *Cathet Cardiovasc Diagn* 1988;15:1–4.

49. Platko WP, Hollman J, Whitlow PL, Franco I. Percutaneous transluminal angioplasty of saphenous vein graft stenosis: long-term follow-up. *J Am Coll Cardiol* 1989;7:1645–1650.

50. Plokker HW, Meester BH, Serruys PW. The Dutch experience in percutaneous transluminal angioplasty of narrowed saphenous veins used for aortocoronary arterial bypass. *Am J Cardiol* 1991;67:361–366.

50a. Douglas JS Jr, Weintraub WS, Liberman HA, Jenkins M, Cohen CL, Morris DC, et al. Update of saphenous graft (SVG) angioplasty: restenosis and long term outcome. *Circulation* 1991;84 [Suppl II]:II-249.

51. Loop FD, Whitlow PL. Coronary angioplasty in patients with previous bypass surgery. *J Am Coll Cardiol* 1990;16:1348–1350.

51a. Webb JG, Myler RK, Shaw RE, Anwar A, Mayo JR, Murphy MC, et al. Coronary angioplasty after coronary bypass surgery: initial results and late outcome in 422 patients. *J Am Coll Cardiol* 1990;16:812–820.

51b. Reeves F, Bonan R, Cote G, Crepeau J, deGuise P, Gosselin G, et al. Long-term angiographic follow-up after angioplasty of venous coronary bypass grafts. *Am Heart J* 1991;122:620–627.

52. Ryan TJ, Faxon DP, Gunnar RM, Kennedy JW, King SB III, Loop FD et al. Guidelines for percutaneous transluminal coronary angioplasty. *J Am Coll Cardiol* 1988;12:529–545.

53. Campeau L, Lesperance J, Bourassa MG. Natural history of saphenous vein aortocoronary bypass grafts. *Mod Concepts Cardiovasc Dis* 1984;53:59–63.

54. Goldman S, Copeland J, Moritz T, Henderson W, Zadina K, Ovitt T, et al. Improvement in early saphenous vein graft patency after coronary artery bypass surgery with antiplatelet therapy: results of a Veterans Administration Cooperative Study. *Circulation* 1988;77:1324–1332.

54a. Bourassa MG. Fate of venous grafts: the past, the present and the future. *J Am Coll Cardiol* 1991;17:1081–1083.

55. Goldman S, Copeland J, Moritz T, Henderson W, Zadina K, Ovitt T, et al. Saphenous vein graft patency 1 year after coronary artery bypass surgery and effects antiplatelet therapy. *Circulation* 1989;80:1190–1199.

56. Kahn JK, Rutherford BD, McConahay DR, Giorgi LV, Johnson WL, Shimshak TM, et al. Early post-operative balloon coronary angioplasty for failed coronary artery bypass grafting. *Am J Cardiol* 1990;66:943–946.

57. Kuntz RE, Piana R, Schnitt SJ, Johnson RG, Safian RD, Baim DS. Early ostial vein graft stenosis: management by atherectomy. *Cathet Cardiovasc Diagn* 1991;24:41–44.

57a. Robertson GC, Simpson JB, Vetter JW, Selmon MR, Doucette JW, Sheehan DJ, et al. Directional coronary atherectomy for ostial lesions. *Circulation* 1991;84[Suppl II]:II-251.

57b. Eigler NL, Douglas JS Jr, Margolis JR, Hestrin L, Litvack FI. Excimer laser coronary angioplasty of arto-ostial stenosis: results of the ELCA Registry. *Circulation* 1991;84[Suppl II]:II-251.

57c. Teirstein P, Stratienko AA, Schatz RA. Coronary stenting for ostial stenoses: initial results and six month follow-up. *Circulation* 1991;84[Suppl II]:II-250.

58. Liu MW, Douglas JS Jr, King SB III, et al. Angiographic predictors of coronary embolization in the PTCA of vein graft lesions. *Circulation* 1989;80[Suppl II]:II-172.

59. de Feyter PJ, Serruys P, van den Brand M, Meester H, Beatt K, Suryapranata H. Percutaneous transluminal angioplasty of a totally occluded bypass graft: a challenge that should be resisted. *Am J Cardiol* 1989;64:88–90.

60. Frumin H, Goldberg M, Rubenfire M, Levine F. Late thrombolysis of an occluded aortocoronary saphenous vein graft. *Am Heart J* 1983;106:401–403.

61. Hartmann J, McKeever L, Teran J, Bufalino V, Marek J, Brown A, et al. Prolonged infusion of urokinase for recanalization of chronically occluded aortocoronary bypass grafts. *Am J Cardiol* 1988;61:189–191.

62. Marx M, Armstrong W, Brent B, Wack J, Bernstein R, Gregoratos G. Transcatheter recanalization of a chronically occluded saphenous aortocoronary bypass graft. *AJR Am J Roentgenol* 1987;148:375–377.

63. Hartmann JR, McKeever LS, Stamato NJ, Bufalino VJ, Marek JC, Brown AS, et al. Recanalization of chronically occluded aortocoronary saphenous vein bypass grafts by extended infusion of urokinase: initial results and short-term clinical follow-up. *J Am Coll Cardiol* 1991;18:1517–1523.

64. Gurley JC, MacPhail BS. Acute myocardial infarction due to thrombolytic reperfusion of chronically occluded saphenous vein coronary bypass grafts. *Am J Cardiol* 1991;68:274–275.

65. McKeever LS, Hartmann JR, Bufalino VJ, Marek JC, Brown AS, Goodwin MJ, et al. Acute myocardial infarction complicating recanalization of aortocoronary bypass grafts with urokinase therapy. *Am J Cardiol* 1989;64:683–685.

66. Coronary Artery Surgery Study (CASS) and their associates. A random trial of coronary artery bypass. Quality of life in patients randomly assigned to treatment groups. *Circulation* 1983;68:951–956.

67. Maynard C, Weaver WD, Litwin P, et al. Acute myocardial infarction and prior coronary artery surgery in the myocardial infarction triage and intervention registry: patient characteristics, treatment, and outcome. *Coronary Artery Dis* 1991;2:443–448.

68. Wiseman A, Waters DD, Walling A, et al. Long-term prognosis after myocardial infarction in patients with previous coronary artery bypass surgery. *J Am Coll Cardiol* 1988;12:873–880.

69. Little WC, Gwinn NS, Burrows MT, Kutcher MA, Kahl FR, Applegate RJ. Cause of acute myocardial infarction late after successful coronary artery bypass grafting. *Am J Cardiol* 1990;65:808–810.

70. Grines CL, Booth DC, Nissen SE, Gurley JC, Bennett KA, O'Connor WN, et al. Mechanism of acute myocardial infarction in patients with prior coronary artery bypass grafting and therapeutic implications. *Am J Cardiol* 1990;65:1292–1296.

71. Kavanaugh KM, Topol EJ. Acute intervention during myocardial infarction in patients with prior coronary bypass surgery. *Am J Cardiol* 1990;65:924–926.

72. Kleiman NS, Berman DA, Gaston WR, Cashion WR, Roberts R. Early intravenous thrombolytic therapy for acute myocardial infarction in patients with prior coronary artery bypass grafts. *Am J Cardiol* 1989;63:102–104.

73. Kahn JK, Rutherford BD, McConahay DR, Johnson W, Giorgi LV, Ligon R, et al. Usefulness of angioplasty during acute myocardial infarction in patients with prior coronary artery bypass grafting. *Am J Cardiol* 1990;65:698–702.

74. Gunnar RM, Bourdillon PD, Dixon DW, Fuster V, Karp RB, Kennedy JW, et al. Guidelines for the early management of patients with acute myocardial infarction. *J Am Coll Cardiol* 1990;16:249–292.

75. Pepine CJ, Allen HD, Bashore TM, Brinker JA, Cohn LH, Dillon JC, et al. ACC/AHA guidelines for cardiac catheterization and cardiac catheterization laboratories. *Circulation* 1991;84:2214–2244.

76. Douglas JS Jr, King SB III, Roubin GS. Technique of percutaneous transluminal angioplasty of the coronary, renal mesenteric, and peripheral arteries. In: Hurst JW, Schlant RC, Rackley CE, Sonnenblick EH, Wenger NK, eds. *The Heart*. 7th ed. New York: McGraw-Hill; 1990:2131–2156.

77. Kahn JK, Hartzler GO: Retrograde coronary angioplasty of isolated arterial segments through saphenous vein bypass grafts. *Cathet Cardiovasc Diagn* 1990;20:88–93.

77a. Leon MB, Ellis SG, Pichard AD, Baim DS, Heuser RR, Schatz RA. Stents may be the preferred treatment for focal aortocoronary vein graft disease. *Circulation* 1991;84[Suppl II]:II-249.

78. Bajaj RK, Roubin GS. Intravascular stenting of the right internal mammary artery. *Cathet Cardiovasc Diagn* 1991;24:252–255.

79. Almagor Y, Thomas J, Colombo A. Balloon expandable stent implantation of a stenosis at the origin of the left internal mammary artery graft. *Cathet Cardiovasc Diagn* 1991;24:256–258.

79a. Brown RIG, Galligan L, Penn IM, Weinstein L. Right internal mammary artery graft angioplasty through a right brachial artery approach using a new custom guide catheter: a case report. *Cathet Cardiovasc Diagn* 1992;25:42–45.

80. Shapira S, Braun S, Puram B, Patel G, Rotman H. Percutaneous transluminal angioplasty of proximal subclavian artery stenosis after left internal mammary to left anterior descending artery bypass surgery. *J Am Coll Cardiol* 1991;18:1120–1123.

81. Ernst S, Bal E, Plokker T, Mast G, Tjon M, Ascoop C. Percutaneous balloon angioplasty (PBA) of a left subclavian artery stenosis or occlusion to establish adequate flow through the left internal mammary artery for coronary bypass purposes. *Circulation* 1991;84[Suppl II]:II-591.

82. Miller RM, Knox M. Patient tolerance of ioxaglate and iopamidol in internal mammary artery arteriography. *Cathet Cardiovasc Diagn* 1992;25:31–34.

83. MacDonald RG, Feldman RL, Conti CR, Pepine CJ. Thromboembolic complications of coronary angioplasty. *Am J Cardiol* 1984;54:916–917.

84. Saber RS, Edwards WD, Holmes DR Jr, Vlieststra RE, Reeder GS. Balloon angioplasty of aortocoronary saphenous vein bypass grafts: a histopathologic study of six grafts from five patients, with emphasis on restenosis and embolic complications. *J Am Coll Cardiol* 1988;12:1501–1509.

85. Saffitz JE, Rose TE, Oaks JB, Roberts WC. Coronary arterial rupture during coronary angioplasty. *Am J Cardiol* 1983;51:902–904.

86. Meier B. Benign coronary perforation during percutaneous transluminal coronary angioplasty. *Br Heart J* 1985;54:33–35.

87. Altman F, Yazdanfar S, Wertheimer J, Ghosh S, Kotler M. Cardiac tamponade following perforation of the left anterior descending coronary system during percutaneous transluminal coronary angioplasty: successful treatment by pericardial drainage. *Am Heart J* 1986;111:1196–1197.

88. Kimbiris D, Iskandrian AS, Goel I, Val PG, Fines P, Robert P, et al. Transluminal coronary angioplasty complicated by coronary artery perforation. *Cathet Cardiovasc Diagn* 1982;8:481–487.

89. Grollier G, Bories H, Commeau P, Foucault J, Potier J. Coronary artery perforation during coronary angioplasty. *Clin Cardiol* 1986;9:27–29.

90. Drummer E, Furey K, Hollman J. Rupture of a saphenous vein bypass graft during coronary angioplasty. *Br Heart J* 1987;58:78–81.

91. Teirstein PS, Hartzler GO. Nonoperative management of aortocoronary saphenous vein graft rupture during percutaneous transluminal coronary angioplasty. *Am J Cardiol* 1987;60:377–378.

92. Namay DL, Roubin GS, Tommaso CL, Warren SG, Douglas JS Jr, King SB III. Saphenous vein graft rupture during percutaneous transluminal angioplasty. *Cathet Cardiovasc Diagn* 1988;14:258–262.

92a. Weintraub WS, Cohen CL, Curling PE, Jones EL, Craver JM, Guyton R, et al. Results of coronary surgery after failed elective coronary angioplasty in patients with prior coronary surgery. *J Am Coll Cardiol* 1990;16:1341–1347.

93. Ghazzal ZMB, Douglas JS Jr, Holmes DR, Ellis SG, Keriakes DJ, Simpson JB, et al. Directional coronary atherectomy of saphenous vein grafts: recent multicenter experience. *J Am Coll Cardiol* 1991;17:219A.

94. Untereker WJ, Litvack F, Margolis JR, Roubin GS, Hartzler GO, White RH, et al. Excimer laser coronary angioplasty of saphenous vein grafts. *Circulation* 1991;84[Suppl II]:II-249.

95. Shimshak TM, Rutherford BD, McConahay DR, Giorgi LV, Johnson WL, Ligon RW. PTCA of internal mammary artery (IMA) grafts—procedural results and late follow-up. *Circulation* 1991;84[Suppl II]:II-590.

Practical Angioplasty,
edited by David P. Faxon.
Raven Press, Ltd., New York © 1993.

CHAPTER 12

Coronary Angioplasty Strategies for the Treatment of Acute Myocardial Infarction

Joseph M. Sutton and Eric J. Topol

The fundamental observation that occlusive coronary artery lesions associated with the onset of acute myocardial infarction are initiated by rupture or fissuring of a stationary atheromatous plaque underlying the intimal layer of the coronary vessel, with subsequent hemorrhage and thrombosis (1–3), has been the impetus for interventional strategies directed at both the intraluminal thrombus and the acutely altered geometry of the underlying lesion. Following the onset of acute myocardial infarction, percutaneous transluminal coronary angioplasty (PTCA) has been used for direct recanalization of the infarct vessel, as an empiric early or deferred strategy for the treatment of residual postthrombolytic lesions, as a fallback procedure for failed reperfusion after administration of a thrombolytic agent, and as an elective strategy reserved for the treatment of demonstrable ischemia after uncomplicated myocardial infarction.

While timely administration of a thrombolytic agent for acute myocardial infarction has unequivocally improved survival, recurrent ischemia and reinfarction are more prevalent in this population, compared with patients receiving a standard medical regimen (4,5). Interventional strategies employing empiric, immediate PTCA for prophylaxis against recurrent ischemia have consistently demonstrated little benefit in the absence of hemodynamic compromise, compared with an empiric, deferred approach (6–10). Among select patients with clinically uncomplicated myocardial infarction, an elective PTCA strategy limited to the treatment of further, spontaneous or provokable ischemia attributable to the residual postthrombolytic infarct stenosis has been as clinically successful as an empiric deferred PTCA approach, suggesting that adjunct mechanical intervention

more than 24 to 48 hr after the onset of acute myocardial infarction is not necessarily mandated (11,12). The necessity of early angiography after the initial commitment to an interventional strategy remains a controversial and unresolved issue, especially when the postthrombolytic clinical course remains uncomplicated (Table 1).

Reviewed here are results of the major clinical trials evaluating the role of coronary angioplasty in the treatment of acute coronary artery occlusion, the optimal timing and overall usefulness of the various interventional strategies, and technical considerations regarding invasive management in the catheterization laboratory during the acute phase of evolving myocardial infarction.

CORONARY ANGIOPLASTY STRATEGIES FOR ACUTE MYOCARDIAL INFARCTION

Direct (Primary) PTCA

Direct recanalization of the infarct coronary artery by mechanical rather than chemical means simultaneously addresses both the occlusive thrombus and underlying stenosis, and is associated with a superior early patency rate of nearly 90%, with few related complications (Table 2) (13–21). Despite these inherent benefits, direct PTCA remains a practical therapeutic option in a minority of facilities where continuous access to an operating catheterization laboratory is available (22). This interventional strategy is available only to patients presenting to hospitals where committed, on-call catheterization and emergency surgical backup teams are available, or to institutions where expeditious transfer to such a facility is feasible.

There have been no large, controlled clinical trials directly comparing intravenous thrombolysis with direct

J. M. Sutton and E. J. Topol: Department of Cardiology, The Cleveland Clinic Foundation, Cleveland, Ohio

TABLE 1. *Overview of coronary angioplasty strategies for acute myocardial infarction*

Strategy	Timing	Advantage	Disadvantage
Direct PTCA	As soon as possible	Avoidance of thrombolytic state High patency rate (nearly 90%) Improved regional wall motion	No randomized trials with IV thrombolysis Requires interventional facilities and personnel Increased risk of abrupt closure (3–14%)
Immediate empiric PTCA	As soon as possible	Improved survival in cardiogenic shock patients compared with failed thrombolysis or successful thrombolysis alone	Trend toward higher mortality rate Higher risk of emergency bypass surgery compared with deferred PTCA No improvement in resting LVEF compared with deferred strategy
Deferred empiric PTCA	1–7 days	Less recurrent ischemia and reinfarction compared with no PTCA	Risk of emergency bypass surgery (3–5%) No improvement of resting LVEF compared with elective PTCA
Elective PTCA	After 7 days	Addresses proven ischemia Possible avoidance of procedure in patients without residual ischemia	Risk of emergency bypass surgery (3–5%) Other potential benefits of open artery lost if no PTCA High-risk anatomy may be missed if no angiogram
Rescue PTCA	60–120 min	Potential myocardial salvage despite thrombolytic failure Improved regional wall motion compared with no PTCA	Requires acute interventional facilities and personnel No large, randomized clinical trials

PTCA, percutaneous transluminal coronary angioplasty; LVEF, left ventricular ejection fraction; IV, intravenous.

PTCA, but a consensus of results may be derived from cumulative experience. This strategy is associated with a 3% to 5% referral for emergency bypass surgery, similar to that observed when empiric, immediate PTCA is performed after successful thrombolysis, which may be partially influenced by the early definition of the underlying coronary disease. In addition to referrals for surgery after acute vessel closure has complicated direct PTCA, patients with underlying severe multivessel disease, left main artery disease or its equivalent, or mechanical complications of acute infarction defined at catheterization (such as ventricular septal defect or papillary muscle necrosis with acute mitral insufficiency) may be identified and triaged to urgent or emergency surgery. Nonetheless, early infarct vessel reocclusion may occur in as many as 9% to 14% of patients undergoing direct PTCA. This occurrence is substantially higher than the reocclusion rates associated with immediate PTCA following successful thrombolysis, and may relate to the unstable thrombogenic and platelet aggregatory milieu present after acute plaque rupture. The ongoing Primary Angioplasty in Myocardial Infarction (PAMI) trial will ran-

TABLE 2. *Direct coronary angioplasty trials*

Study (reference)	n	Successful PTCA (%)	Early mortality (%)	Emergency CABG (%)	Early reocclusion (%)	Late reocclusion (%)
Holmes et al. (13)	11	91	0	0	0	NR
Linnemeier et al. (14)	31	87	NR	0	NR	NR
Hartzler et al. (15)	222	91	7.0	3.6	10	NR
O'Neill et al. (16)	29	85	7.0	0	3.6	NR
Topol et al. (17)	47	86	6.3	0	3	13
Rothbaum et al. (18)	75	89	6.3	2.6	NR	17
Kimura et al. (19)	58	88	NR	NR	14	2
Sriram et al. (20)	8	87	0	0	0	0
Kahn et al. (21)	250	95	1.0	1.2	NR	9

n, number of patients; NR, not reported; PTCA, percutaneous transluminal coronary angioplasty; CABG, coronary artery bypass graft surgery.

dom a projected 400 patients with acute myocardial infarction to treatment with either direct angioplasty or intravenous tissue-type plasminogen activator (t-PA). The forthcoming analysis will prospectively compare the combined mortality and recurrent ischemia rates associated with each strategy, as well as provide a comparative assessment of left ventricular function, bleeding complications, and cost differences. The direct PTCA approach in this trial has been associated with a similar 85% early success rate among the subset of patients over 70 years old who are currently enrolled.

The clinical outcome of direct PTCA may be influenced by characteristics of the infarct vessel targeted. The procedure may be less successful when the left circumflex artery is targeted, where a 6% to 8% lower success rate is reported, compared with treatment of the left anterior descending or right coronary artery infarct vessels (21). Further, significantly higher incidences of paroxysmal bradycardia and hypotension have been observed at the time of recanalization of the right coronary artery by direct angioplasty, possibly due to the vagus-mediated Bezhold-Jarisch reflex (21,23). Overall intraprocedural events, including death, malignant arrhythmias, cardiogenic shock, and referral for emergency bypass surgery, are more common in the absence of baseline antegrade flow. Kahn and colleagues reported a 29% intraprocedural rate of these events when the baseline flow was Thrombolysis In Myocardial Infarction (TIMI) grade 0 or 1, compared with a lower incidence of 2% when the baseline flow was TIMI grade 2 or 3 ($p < 0.001$) (21). This observation may relate to the excess burden of thrombus present at the time of the intervention, when treating total or subtotal occlusions. Substantially more thrombus associated with persistent total or subtotal occlusion, compared with spontaneous restoration of flow attributable to autothrombolysis.

Direct PTCA continues to have merit as an alternative to thrombolytic therapy in certain subsets of patients, particularly those patients with a contraindication to thrombolytic therapy, such as recent trauma, surgery, or stroke. Further, patients who can be taken to the catheterization laboratory very early after the onset of symptoms, for example, hospitalized patients developing acute myocardial infarction while the catheterization laboratory is operational, may benefit from direct PTCA, avoiding the inherent delay of preparation and initiation of thrombolytic drug infusions, and affording a superior (approximately 90%) early patency rate within a minimum of 75 to 90 min after triage to direct angioplasty (16). For a majority of patients, however, such timely transfer to a catheterization laboratory is not possible, and more rapid recanalization has been achieved with prompt initiation of thrombolytic therapy, with 70% to 80% of patients experiencing reperfusion within 60 to 90 min of treatment with t-PA (22,24–27).

Finally, the direct angioplasty approach may be bene-ficial for patients in whom the diagnosis of acute infarction is ambiguous because of a vague history or patients who show the presence of baseline electrocardiographic abnormalities such as left bundle branch block, left ventricular hypertrophy, or previous myocardial infarction (Fig. 1). The diagnosis can be readily established at angiography, and prompt intervention may be initiated thereafter, while unnecessary thrombolytic therapy and its associated risks can be avoided if a diagnosis of acute myocardial infarction is excluded.

Empiric (Immediate and Deferred) PTCA

After successful thrombolysis, a substantial ($\geq 70\%$) residual stenosis persists in a majority of patients at early angiography (28–30), and in patients undergoing subse-

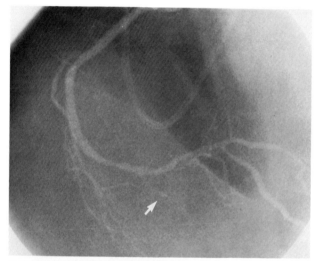

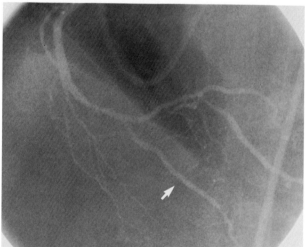

FIG. 1. Direct coronary angioplasty. A 66-year-old man with prior lateral wall myocardial infarction underwent cardiac catheterization for evaluation of 3 hr of continuous substernal pressure, without diagnostic electrocardiographic changes. Acute posterior wall infarction was diagnosed after definition of an occluded right posterior descending artery with persistent contrast staining and an angiographic filling defect. Results after primary or direct angioplasty are demonstrated.

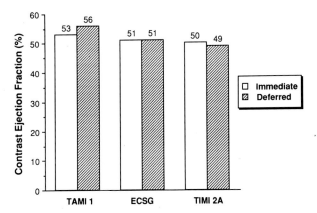

FIG. 2. Randomized trials of immediate versus deferred angioplasty. No differences in global left ventricular function at the time of hospital discharge were observed when patients were randomized to empirical adjunct therapy with either immediate or deferred angioplasty in the Thrombolysis and Angioplasty in Myocardial Infarction (TAMI) trial, the European Cooperative Study Group (ECSG) trial, or phase 2A of the Thrombolysis in Myocardial Infarction (TIMI-2A) study.

quent serial angiography, a limited 15% improvement in this residual stenosis has been noted after 7 to 10 days (26). Empiric balloon dilatation of the postthrombolytic residual stenosis for prophylaxis against recurrent ischemia or reinfarction is a nonselective strategy designed to address the overall higher group incidence of recurrent ischemia and reinfarction observed after thrombolytic intervention, compared with standard medical therapy (4,5). The optimal timing of empiric PTCA after successful thrombolytic therapy for acute myocardial infarction has been assessed in several large clinical trials to date, and no significant advantage in mortality or global left ventricular function has been defined when comparing an immediate with a deferred strategy (Fig. 2) (8,10,26,31).

Immediate angioplasty is a strategy of empiric angioplasty as soon as successful thrombolysis can be confirmed at early angiography, while a deferred angioplasty strategy has been applied empirically from 18 hr to 7 days after thrombolysis (Table 3). In phase 1 of the Thrombolysis and Angioplasty in Myocardial Infarction (TAMI-1) study (26), patients were randomly assigned to undergo immediate PTCA after 90-min angiographic assessment (99 patients), or deferred PTCA (98 patients) 7 days later. The study found no significant differences between the two cohorts with respect to procedural success rate (90% immediate; 98% deferred), early reocclusion (11% immediate; 13% deferred), or global left ventricular ejection fraction (LVEF) (52% immediate; 55% deferred). Further, late analysis revealed a similar degree of left ventricular recovery, with a mean increment in LVEF of 1.1% for the immediate group, and 1.3% for the deferred cohort.

TABLE 3. Immediate versus delayed angioplasty trials

	TAMI-1	TIMI-2 Pilot	TIMI-2A	ECSG
Patients (n)	197	286	389	367
t-PA therapy				
Time to treatment (hr)	2.9	2.7	2.9	2.6
t-PA dose (mg)	150	150	100, 150[a]	150
Reperfusion successful (%)	75.0	85.5	78.5	89.0
PTCA therapy				
Immediate PTCA				
Patients (n)	99	33	137[c]	183
Timing after t-PA (hr)	1–1.5	2.0	2.0	0.1–2.8
LVEF (%)				
Early	52.0	NR	NR	NR
Late	53.2	NR	50.0	51.0
Reocclusion (%)	11.0	8.0	NR	12.5
Mortality (%)	4.0	9.1	3.6	7.0
Delayed PTCA				
Patients (n)	98	128[d]	102[e]	184
Timing after t-PA	7–10 days	18–48 hr	18–48 hr	18–48 hr
LVEF (%)				
Early	55.0	NR	NR	NR
Late	56.4	NR	49.0	51.0
Reocclusion (%)	13.0	14.0	NR	11.0
Mortality (%)	1.0	6.3	5.9	3.0

NR, not reported; PTCA, percutaneous transluminal coronary angioplasty; LVEF, left ventricular ejection fraction; t-PA, tissue-type plasminogen activator.

[a] The first third of patients received 150 mg; the last two-thirds received 100 mg t-PA.

[b] Patient numbers are expressed in terms of those actually undergoing PTCA.

[c] 70% of 195 patients randomized.

[d] 58% of 220 patients randomized.

[e] 53% of 194 patients randomized.

There were several disadvantages associated with the empiric, immediate PTCA strategy in this study. First, the deferred approach allowed additional time for late thrombolysis beyond the 90-min time of randomization, and an additional 15% of patients were found to have minimal residual disease 7 days later, a finding which eliminating the need for the procedure and its inherent risks (Fig. 3). Second, although coronary artery bypass referral rates were similar (14.7% immediate; 15.5% deferred), emergency bypass surgery was required more often after immediate PTCA, often precluding the careful dissection necessary for optimal internal mammary artery grafting.

Finally, there was a higher, although not statistically significant, mortality rate for the immediate (4%) versus the deferred strategy (1%). The trend in higher mortality among patients subjected to immediate PTCA was also observed in the TIMI-2 pilot trial (8) and the subsequent TIMI-2A trial (31); however, only the European Cooperative Study Group (ECSG) trial found a statistically significant difference, perhaps because of the unprecedented adherence to the randomized intended treatment (10).

Unlike the TAMI-1 trial, both the ECSG and the TIMI groups randomized patients to either immediate or deferred PTCA without prior definition of the underlying residual coronary anatomy. The ECSG randomized 183 patients to immediate PTCA, and an impressive majority (93%) of those patients underwent the intended procedure. This is in contrast to the 68% of randomized patients who actually underwent immediate PTCA in the TAMI-1 trial, and the limited 70% adherence to the intended immediate PTCA strategy in the TIMI-2A study. Overall, only 52% of all patients randomized to immediate PTCA in both the TAMI-1 and

TIMI-2A trials actually underwent the procedure, after allowing for exclusion from the intended therapy. This relatively selective adherence to the intended therapy may have limited the impact of the immediate PTCA strategy on mortality.

In the TIMI-2 pilot study, 33 patients were randomly assigned to undergo immediate PTCA 1 hr after thrombolytic therapy, while a substantially larger group of 253 patients underwent empiric deferred PTCA 18 and 48 hr after initiating therapy (8). Although only 58% of the deferred PTCA cohort (128 of 253 patients) actually underwent the planned procedure, a slightly higher mortality rate was found among the smaller group of patients undergoing immediate PTCA (9.1%), compared with the 6.3% mortality rate observed among patients in the deferred group. These data were subsequently supported by the more equitable TIMI-2A trial. In this trial, 195 postthrombolytic patients were randomly assigned to undergo immediate PTCA within 2 hr of therapy, while 194 patients were randomized to deferred PTCA between 18 and 48 hr after enrollment. Again, mortality was higher among patients randomized to undergo PTCA within 2 hr (7.2%; 14 of 195 patients), than among patients assigned to the deferred strategy at 18 to 48 hr (5.7%; 11 of 194 patients). Of note, only 70% of randomized patients underwent immediate PTCA, while 53% of patients in the deferred cohort actually underwent the intended subsequent intervention.

A common pitfall of the large, clinical trails is the discrepancy between randomized treatment intent and actual treatment rendered (Fig. 4). While there were 14 deaths in the TIMI-2A immediate PTCA cohort, only 5 of these 14 patients (36%) actually underwent the intended procedure, while 6 of the 11 patients who died in the deferred PTCA group (55%) actually underwent the

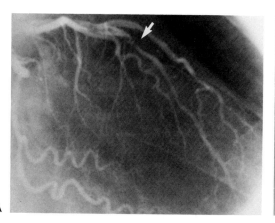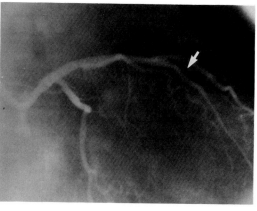

A   B

FIG. 3. (A) Residual stenosis improvement. After intravenous thrombolytic therapy for acute anterior wall myocardial infarction, this 49-year-old woman was found to have a patent infarct vessel, with a complex lesion within the mid left anterior descending artery and brisk antegrade flow. Her chest pain had resolved, although there was persistent ST-segment elevation in the anterior precordial electrocardiographic leads. **(B)** Follow-up angiogram after 5 days of conservative management and continuous heparin infusion shows resolution of the intraluminal filling defect, with a persistent disruption of the intima at the site of a minimal stenosis (arrow). Subsequent exercise stress testing demonstrated no provokable ischemia.

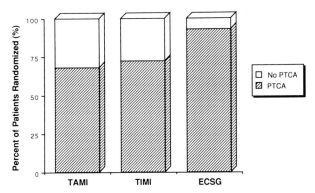

FIG. 4. Randomized intention to treat with immediate angioplasty. Adherence to the intended treatment strategy was possible in 68% of patients randomized to immediate angioplasty in the Thrombolysis and Angioplasty in Myocardial Infarction (TAMI) trial among 70% of patients in phase 2A of the Thrombolysis in Myocardial Infarction (TIMI-2A) study. In the European Cooperative Study Group (ECSG) trial, an unprecedented 93% of those patients randomized to an immediate angioplasty strategy actually underwent the intended procedure, despite treatment commitment prior to definition of the coronary anatomy, with a mortality rate that reached statistical significance with this strategy compared with a deferred approach.

planned angioplasty; two of the deaths occurred in patients undergoing emergency PTCA beyond the study protocol. Thus, 56% (14 of the total 25) of the reported early deaths occurred in patients who did not undergo angioplasty at any time during the trial, regardless of the initial randomization to immediate or deferred treatment intention. The efficacy assessment of a treatment strategy may vary substantially from an intent-to-treat analysis when the randomized intended protocol is adhered to in a limited manner with liberal allowance for crossover to the alternate strategy.

Despite the higher mortality rate and more frequent referral for emergency coronary bypass surgery compared with a deferred strategy, immediate PTCA may improve the prognosis of patients presenting with cardiogenic shock despite successful thrombolysis. Cardiogenic shock continues to have an associated 78% to 85% mortality rate (32), although this may improve following acute recanalization of the coronary infarct vessel (33). Cumulative data from the Intracoronary Streptokinase Registry demonstrate an associated lower mortality rate (42% mortality) after successful thrombolytic therapy in patients with cardiogenic shock, compared with failed reperfusion (84% mortality) (34).

Comparable results have not been achieved after administration of intravenous thrombolytic therapy alone. In the large GISSI (4) trial, no significant reduction in mortality among patients with cardiogenic shock was demonstrated after intravenous streptokinase (4,5). This may be due to delayed peak activity at the targeted thrombus site when this agent is administered by the intravenous route, or to a decrease in local delivery of the drug to the thrombus site, as a result of circulatory collapse, compared with the direct local administration of the drug by an intracoronary route. Another possible explanation for this response discrepancy is that mechanical perforation of the thrombus with a guidewire was reported in many cases included in the intracoronary streptokinase registry (34). In patients with sustained cardiogenic shock after intravenous thrombolytic therapy, Lee and colleagues (33) reported a 75% mortality rate associated with unsuccessful reperfusion. After successful adjunct PTCA, mortality was reduced to 17% in this subset of patients, and improved survival rates with fewer heart failure symptoms and related arrhythmic events have been observed after 2- to 4.5-year follow-up (35).

Since there is an established trend toward higher mortality, more frequent coronary artery bypass surgery referral, and lack of any demonstrable influence on global left ventricular function, the only current indication for immediate PTCA is the treatment of persistent cardiogenic shock. Deferred PTCA, with a delay of several days before adjunct mechanical intervention, provides a more favorable environment for an uncomplicated procedure. This benefit is likely attributable to the resolution of the acute thrombogenic milieu at the target lesion encountered during the acute phase of myocardial infarction.

Elective PTCA

Deferred PTCA is a nonselective, empiric strategy of adjunct mechanical treatment of the late residual stenosis following successful thrombolytic therapy. The selective triage of postthrombolytic patients to delayed adjunct PTCA only for the treatment of subsequent spontaneous or provokable ischemia is an elective PTCA strategy aimed at demonstrable residual physiological ischemia, rather than at the anatomical lesion itself.

In the Johns Hopkins trial of deferred versus elective PTCA, 85 patients received either intravenous t-PA or placebo (36). Patients with suitable coronary anatomy were randomly assigned to undergo empiric, deferred PTCA on the third day after medical treatment, or to await further intervention until after the conclusion of the 10-day study. Gated blood pool analysis revealed no significant differences in improvement of resting left ventricular ejection fraction by the end of the study, with a mean improvement of 1.1% in the deferred PTCA group and 1.9% among patients in the elective group, when the values were compared with baseline studies obtained upon patient enrollment. However, these investigators reported a lower rate of recurrent ischemia and reinfarction after deferred PTCA (5%) compared with the conservatively managed group (19%); two of the patients (5%) awaiting an elective procedure underwent emergency

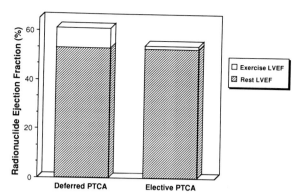

FIG. 5. Deferred versus elective angioplasty. More ischemia was noted with medical management and postponement of angioplasty in the Johns Hopkins trial, compared with a deferred, empiric angioplasty strategy. Radionuclide left ventricular ejection improved by 8.1% with exercise after deferred angioplasty, compared with a 1.2% augmentation of global left ventricular ejection fraction following conservative management.

PTCA during the course of the study. Further, provokable ischemia during an exercise-gated blood pool scan was more common in the elective group. A limited rise in mean ejection fraction during exercise of 1.2% was observed among patients awaiting an elective procedure, compared to a mean 8.1% augmentation with exercise among patients who underwent deferred PTCA (Fig. 5).

The liberal use of empiric PTCA in the TAMI-1 trial was associated with a 1% and 3.7% mortality rate at 1- and 3-year follow-up respectively. Survival among these patients compares favorably with late deaths reported with less invasive strategies. Among the 11,800 patients enrolled in the GISSI megatrial of intravenous strepto-

kinase, only 0.3% of patients underwent subsequent angioplasty. Mortality at 1 year was 8.7% in this trial; a similar 8.3% mortality rate was reported at 2 years in the noninvasive International Study of Infarct Survival (ISIS)-2 study (Fig. 6) (5,36). Without specifically targeting demonstrable ischemia, this improved survival may have resulted from an unusually high incidence of residual ischemia in the TAMI-1 cohort; however, the incidence of demonstrable postthrombolytic ischemia was limited to 19% in both the Johns Hopkins trial and phase 2B of the TIMI trial at the time of 6-week stress testing (11,37). The additional improvement in survival attributable to empiric, deferred PTCA in the absence of residual ischemia may conceivably relate to preservation of left ventricular wall integrity due to the promotion of healing and remodeling of the necrotic myocardium by an increased local influx of nutrients. Survival may be further influenced by improved flow to potential collateral conduits supplying ischemic myocardium distant from the infarct zone, and establishing a reliable route for the local delivery of antiarrhythmic or inotropic agents to surviving myocardium at the watershed periphery of the infarct.

The higher rate of recurrent ischemia and reinfarction observed after administration of a thrombolytic agent alone mandates careful clinical observation for residual ischemia and reocclusion. This continued vigilance does not require immediate transfer to an institution with an interventional team, but requires easy access to such a facility. Some authorities suggest that early diagnostic catheterization is unnecessary after thrombolytic therapy for acute myocardial infarction, and that in the absence of subsequent, demonstrable ischemia, the patient

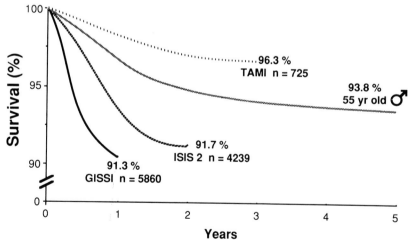

FIG. 6. Empiric angioplasty and survival. Long-term outcome of four different cohorts. Follow-up at 3 years in 725 patients enrolled in the TAMI trials demonstrated a 96.3% survival rate after liberal application of immediate or rescue angioplasty, which compares favorably with the United States 55-year-old male population, in whom there is a 93.8% survival rate at 5 years, according to United States vital statistics data. In comparison, there was substantially higher short-term mortality in the two megatrials of thrombolysis alone, with an 8.7% 1-year out-of-hospital mortality rate in the GISSI trial (4), and an 8.3% 2-year out-of-hospital mortality rate among patients in the ISIS-2 trial. From Topol EJ (82), with permission. TAMI, Thrombolysis and Angioplasty in Myocardial Study.

may be managed conservatively (11,38). In the TIMI-2B trial, 3,262 patients were randomly assigned to two treatment groups: 1,636 patients were randomized to a treatment intended to include delayed catheterization and empiric deferred PTCA between 18 and 48 hours after thrombolytic therapy, and 1,626 patients were managed conservatively, with no follow-up catheterization unless spontaneous or provokable postinfarction ischemia occurred (11).

There were no significant differences in the primary endpoints of death or reinfarction at 42 days, between the conservative and invasive management groups; however, the conservative strategy was associated with a significantly higher incidence of provokable ischemia at both predischarge and 6-week follow-up stress testing (Table 4). By the time of the 6-week stress gated blood pool scan, a significant difference in the augmentation of global left ventricular function during exercise favored the deferred PTCA strategy (3.3% improvement with exercise in the invasive, versus 2.3% among patients in the conservatively managed cohort); these findings were similar to those of the Johns Hopkins investigators (37).

Early reocclusion in the TIMI-2B study occurred in 68 patients (7.7%) who, by study design, underwent PTCA between 18 and 48 hrs after infarction, while recurrent ischemia within the first 14 days of the study was experienced by 420 patients (26%) who were managed conservatively, with 25 of these patients suffering reinfarction (11%). Of the 432 patients (50%) from the conservatively managed group who were triaged to elective PTCA, 216 patients underwent the procedure within the first 14 days of the trial. There were 50 patients from the invasive group who had continued, overt ischemia despite thrombolytic therapy and who underwent emergency PTCA before the intended 18- to 48-hr catheterization, with an unusually low 80% successful recanalization rate. Subsequently, 12% of these patients experienced reocclusion, 6% reinfarcted, and one patient died. Because of the delayed 18- to 48-hr angiographic assessment, rescue PTCA for less clinically apparent persistent ischemia was not rendered to all patients with failed thrombolysis; the potential impact of this strategy among the 177 patients (12%) excluded from PTCA because of a closed infarct related artery was not assessed. Importantly, patients with total occlusion of the infarct vessel were excluded from proceeding with PTCA within the protocol of the study.

Considerable inhomogeneity within the two treatment strategies was noted by the end of the trial. Of note, the conservative strategy was designed to incorporate elective catheterization when clinically necessary, while the invasively managed group was committed to deferred PTCA by protocol if physically possible. The incidence of referral for early catheterization was 33% (532 patients) among patients in the intended noninvasive group, and 432 patients (27%) underwent revascularization by PTCA or bypass surgery by the end of the 42-day study. Importantly, many of the patients with provokable ischemia at the end of the trial may have required late elective or emergency revascularization after the end of the study, an occurrence further misrepresenting the ultimate treatment distribution, and the late morbidity and mortality rates between the two cohorts. As illustrated in Fig. 7, only 60% of patients included in the invasive management group actually underwent the intended procedure.

Stricter adherence to the intended treatment was possible in a study of 800 patients randomly assigned to a conservative (n = 403) versus an invasive (catheterization within 48 hr, deferred PTCA within 7 days) strategy (n = 397) after intravenous anistreplase treatment conducted by the Should We Intervene Following Thrombolysis (SWIFT) study group (Fig. 8) (38). By the time of 12-month follow-up, additional postdischarge invasive procedures were infrequent, including diagnostic angiography (20 invasive vs. 57 conservative patients; $p < 0.001$), PTCA (4 invasive vs. 16 conservative patients; $p = 0.011$) and bypass surgery (10 invasive vs. 24 conservative patients; $p = 0.022$). At the end of the 12-month study, mortality (5.8% invasive vs. 5.0% for conservative management) and reinfarction rates (15.1% invasive vs. 12.9% for conservative management) were similar. Fur-

TABLE 4. *TIMI-2B trial of empiric deferred PTCA versus conservative elective intervention*

	Invasive strategy	Conservative strategy
Clinical Characteristics		
Emergency PTCA (<18 hr)	50 (3.1%)	NA
Deferred PTCA (18–48 hr)	878 (54%)	NA
No PTCA by day 42	518 (32%)	1364 (84%)
CABG surgery	195 (11.9%)	170 (10.5%)
Primary endpoints		
Death or reinfarction	178 (10.9%)	158 (9.7%)
Death	5.2%	4.7%
Reinfarction	5.9%	5.4%
Secondary endpoints		
Early positive stress (≤42 days)	12.8%*	17.7%*
Late positive stress (6 weeks)	16.8%**	19.4%**
Resting LVEF at discharge	50.5%	49.9%
ΔLVEF at discharge	3.7%	3.1%
Resting LVEF at 6 weeks	50.0%	50.4%
ΔLVEF at 6 weeks	3.3%***	2.3%***

* $p < 0.001$.
** $p = 0.09$.
*** $p = 0.02$.
LVEF, left ventricular ejection fraction; ΔLVEF, (stress − resting) ejection fraction; CABG, coronary artery bypass graft; NA, not applicable.

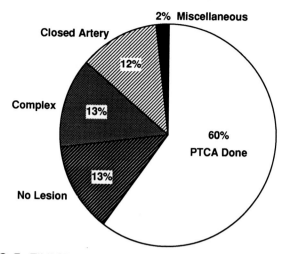

FIG. 7. TIMI-2B invasive strategy. The distribution of actual treatment rendered among 1,636 patients randomized to the invasive strategy at 48 hr of the Thrombolysis in Myocardial Infarction (TIMI) phase 2B study. A significant proportion of randomized patients (40%) did not undergo the intended treatment strategy. A closed artery, due to thrombolytic failure or unrecognized reocclusion, excluded 12% of patients from late revascularization.

ther, there were no differences in the incidence of subsequent angina pectoris, and resting mean left ventricular ejection fraction was similar between the two groups (52% vs. 51% for invasive vs. conservative cohorts respectively). Like the TIMI-2B study, the SWIFT investigators were not obliged by protocol to approach a closed artery, and the delayed catheterization (≤48 hr) did not allow rescue angioplasty for failed thrombolysis.

An elective, wait-and-see conservative strategy reserved for the treatment of spontaneous or provokable

ischemia after thrombolytic therapy can yield mortality rates and left ventricular systolic function similar to that achieved with empiric, immediate PTCA when it applied indiscriminately to all approachable postthrombolytic lesions. Although subsequent ischemia is more frequent during conservative management, careful clinical vigilance and appropriate, timely referral for further intervention is a comparable and somewhat less expensive strategy prior to hospital discharge (Fig. 9). A difference of $1,363 in hospital costs was noted by the TIMI-2B investigators between the more costly invasive strategy and the less expensive conservative management approach (25). However, long-term cost analysis is necessary as the conservatively managed patients accrue additional expenses related to close clinical follow-up, continued medication, recurrent hospital admissions, and late interventional procedures. Unequivocally, in the presence of a patent infarct artery, elective PTCA only for demonstrable ischemia beyond the acute 6- to 12-hr postthrombolysis phase is widely accepted. The impetus for early angiography, however, to identify high risk coronary anatomy in need of urgent bypass surgery, or to identify failed thrombolysis or to allow treatment with rescue PTCA, remains the focus of intense clinical debate.

Rescue PTCA

The application of PTCA in a persistently occluded infarct-related artery after failure of a thrombolytic agent is not synonymous with direct angioplasty (39). A major pitfall of thrombolytic therapy with presently available agents is the limited 50% to 75% efficacy, and synergy

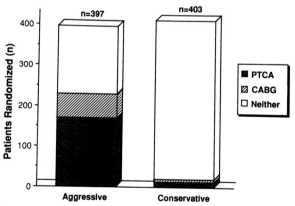

FIG. 8. SWIFT treatment intent. Adherence to the intended treatment strategy was similar in the Should We Intervene Following Thrombolysis? (SWIFT) trial. Delayed catheterization at 48 hr in the aggressively managed group did not allow assessment of a rescue angioplasty (PTCA) strategy. Deferred PTCA was associated with similar survival and left ventricular function at the time of 1-year follow-up; adherence to the conservative strategy was relatively strict, with crossover limited to PTCA in 12 patients and coronary artery bypass graft surgery (CABG) in 7 patients.

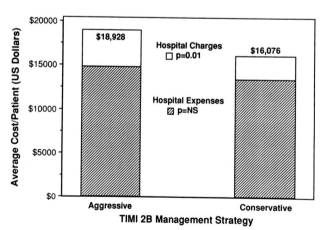

FIG. 9. TIMI-2B Strategy Cost Comparison. Although the total hospital charges associated with deferred angioplasty were significantly higher compared with the conservative management strategy, the total expenses accrued by the hospital were similar with a mean expense of $14,755 for the aggressive, versus $13,142 for the conservative management approach. This difference largely reflects the wide variability of professional fees and institutional profit margins. TIMI, thrombolysis in myocardial infarction.

has not been observed when combining agents with rapid and intermediate peak activities (40). Further, there is currently no reliable (both sensitive and specific) clinical or electrocardiographic indicator of thrombolytic success (41). The use of PTCA as an adjunct, fallback method of infarct vessel recanalization when thrombolytic therapy is ineffectual is referred to as rescue angioplasty (42–48). This strategy requires access to the same comprehensive interventional cardiac facilities as direct PTCA, but the delay in therapy inherent in hospital transfer is potentially avoided by the early administration of a thrombolytic agent. At present, the 25% to 50% of patients resistant to thrombolytic therapy are identified by acute catheterization—until a definitive, timely noninvasive marker for reperfusion is devised—and the infarct vessel is recanalized mechanically by PTCA to limit myocardial necrosis.

Rescue PTCA has been implemented in few clinical trials to date (Table 5). Patients in whom thrombolytic therapy fails to recanalize the infarct vessel have an especially poor prognosis (43). Fung and colleagues (42) were the first to observe improved left ventricular systolic function following rescue PTCA after failed thrombolysis with intravenous streptokinase. This observation has been persistent throughout the TAMI trials. Cumulative experience with 169 patients undergoing successful rescue PTCA for failed thrombolysis has demonstrated improvement in left ventricular ejection fraction and regional wall motion compared with patients in whom the fallback mechanical intervention is technically unsuccessful (48). However, the improvement in regional wall motion is not comparable to that achieved with successful thrombolysis alone (49).

In phase 1 of the TAMI trial, 86 of the 96 patients (90%) found to be resistant to thrombolysis were triaged to rescue PTCA. Overall mortality proved to be highest among patients in this subgroup (10.4%), with an exceptional mortality rate of 44% among the 9 patients in whom the attempted procedure was completely unsuccessful (43). Mortality was substantially altered after a partially successful result (14% with 50% or more residual stenosis), and further diminished (6%) when the procedure was completely successful. Although there were no deaths among the patients who had an occluded vessel after thrombolytic therapy and who did not undergo rescue PTCA, this disproportionate mortality may have occurred because 6 of the 10 patients excluded from the procedure were found to have small, branch vessel infarct lesions with associated limited myocardial necrosis, and 2 patients had late thrombolysis just beyond the time of the 90-min angiogram. Only the remaining 2 patients were excluded from PTCA due to technically unapproachable disease. Despite partial or complete initial angiographic success, the reocclusion rate for these patients was 29%.

Clinical outcome among the 23 rescue PTCA patients after combined intravenous thrombolytic therapy with t-PA (1.0 mg/kg) and 0.5 to 2.0 million units of urokinase in the second phase of the TAMI trial was more favorable. There were no deaths prior to discharge, or at the time of 1-year follow-up, and the high reocclusion rate of the TAMI-1 trial was not reproducible, with a lower 7% reocclusion rate being observed after combination therapy. Because of the differing thrombolytic regimens, the results may not be comparable; rescue PTCA outcome may be dependent upon the thrombolytic regimen administered prior to the procedure. Nonetheless, rescue PTCA has been associated with a notably lower procedural success rate (70% to 90% success) compared with direct or elective PTCA (90% to 95% success), and reocclusion after this interventional strategy appears to be extraordinarily high, ranging from 14% to nearly 30%. In an alarming number of otherwise uncomplicated cases, rescue PTCA of a persistently occluded right coronary artery has initiated paroxysmal ventricular fibrillation and bradydysrhythmias (23). This sudden clinical deterioration merits an especially cautious approach when targeting infarct-related lesions within this vessel.

Thrombolytic failure remains a common, problematic, and often clinically occult phenomenon, requiring early catheterization of nearly all patients to be accurately diagnosed. The merits of rescue PTCA remain un-

TABLE 5. *Rescue coronary angioplasty*

Study (references)	Agent(s)	n	PTCA success (%)	Reocclusion (%)	ΔEF[a]	Mortality (%)
Fung et al. (43)	SK	13	92	16	+10	7.6
Califf et al./TAMI-1 (44)	t-PA	86	73	29	−1	10.4
Topol et al./TAMI-2 (41)	t-PA + UK	22	86	4	+5	0
Baim et al. (45)	t-PA	37	92	26	NR	5.4
O'Connor et al. (46)	SK	90	89	14	−1	17.0
Grines et al. (47)	t-PA + SK	10	90	NR	+5	NR
Holmes et al. (48)	SK	34	71	NR	NR	3.0

[a] Change in left ventricular ejection fraction from baseline to 7 days.
NR, not reported; EF, ejection fraction; SK, streptokinase; t-PA, tissue-type plasminogen activator; UK, urokinase.

clear, but the potential salvage of myocardium which accompanies early recanalization of the infarct within 6-hr, even when failed thrombolysis, warrants further, prospective clinical investigation.

EARLY CATHETERIZATION AND ADJUNCT MECHANICAL INTERVENTIONS

Rationale

The decision to perform early catheterization in patients presenting with acute myocardial infarction is predicated on the limited efficacy of currently available thrombolytic regimens, the inherent risks of thrombolytic agents in certain subsets of patients, and the establishment of early prognosis. Cardiac catheterization in the acute phase of myocardial infarction is unequivocally justified in the presence of persistent ischemia or cardiogenic shock following administration of a thrombolytic agent, or as a primary investigative procedure when the diagnosis is uncertain and the patient is at high risk for hemorrhagic complications from thrombolytic therapy. Early definition of the coronary anatomy can allow for triage to direct or rescue PTCA, or to emergency coronary bypass surgery. There is intense controversy regarding the optimal management of the hemodynamically stable patient with suspected, but unconfirmed, reperfusion after administration of a thrombolytic. Fueling the controversy is the limited accuracy of frequently used noninvasive clinical indices of thrombolytic success.

In the TAMI-I study, improvement of initial ST-segment changes was associated with an 84% probability of a patent infarct vessel, but occurred in only 38% of patients experiencing successful reperfusion, while complete normalization of the ST-segment was associated with a patent infarct artery in 96% of cases, but occurred in only 6% of patients with an open artery at acute catheterization (27). Similarly, the probability of a patent infarct artery was 71% when chest pain symptoms improved, and increased to 84% when chest pain completely resolved; however, these indices were observed in only 51% of patients with chest pain improvement, and 29% with chest pain resolution, in the presence of angiographically confirmed reperfusion (27). Beyond myocardial salvage, experimental models have demonstrated that reperfusion, even after the acute phase of myocardial infarction, can promote infarct healing, as well as prevent infarct expansion and ventricular aneurysm formation (50–53). Early angiography remains the only highly sensitive and specific indicator of infarct vessel patency. The identification of patients who may benefit from more aggressive adjunct mechanical intervention effecting additional myocardial salvage requires further investigation. In both the TIMI-2B and

SWIFT trials (11,12), the effect of mechanical intervention for failed thrombolysis was not assessed, since patients with persistent total occlusion of the infarct vessel were excluded from PTCA.

Early and late prognosis may be assessed by angiographic parameters determined at early cardiac catheterization. The definition of multivessel disease at early angiography among patients in the TAMI trials was associated with an in-hospital mortality rate of 12%, compared with the 4% mortality observed among patients with single-vessel disease (54). Patients with severe, multivessel disease, or left main coronary artery stenosis defined at early angiography, may be referred for urgent bypass surgery. Certainly, knowledge of such high-risk anatomy can heighten the clinical vigilance for ongoing or recurrent ischemia after thrombolytic therapy.

Although early, postthrombolytic exercise testing is advocated to focus subsequent referral for elective PTCA on the subset of patients most likely to benefit from the procedure (11,12), Simoons and colleagues found that event rates among 533 patients followed for 5 years after reperfusion therapy were not predicted by a positive functional study (55). By regression analysis, these investigators found that age, prior infarction, ejection fraction, the severity of residual stenosis in the infarct-related artery, as well as the number of diseased vessels, were the key indices of late prognosis; the latter two predictors are definable only at cardiac catheterization. We have found that a negative postthrombolytic stress test correlates best with greater myocardial necrosis; inadequate myocardial salvage despite treatment, rather than optimal therapy with no residual ischemia, may be the most likely explanation for such a clinical course (56).

Care must be taken to avoid empiric, a priori PTCA of the residual stenosis, since the angiogram confers anatomical but not physiological information about the residual infarct lesion. Early recurrent ischemic events are not predicted by the severity of the residual stenosis after thrombolytic therapy (57,58), but there may be a temptation to triage the patient to empiric PTCA or bypass surgery on the basis of the angiographic appearance of the postthrombolytic residual stenosis. This "reperfusion momentum" may predispose to unnecessary intervention and its inherent risks (59,60).

Clinical Assessment

Prior to undertaking emergency direct or rescue PTCA in the setting of acute myocardial infarction, a thorough evaluation of the patient's clinical status is mandated. If the patient is hypotensive with a systolic pressure of less than 90 mmHg on presentation, right heart catheterization to determine baseline right atrial, pulmonary artery, and pulmonary artery wedge pressures is necessary to distinguish severe left heart failure from hypovolemia, ventricular rupture with tamponade physiology, or, in the presence of ST-segment changes in the inferior or posterior electrocardiographic leads, right ventricular infarction. Left ventricular pump failure may benefit from diuresis, initiating inotropic agents or placement of an intraaortic balloon pump, while hypotension associated with hypovolemia, tamponade, or right ventricular infarction may improve with volume expansion. Sequential pacing of the right atrium and ventricle may be indicated in the presence of acute right ventricular infarction, especially if high grade AV nodal block or bradycardia are observed. Pacing of the right atrium, in the presence or right ventricular infarction without atrial involvement, can increase right heart forward output by as much as 20% to 30%.

If impaired left ventricular function is defined, contralateral femoral arterial access with a small (5 French) sheath should be established if an intraaortic balloon pump is not placed prophylactically. When targeting the right coronary artery for direct or rescue PTCA, venous access should be anticipated for rapid volume infusion, or temporary right ventricular pacing, to counteract the sudden vasovagal reaction often associated with intervention within this vessel (21,23). For the treatment of transient hypotension, unresponsive to fluid bolus, the intravenous infusion of dopamine or norepinephrine should be promptly initiated. Both agents cause a rapid rise in systolic blood pressure due to both peripheral vasoconstriction and increased cardiac output secondary to tachycardia. We have routinely used bolus administration of metaraminol for treatment of such events. This agent's pressor effect is due predominantly to peripheral vasoconstriction, without associated tachycardia, or even a paradoxical reflex bradycardia response, and thus there is less increase in myocardial oxygen demand than is observed with the use of either dopamine or norepinephrine.

Although mechanical disruption of the intima or media of the target PTCA vessel cannot presently be prevented or altered by pharmacological agents, modification of the resultant platelet and fibrin response can prevent subsequent acute thrombotic occlusion (61–63). In a study by Schwartz and the Montreal Heart Institute (63), 366 patients were randomly assigned to pretreatment with either combined oral aspirin (330 mg/day) and dipyridamole (75 mg three times a day) or with placebo, prior to elective PTCA. The incidence of acute occlusion resulting in Q-wave myocardial infarction in the trial was 6.9% in the placebo group, and only 1.6% among patients treated with the antiplatelet regimen. In the patient presenting for acute angioplasty in the setting of acute myocardial infarction, who is not premedicated with daily aspirin, immediate administration of at least 160 mg of chewable, noncoated aspirin is mandated

prior to the procedure. This route of administration facilitates early, gastric absorption of the drug. Although adjunct administration of dextran, another antiplatelet agent, has potential benefit in the previously untreated patient, the maximal antiplatelet effect of this agent does not peak until 4 to 6 hr after infusion (64), and little clinical efficacy has been observed with this agent even when it is administered as much as 30 min before balloon dilatation (65).

Heparin has been reported to inhibit platelet aggregation (66); however, in patients without gross intimal dissection of the target vessel, Ellis and associates found no effect on reocclusion when heparin administration was continued for 18 to 24 hr after the procedure (67), and a similar lack of benefit has been reported when patients with uncomplicated intimal dissection are treated (68). Finally, the use of intravenous nitrates, if hemodynamically tolerated, may provide additional antiplatelet activity (69). Thus, until more specific and rapidly acting antiplatelet agents are developed and tested, early determination of the patient's antiplatelet therapy and prompt administration of aspirin, dextran (if PTCA can be deferred for a few hours), and possibly intravenous nitrates may optimize the clinical result. Prolonged heparin therapy is unnecessary unless a large intimal dissection with associated intraluminal filling defect is produced at the target site.

Equipment Selection

Judicious selection of angioplasty equipment, and an appreciation of the injury potential of overzealous use or misuse of the guide catheter, guidewire, or balloon catheter are essential for procedural success. Because of the increased stiffness required for backup support, the guide catheter can cause direct trauma to the ostial or proximal coronary arteries (Fig. 10). Because of this propensity, newer guide catheters are increasingly incorporating a softer tip material. Selection of guide catheters, as well as their diagnostic counterparts, is based primarily the target artery and its angle of origin, to allow atraumatic, coaxial intubation of the coronary ostium.

Unique to the selection of a guide catheter, however, is the need for adequate backup support to allow the successful advancement of the intraluminal equipment. In general, catheters that tend to jump into position, such as the multipurpose or Amplatz design, should be avoided unless exceptional backup is required to cross the target lesion with the balloon catheter. Diffuse lesions, excessive proximal tortuosity of the infarct artery, bifrication lesions, distal lesions, calcified vessels, and total occlusions are anatomical characteristics that are likely to require additional guide catheter support to facilitate crossing the target stenosis. Active support augmentation refers to deep seating the guide into the artery with

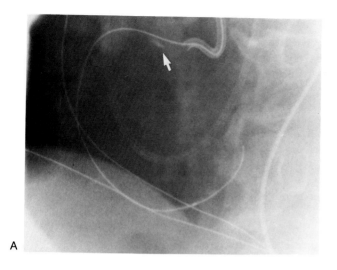

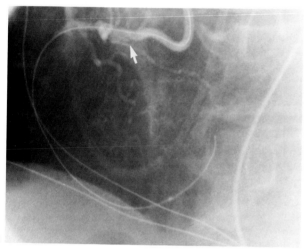

FIG. 10. A: Guide catheter dissection. Intimal dissection of the proximal right coronary artery occurred after deep seating of an Amplatz guide catheter was required to cross a total midvessel occlusion (*arrow*). **B**: Persistent contrast staining (*arrow*) was observed during small test injections under fluoroscopy to visualize guidewire probing of the obstruction.

or without torquing the catheter into an Amplatz configuration (Amplatzing), and risks trauma to the ostium of the target vessel. This method is contraindicated in the presence of severe ostial disease, as well as in vessels with small ostia whose diameter is less than that of the guide catheter. Passive support results from intraaortic stabilization or buttressing of the catheter and varies with the type of curve and the stiffness of the guide catheter shaft. The selection of a left Amplatz with a short tip, Arani double loop, or an El Gamal (especially for bypass graft lesions) catheter can afford additional support from the contralateral aortic wall without the need for deep seating the guide into the proximal vessel.

Percutaneous transluminal coronary angioplasty of the left anterior descending artery may be facilitated by use of an undersized left Judkins catheter, which will

subselectively direct the equipment superiorly and into the vessel; however, deep seating of the undersized catheter must be approached with particular caution to avoid trauma to the left main trunk. Similar care must be taken when disengaging the Amplatz catheter and the operator must remember to advance and torque the shaft to free the tip under fluoroscopic guidance before withdrawing the catheter.

Guidewire selection should always begin with the most flexible model available, with progression to the stiffer wire designs only after several thoughtful, failed attempts to cross the stenosis. The choice of wire type and diameter may be influenced by the lesion to be targeted. For severe, distal vessel lesions, a 0.010-mm system can minimize the profile for crossing the lesion, while a 0.018-mm guidewire may provide additional forward support for tracking across a stenosis within a more proximal, tortuous vessel segment. Unless the infarct vessel is small ($\leq$2.0 mm in diameter), or unless the lesion proves extremely difficult to cross, an over-the-wire system is generally more desirable than a fixed-wire system when PTCA is performed in the setting of acute myocardial infarction. Guidewire position across the stenosis (purchase) is maintained in the event of acute closure, providing a channel for rapidly recrossing the obstruction. The use of tapered guidewires, without a discrete transition zone can aid entry into an angulated left circumflex artery or side branch vessel, preventing prolapse of the wire into the main channel; however, these wires are radiopaque, and can impair visualization of the angiographic result. Guidewire trauma remains a well-recognized cause of intimal dissection, especially in the presence of long or eccentric lesions. Forceful probing of the lesion should be avoided, and freedom of the guidewire tip within the vessel lumen ensured by floroscopic observation as the tip crosses the lesion to circumvent this complication.

Balloon catheter selection depends upon artery size and balloon material requirements. Successful balloon sizing is determined by the native artery diameter and the initial minimal luminal diameter of the stenosis. Initially, if crossing the stenosis proves difficult, preliminary dilatation with a smaller balloon catheter that can readily cross the stenosis may allow subsequent positioning of the desired balloon size for a series of optimal inflations. The importance of proper balloon sizing was emphasized by Roubin and associates who conducted a study that was halted prematurely because of significant differences in clinical outcome among 336 patients randomly assigned to undergo PTCA with a large balloon (n = 169; balloon/artery diameter ratio = 1.13 $\pm$ 0.14), or a balloon that was slightly smaller than artery diameter (n = 167; balloon/artery diameter ratio = 0.93 $\pm$ 0.12) (70). In this abbreviated trial, referral for emergency bypass surgery and the incidence of myocardial infarction (MI) was higher when the balloon was oversized, (large balloon: surgery; MI = 7.7%) than when the patient was assigned to the smaller balloon group (small balloon: surgery referral = 3.6%; MI = 3.0%). Undersizing, with a balloon:artery diameter ratio of less than 0.9 was associated with more severe residual stenosis and a higher rate of restenosis in a subsequent, smaller study by Nichols and colleagues (71). These investigators confirmed that there was a higher rate of dissection complicating PTCA when oversized balloons with balloon: artery diameter ratios in excess of 1.3 were used. The combination of high inflation pressure and balloon oversizing has produced more extensive intimal hyperplasia and luminal renarrowing by histological analysis in animal models (72). Thus, proper balloon sizing for optimal short- and long-term results should approximate the native vessel diameter as closely as possible.

The choice of balloon material depends upon the required properties of compliance (the change in diameter accompanying changes in inflation pressure), and conformability (assuming the vessel contour without straightening angulated or curved segments). The polyolefin balloons (POC) are more compliant than the polyethylene or polyethylene terephthalate (PET) materials, and are useful when the vessel size is intermediate between two standard balloon sizes, since balloon diameter increases at higher inflation pressures. The polyolefin material also allows dilation of several lesions within varying-sized coronary artery segments, providing variable but relatively predictable balloon sizing according to the inflation pressure. Polyolefin material has an obvious disadvantage when addressing an indurated lesion. First, the polyolefin material has a mean balloon burst rating between 10 and 12 atmospheres, which prohibits higher inflation pressures to deliver increased radial force to the lesion. Second, because of the material's compliance, dilation at higher inflation pressures carries a distinct risk of oversizing the effective balloon diameter relative to the artery size. The PET balloon material is less compliant and more durable, allowing safe inflation at high pressures (15 to 20 atmospheres), with considerably less variability in balloon size. A balloon of PET material should be selected when the targeted vessel segment appears heavily calcified, and high-pressure inflations are anticipated. Although balloon size titration to the precise vessel diameter is not readily accomplished with PET material, the availability of quarter-sized balloon diameters allows better matching of balloon to artery diameter. The conformability of PET is higher than that of POC; for stenoses within highly angulated vessel segments, this material has been reported to reduce the incidence of intimal dissection and acute closure by 39% in one retrospective analysis (73). Despite ideal equipment selection, the single most important factor influencing procedural success remains operator experience (74).

Subsequent Management

Coadministration of heparin with t-PA does not enhance reocclusion reperfusion (75); however, early initiation of continuous heparin infusion can prevent thrombotic reocclusion after successful thrombolysis. In a randomized trial of 205 patients treated with t-PA and either intravenous heparin or aspirin (80 mg/day), infarct vessel patency at 18 hr was 82% in the heparin group, versus 52% among patients receiving adjunctive aspirin alone ($p < 0.001$) (76). In the National Heart Foundation of Australia study, 202 patients receiving t-PA and adjunctive heparin were randomly assigned, after 24 hr, to continue heparin therapy, or were switched to aspirin (300 mg/day) and dipyridamole (300 mg/day) (77). Coronary arteriography 7 days after thrombolytic therapy revealed the same 80% patency rate with both strategies. Intravenous heparin should be continued for at least 24 hr after thrombolytic therapy, independent of early PTCA results.

Sheath removal after thrombolysis and early PTCA is necessarily postponed for 24 hr in the absence of access site hemorrhage. Interim hemorrhage from the femoral access site can usually be remedied by upsizing the sheath by sterile exchange to a larger sheath size over a guidewire. If significant bleeding continues, referral for vascular surgery with direct closure of the puncture site during continued heparin infusion is occasionally necessary. If heparin therapy is desired for more than 24 hr after PTCA because of a poor angiographic result, heparin infusion can be reduced to 400 IU/hr until activated clotting time (ACT) falls below 175 to 190 sec, or APTT is less than 50 sec. Sheath removal and hemostasis can be readily achieved at this time by manual compression, and heparin therapy can resume thereafter, with a low-dose bolus of 2,000 to 3,000 IU. The intravascular sheaths should not remain electively in place for more than 24 hr. Intraaortic balloon pump placement may have a distinct role in maintaining coronary artery patency, either after successful thrombolytic therapy in the presence of residual thrombus (78), or after a suboptimal PTCA result, by increasing diastolic coronary artery pressure and flow (79). If the lesion appears at especially high risk for early reocclusion due to a suboptimal result or a significant dissection with diminution of flow, such adjunctive mechanical support should be considered at the time of the final angiographic assessment.

CONCLUSIONS

Coronary artery angioplasty in the setting of acute myocardial infarction has merit as a direct or primary strategy in patients who can be taken rapidly to the catheterization laboratory, in whom the diagnosis is uncertain, or who have a contraindication to thrombolytic therapy. Among patients with an uncomplicated infarction, a conservative strategy of medical management and elective PTCA reserved for the treatment of subsequent spontaneous or provokable ischemia has been as effective (or ineffective) as a more aggressive deferred, empiric strategy, and yields similar mortality and global left ventricular function.

Immediate, empiric PTCA is presently reserved for the treatment of persistent cardiogenic shock, despite successful thrombolysis. Immediate PTCA improves both short- and long-term survival in this particular clinical setting, but is associated with an increased risk of acute closure with referral for emergency coronary artery bypass surgery, and an overall trend toward higher mortality compared with a deferred strategy. The role of rescue PTCA for the acute, mechanical recanalization of the infarct vessel that proves resistant to thrombolytic therapy remains controversial. Late survival after the liberal use of adjunct PTCA following thrombolytic therapy is notably improved, compared with the late followup mortality rate reported when a conservative, thrombolysis-only regimen is used (Fig. 6).

The current challenge is to determine the appropriate timing and clinical patient profile to optimize the benefit of further adjunct PTCA after administration of a thrombolytic agent. In the large clinical trials of immediate and rescue PTCA, patients could undergo adjunct mechanical revascularization as late as 4.4 hr after presentation in the TAMI trial, 4.7 hr in the TIMI-2 pilot study, 4.6 hr in TIMI-2A, 5.2 hr in TIMI-2B, 5.7 hr in the Johns Hopkins trial, and 3.3 hr in the European Cooperative study. The timing of early PTCA in these trials may have restricted myocardial salvage because of late interruption of the ongoing wavefront of necrosis (Fig. 11) (80). Further, many of the trials promoted PTCA of residual lesions widely held to be of limited hemodynamic significance, with patients undergoing PTCA for 60% residual lesions in the TIMI and European Cooperative studies, and as little as 50% residual luminal diameter narrowing in the TAMI trials. Earlier adjunct PTCA, or limiting triage to more critical, flow-limiting residual lesions may yield different clinical results.

Among a consecutive series of 500 patients undergoing immediate or rescue PTCA for acute myocardial infarction, Ellis and associates found that the major determinants of mortality were an age of more than 65 years, a baseline left ventricular ejection fraction of 30% or less, systolic blood pressure less than 100 mmHg, failed PTCA with a closed artery despite the attempted procedure, and referral for emergency bypass surgery (81). Only patients in whom the attempted acute PTCA was successful, particularly those patients presenting with anterior infarction, demonstrated improved survival with early PTCA. Although there was an insignificant trend toward lower mortality when patients with inferior in-

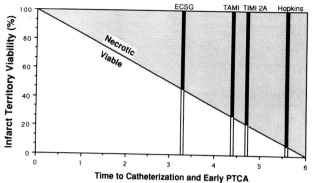

FIG. 11. Early PTCA and the wavefront phenomenon of necrosis. Following coronary artery occlusion in the dog, an advancing wavefront of myocardial necrosis is observed, with completion of the infarction noted after about 6 hr of infarct vessel occlusion. Myocardial viability within the infarct zone diminishes with longer duration of occlusion. Theoretically, assessment of acute angioplasty for the treatment of myocardial infarction in the large clinical trials has occurred relatively late into the event, with limited myocardial salvage expected after later adjunct mechanical intervention. More substantial differences in patients outcome may be observed with earlier treatment. Patients could undergo mechanical revascularization as late as 3.3 hr after symptom onset in the European Cooperative Study Group (ECSG) trial, 4.4 hr in the Thrombolysis and Angioplasty in Myocardial Infarction (TAMI) trial, 4.6 hr in phase 2A of the Thrombolysis in Myocardial Infarction (TIMI-2A) study, and 5.7 hr in the Johns Hopkins study. Deferred, aggressive angioplasty was scheduled as late as 48 to 52 hr after symptom onset in the TIMI-2B and SWIFT trials.

farction underwent early PTCA, left ventricular ejection fraction improved significantly when these patients underwent a successful procedure. The presence of collateral flow to the infarct vessel, and a baseline ejection fraction of 40% or less also proved predictive of improved left ventricular function after successful PTCA. Thus, focusing treatment with early angioplasty upon select patients may optimize the survival benefit observed with liberal, unselective application of this strategy. Refining the indications for earlier, adjunct mechanical intervention may potentiate myocardial salvage in patients likely to benefit from such a strategy, while preventing further, unnecessary intervention among patients whose clinical course would be unaltered by the procedure. Elective PTCA is a utilitarian, cost-effective strategy after successful thrombolytic therapy for acute myocardial infarction; however, elective adjunctive PTCA can be advanced from a post hoc treatment for residual, periinfarct ischemia to an earlier, pivotal myocardial salvage procedure as further clinical investigation defines the optimal timing, thrombolytic milieu, and presenting clinical characteristics that are conducive to improving survival and reducing the incidence of recurrent ischemia and repeated hospital admissions.

REFERENCES

1. Davies MJ, Thomas A. Thrombosis and acute coronary artery lesions in sudden cardiac ischemic death. *N Engl J Med* 1984;310:1137–1142.
2. Davies MJ, Thomas A. Plaque fissuring—the cause of acute myocardial infarction, sudden ischemic death, and crescendo angina. *Br Heart J* 1985;53:363–368.
3. DeWood MA, Spores J, Notske R, Mouser LT, Burroughs R, Golden MS, Lang HT. Prevalence of total coronary occlusion during the early hours of transmural myocardial infarction. *N Engl J Med* 1980;303:897–902.
4. Gruppo Italiano per lo Studio della Streptochinasi nell'Infarcto Miocardio (GISSI). Effectiveness of intravenous thrombolytic treatment in acute myocardial infarction. *Lancet* 1986;1:397–402.
5. Gruppo Italiano per lo Studio della Streptochinasi nell'Infarcto Miocardio (GISSI). Long-term effects of intravenous thrombolysis in acute myocardial infarction: final report of the GISSI study. *Lancet* 1987;2:871–874.
6. Topol EJ, Califf RM, George BS. The Thrombolysis and Angioplasty in Myocardial Infarction (TAMI) group. A randomized trial of immediate versus delayed angioplasty after intravenous tissue plasminogen activator in acute myocardial infarction. *N Engl J Med* 1987;317:581–588.
7. Topol EJ, Califf RM. The Thrombolysis and Angioplasty in Myocardial Infarction (TAMI) group. Thrombolysis and angioplasty in myocardial infarction (TAMI) trial. *J Am Coll Cardiol* 1987;10:65B–74B.
8. The TIMI Study Group. The Thrombolysis In Myocardial Infarction (TIMI) Phase II pilot study: tissue plasminogen activator followed by percutaneous transluminal coronary angioplasty. *J Am Coll Cardiol* 1987;10:51B–64B.
9. The TIMI Research Group. Immediate vs. delayed catheterization and angioplasty following thrombolytic therapy for acute myocardial infarction: TIMI IIA results. *JAMA* 1988;260:2849–2858.
10. Simoons ML, The European Cooperative Study Group for Recombinant Tissue-type Plasminogen Activator. Thrombolysis with tissue plasminogen activator in acute myocardial infarction: No additional benefit from immediate percutaneous coronary angioplasty. *Lancet* 1988;1:197–203.
11. The TIMI Study Group. Comparison of invasive and conservative strategies after treatment with intravenous tissue plasminogen activator in acute myocardial infarction. *N Engl J Med* 1989;320:618–627.
12. de Bono DP, Pocock SJ, the SWIFT Investigators Group. The SWIFT study of intervention versus conservative management after anistreplase thrombolysis. *Br Med J* 1991;302:555–560.
13. Holmes DR, Smith HC, Vlietstra RE, Nishimura A, Reeder GS, Bove AA, Bresnahan JF, Chesebro JH, Piehler JM. Percutaneous transluminal coronary angioplasty, alone or in combination with streptokinase therapy, during acute myocardial infarction. *Mayo Clin Proc* 1985;60:449–456.
14. Linnemeier TJ, Rothbaum DA, Landin RJ, Noble J. Percutaneous transluminal coronary angioplasty versus thrombolytic therapy in acute myocardial infarction. *Circulation* 1985;72[Suppl III]:III456–462.
15. Hartzler GO, McConahay DR, Johnson WL Jr. Direct balloon angioplasty in acute myocardial infarction: without prior use of streptokinase. *J Am Coll Cardiol* 1986;7:149A.
16. O'Neill W, Timmis G, Bourdillon P, Lai P, Ganghadarhan V, Walton J, Ramos R, Laufer N, Gordon S, Schork MA, Pitt B. A prospective randomized clinical trial of intracoronary streptokinase versus direct coronary angioplasty for acute myocardial infarction. *N Engl J Med* 1986;314:812–828.
17. Topol EJ, O'Neill WW, Lai P, Fung A, Bourdillon PVD. Sequential intravenous thrombolysis and coronary angioplasty versus direct PTCA therapy for acute myocardial infarction. *J Am Coll Cardiol* 1986;7:18A.
18. Rothbaum DA, Linnemeier TJ, Noble RJ. Emergency percutaneous transluminal coronary angioplasty in acute myocardial infarction. *J Am Coll Cardiol* 1986;7:149A.
19. Kimura T, Nosaka H, Ueno K, Nobuyoshi M. Role of coronary angioplasty in acute myocardial infarction. *Circulation* 1986;74:11–22.
20. Sriram R, Mullen GM, Foschi A, Bicoff JP. Percutaneous transluminal coronary angioplasty in acute myocardial infarction without prior thrombolytic therapy. *Am J Cardiol* 1988;55:842–853.
21. Kahn JK, Rutherford BD, McConahay DR, Johnson WL, Giorgi LV, Shimshak TM, Ligon RW, Hartzler GO. Catheterization laboratory events and hospital outcome with direct angioplasty for acute myocardial infarction. *Circulation* 1990;82:1910–1915.
22. Topol EJ, Bates ER, Walton JA Jr, Baumann G, Wolfe S, Maino J, Bayer L, Gorman L, Kline EM, O'Neill WW, Pitt B. Community hospital administration of intravenous tissue plasminogen activator in acute myocardial infarction: improved timing, thrombolytic efficacy and ventricular function. *J Am Coll Cardiol* 1987;10:1173–1177.
23. Gacioch GM, Topol EJ. Sudden, paradoxical clinical deterioration during angioplasty of the occluded right coronary artery in acute myocardial infarction. *J Am Coll Cardiol* 1989;14:1202–1209.
24. The TIMI Study Group. The thrombolysis in myocardial infarction (TIMI) trial: phase 1 findings. *N Engl J Med* 1985;312:932–936.
25. Charles ED, Rogers WJ, Reeder GS, Chesebro JH. Economic advantages of a conservative strategy for acute myocardial infarction management: rt-PA without obligatory PTCA. *J Am Coll Cardiol* 1989;13:152A(abst).
26. Topol EJ, Califf RM, George BS. The Thrombolysis and Angioplasty in Myocardial Infarction (TAMI) group. A randomized trial of immediate versus delayed angioplasty after intravenous tissue plasminogen activator in acute myocardial infarction. *N Engl J Med* 1987;317:581–588.
27. Topol EJ, Califf RM. The Thrombolysis and Angioplasty in Myocardial Infarction (TAMI) group. Thrombolysis and angioplasty in myocardial infarction (TAMI) trial. *J Am Coll Cardiol* 1987;10:65B–74B.
28. Serruys WW, Wijns W, vanden Brand M. Is transluminal angioplasty mandatory after successful thrombolysis? *Br Heart J* 1983;50:257.
29. Schroder R, Vohringer H, Linderer T, Biamino G, Bruggemann T, Leitner EV. Follow-up after coronary arterial perfusion with intravenous streptokinase in relation to residual myocardial infarct artery narrowings. *Am J Cardiol* 1985;55:313–317.
30. Meyer J. Thrombolysis in acute myocardial infarction: what about the underlying coronary stenosis? *Int J Cardiol* 1983;3:447–450.
31. The TIMI Research Group. Immediate vs. delayed catheterization and angioplasty following thrombolytic therapy for acute myocardial infarction: TIMI IIA results. *JAMA* 1988;260:2849–2858.
32. Goldberg RJ, Gore JM, Alpert JS, Osganian V, De Groot J, Bade J, Chen Z, Frid D, Dalen JE. Cardiogenic shock after acute myocardial infarction: incidence and mortality from a community-wide perspective, 1975 to 1988. *N Engl J Med* 1991;325:1117–1122.
33. Lee L, Bates ER, Pitt B, Walton JA, Laufer N, O'Neill WW. Percutaneous transluminal coronary angioplasty improves survival in acute myocardial infarction complicated by cardiogenic shock. *Circulation* 1988;78:1345–1351.
34. Kennedy JW, Gensini GG, Timmis GC, Maynard C. Acute myocardial infarction treated with intracoronary streptokinase: a report for the Society for Cardiac Angiography. *Am J Cardiol* 1985;55:871–877.
35. Lee L, Erbel R, Brown TM, Laufer N, Meyer J, O'Neill WW. Multicenter registry of angioplasty therapy of cardiogenic shock: initial and long-term survival. *J Am Coll Cardiol* 1991;17:599–603.
36. ISIS-2 Collaborative Group. Randomized trial of intravenous streptokinase, oral aspirin, both, or neither among 17,187 cases of suspected acute myocardial infarction. *Lancet* 1988;2:349–360.
37. Guerci AD, Gerstenblith G, Brinker JA, Chandra NC, Gottlieb SO, Bahr RD, Weiss JL, Shapiro EP, Flaherty JT, Bush DE, Chew PH, Gottlieb SH, Halperin HR, Ouyang P, Walford GD, Bell WR, Fatterpaker AK, Llewellyn M, Topol EJ, Healy B, Siu CO, Becker LC, Weisfeldt ML. A randomized trial of intravenous tissue plasminogen activator for acute myocardial infarction with subse-

quent randomization to elective coronary angioplasty. *N Engl J Med* 1987;317:1613–1618.

38. SWIFT: Should We Intervene Following Thrombolysis Trial Study Group. SWIFT trial of delayed elective intervention v. conservative treatment after thrombolysis with anistreplase in acute myocardial infarction. *Br Med J* 1991;302:555–560.
39. Meier B. Balloon angioplasty for acute myocardial infarction: was it buried alive? *Circulation* 1990;82:2243–2245(editorial).
40. Topol EJ, Califf RM, George BS, Kereiajes DJ. Coronary arterial thrombolysis with combined infusion of recombinant tissue-type plasminogen activator and urokinase in patients with acute myocardial infarction. *Circulation* 1988;77:1100–1107.
41. Kircher B, Topol EJ, Schork MA, Kline E, Pitt B, O'Neill WW. Noninvasive prediction of infarct vessel recanalization status after intravenous tissue plasminogen activator or streptokinase. *Clin Res* 1986;34:315–321A.
42. Fung AY, Lai P, Topol EJ. Value of percutaneous transluminal coronary angioplasty after unsuccessful intravenous streptokinase therapy in acute myocardial infarction. *Am J Cardiol* 1986;58:686–691.
43. Califf RM, Topol EJ, George BS. Characteristics and outcome of patients in whom reperfusion with intravenous tissue-type plasminogen activator fails: results of the Thrombolysis and Angioplasty in Myocardial Infarction (TAMI) I trial. *Circulation* 1988;77:1090–1099.
44. Baim DS, Diver DJ, Knatterud GL, the TIMI II-A Investigators. PTCA 'salvage' for thrombolytic failures—implications from TIMI II-A. *Circulation* 1988;78[Suppl II]:112.
45. O'Connor CM, Mark DB, Hinohara T, et al. Rescue angioplasty after failure of intravenous streptokinase in acute myocardial infarction: in-hospital and long term outcomes. *J Invas Cardiol* 1989;1:85–95.
46. Holmes DR, Gersh BJ, Bailey KR, et al. "Rescue" percutaneous transluminal coronary angioplasty after failed thrombolytic therapy—4 year follow-up. *J Am Coll Cardiol* 1989;13:193A.
47. Grines CL, Nissen SE, Booth DC, Branco MC, Bennett KA, DeMaria AN. Efficacy, safety and cost effectiveness of a new thrombolytic regimen for acute myocardial infarction using half dose tPA with full dose streptokinase. *Circulation* 1988;78[Suppl I]:II304 (abst).
48. Abbottsmith CW, Topol EJ, George BS, Stack RS, Kereiakes DJ, Candela RJ, Anderson LC, Harrelson-Woodlief SL, Califf RM. Fate of patients with acute myocardial infarction with patency of the infarct-related vessel achieved with successful thrombolysis versus rescue angioplasty. *J Am Coll Cardiol* 1990;16:770–778.
49. Sutton JM, Califf RM, Woodlief L, Higby NA, Karnash SL, Schwaiger M, Topol EJ. Thrombolytic therapy and immediate catheterization for triage to rescue angioplasty: is improved infarct zone wall motion after rescue angioplasty sustained at six weeks? *J Am Coll Cardiol* (in press).
50. Hochman JS, Choo H. Limitation of myocardial infarct expansion by reperfusion independent of myocardial salvage. *Circulation* 1987;75:299–306.
51. Hale SL, Kloner RA. Left ventricular topographic alterations in the completely healed rat infarct caused by early and late coronary artery reperfusion. *Am Heart J* 1988;116:1508–1513.
52. Califf RM, Topol EJ, Gersh BJ. From myocardial salvage to patient salvage in acute myocardial infarction: the role of reperfusion therapy. *J Am Coll Cardiol* 1989;14:1382–1388.
53. Braunwald E. Myocardial reperfusion, limitation of infarct size, reduction of left ventricular dysfunction and improved survival. Should the paradigm be expanded? *Circulation* 1989;79:441–444.
54. Topol EJ, Ellis SG, George BS. The pivotal role of multivessel coronary artery disease and the remote zone in the reperfusion era. *J Am Coll Cardiol* 1989;13:92A(abst).
55. Simoons ML, Vos J, Tijssen JG. Long-term benefit of early thrombolytic therapy in patients with acute myocardial infarction: 5 year follow-up of a trial conducted by the Interuniversity Cardiology Institute in the Netherlands. *J Am Coll Cardiol* 1989;14:1609–1615.
56. Sutton JM, Topol EJ. The significance of a paradoxical negative exercise tomographic thallium test in the presence of a critical residual stenosis after thrombolysis for evolving myocardial infarction. *Circulation* 1991;83:1278–1286.
57. Little WC, Constantinescu M, Applegate RJ. Can coronary angiog-

raphy predict the site of a subsequent myocardial infarction in patients with mild-to-moderate coronary artery disease? *Circulation* 1988;78:1157–1166.
58. Ellis SG, Topol EJ, George BS. Recurrent ischemia without warning. Analysis of risk factors for in-hospital ischemic events following successful thrombolysis with intravenous tissue plasminogen activator. *Circulation* 1989;80:1159–1165.
59. Holmes DR Jr, Topol EJ. Reperfusion momentum: lessons from the randomized trials of immediate coronary angioplasty for myocardial infarction. *J Am Coll Cardiol* 1989;14:1572–1578.
60. Topol EJ, Holmes DR Jr, Rogers WJ. Coronary angiography after thrombolytic therapy for acute myocardial infarction. *Ann Intern Med* 1991;114:877–885.
61. Cunningham DA, Kumar B, Siegal BA, Gilula LA, Totty WG, Welch MJ. Aspirin inhibition of platelet deposition at angioplasty sites: demonstration by platelet scintigraphy. *Radiology* 1984;151:487–490.
62. Barnathan ES, Schwartz JS, Taylor L. Aspirin and dipyridamole in the prevention of acute coronary thrombosis complicating coronary angioplasty. *Circulation* 1987;76:125–136.
63. Schwartz L, Bourassa MG, Lesperance J. Aspirin and dipyridamole in the prevention of restenosis after percutaneous transluminal coronary angioplasty. *N Engl J Med* 1988;318:1714–1719.
64. Bygdeman S, Eliasson R, Guilbring B. Effect of dextran infusion on the adenosine phosphate-induced adhesiveness and spreading capacity of human blood platelets. *Thromb Diath Haemorrh* 1966;15:451–456.
65. Swanson KT, Vlietstra RE, Holmes DR. Efficacy of adjunctive dextran during percutaneous transluminal coronary angioplasty. *Am J Cardiol* 1984;54:447–448.
66. Saba HI, Saba SR, Morelli GA. Effect of heparin on platelet aggregation. *Am J Hematol* 1984;17:295–306.
67. Ellis SG, Roubin GS, Wilentz J, Douglas JS, King SB. Effect of 18–24 hour heparin administration for prevention of restenosis after uncomplicated coronary angioplasty. *Am Heart J* 1989;117:777–782.
68. Walford GD, Midei MM, Aversano TR, Gottlieb SO, Chew PH, Siu CO, Brin KP, Brinker JA. Heparin after PTCA: increased early complications and no clinical benefit. *Circulation* 1991;84(II):592(abst).
69. Lam JYT, Chesebro JH, Fuster V. Platelets: vasoconstriction and nitroglycerin during arterial wall injury—a new antithrombotic role for an old drug. *Circulation* 1988;78:712–716.
70. Roubin GS, Douglas JS Jr, King SB III, Lin S, Hutchison N, Thomas RG, Gruentzig AR. Influence of balloon size on initial success, acute complications, and restenosis after percutaneous transluminal coronary angioplasty. A prospective randomized trial. *Circulation* 1988;78:557–565.
71. Nichols AB, Smith R, Berke AD, Shlofmitz RA, Powers ER. Importance of balloon size in coronary angioplasty. *J Am Coll Cardiol* 1989;13:1094–1100.
72. Sarembock IJ, LaVeau PJ, Sigal SL, Timms I, Sussman J, Haudenschild C, Ezekowitz MD. Influence of inflation pressure and balloon size on the development of intimal hyperplasia after balloon angioplasty. *Circulation* 1989;80:1029–1040.
73. Ellis SG, Topol EJ. Results of percutaneous transluminal coronary angioplasty of high-risk angulated stenoses. *Am J Cardiol* 1990;66:932–937.
74. Hamad N, Prichard AD, Lyle HRP, Lindsay J. Results of percutaneous transluminal coronary angioplasty by multiple, relatively low frequency operators: 1986–1987 experience. *Am J Cardiol* 1988;61:1229–1231.
75. Topol EJ, George BS, Kereiakes DJ. A randomized controlled trial of intravenous tissue plasminogen activator and early intravenous heparin in acute myocardial infarction. *Circulation* 1989;79:281–286.
76. Hsai J, Hamilton WP, Leiman N, Roberts R, Chaitman BR, Ross AM. A comparison between heparin and low dose aspirin as adjunctive therapy with tissue plasminogen activator for acute myocardial infarction. *N Engl J Med* 1990;323:1433–1437.
77. National Heart Foundation of Australia Coronary Thrombolysis Group. A randomized comparison of oral aspirin/dipyridamole versus intravenous heparin after rt-PA for acute myocardial infarction. *Circulation* 1989;80[Suppl II]:II-114.
78. Ohman EM, Califf RM, George BS, Quigley PJ, Kereiakes DJ,

Harrelson-Woodlief L, Candela RJ, Flanagan C, Stack RS, Topol EJ. The use of intraaortic balloon pumping as an adjunct to reperfusion therapy in acute myocardial infarction. *Am Heart J* 1991;121:895–901.

79. Ishihara M, Sato H, Tateishi H, Uchida T, Dote K. Intraaortic balloon pumping as the postangioplasty strategy in acute myocardial infarction. *Am Heart J* 1991;122:385–389.

80. Reimer KA, Lowe JE, Rasmussen MM, Jennings RB. The wavefront phenomenon of ischemic cell death: myocardial infarct size vs. duration of coronary occlusion in dogs. *Circulation* 1977;56:786–794.

81. Ellis SG, O'Neill WW, Bates ER, Walton JA, Nabel EG, Werns SW, Topol EJ. Implications for patient triage from survival and left ventricular functional recovery analyses in 500 patients treated with coronary angioplasty for acute myocardial infarction. *J Am Coll Cardiol* 1989;13:1251–1259.

82. Topol EJ. Thrombolytic intervention. In: Topol EJ, ed. *Textbook of Interventional Cardiology.* Philadelphia: WB Saunders; 1990

Practical Angioplasty,
edited by David P. Faxon.
Raven Press, Ltd., New York © 1993.

CHAPTER 13

Assessment of Early and Late Success After Percutaneous Transluminal Coronary Angioplasty

Walter R. M. Hermans, David P. Foley, Benno J. Rensing,
Carlo di Mario, and Patrick W. Serruys

Since its introduction by Andreas Gruentzig in 1977 as an alternative to coronary artery bypass grafting (CABG), percutaneous transluminal coronary angioplasty (PTCA) has emerged as a widely accepted treatment modality for patients with coronary artery disease (1). In 1991 alone, more than 400,000 patients have been treated worldwide, and most likely the annual number will increase further. Major improvements in angioplasty hardware and operator experience, have resulted in a high primary success rate (more than 90%) and low complication rate (4% to 5%: death, nonfatal myocardial infarction, acute bypass operation) despite extension of the indication to include patients with unstable angina, multivessel disease, and totally occluded vessels (2).

Despite the therapeutic success of coronary angioplasty, the exact mechanism of dilatation remains speculative and apparently involves multiple processes, including endothelial denudation, cracking and splitting or disruption of the intima and atherosclerotic plaque, dehiscence of the intima and plaque from the underlying media, and stretching or tearing of the media with persistent aneurysmal dilatation of the media and adventitia (3–7). Furthermore, the mechanisms of vessel wall reaction to the induced injury are only partially understood.

A patient treated with coronary angioplasty is at risk for two major coronary events: abrupt vessel closure and recurrence of stenosis.

WRM Hermans, DP Foley, BJ Rensing, C di Mario, and PW Serruys: Catheterization Laboratory, Thoraxcenter, Erasmus University, Rotterdam, The Netherlands.

Abrupt Vessel Closure

The reported incidence of acute coronary artery occlusion varies, depending on the definition, from 2% to 11% (8,9,10). It is the major cause of in-hospital PTCA-related morbidity and mortality and has restricted application of this technique to centers where surgical standby can be provided or is readily accessible. The mechanisms of abrupt coronary artery occlusion are multifactorial and include (i) mechanical obstruction due to intimal dissection, (ii) elastic recoil following dilatation, (iii) platelet adhesion and aggregation with ensuing intracoronary thrombus formation, (iv) subintimal hemorrhage, and (v) vasoconstriction or frank spasm of the disease-free wall (3,7,11–14). It is not always possible to distinguish between these mechanisms by angiography, and they often occur in combination. However, it is likely that occlusive dissection accounts for the vast majority of abrupt coronary artery occlusion. Although acute coronary occlusion during PTCA is unpredictable in the individual patient, it appears that gender (female), symptomatic status (unstable angina) and the severity, extent, and complexity of coronary artery lesions are important preprocedural factors (8–10).

Recurrence of Stenosis

One of the main areas of interest in interventional cardiology, at present, is the understanding, and ultimate prevention, of restenosis after coronary angioplasty. Recurrence of stenosis after initially successful PTCA is the major limitation of PTCA and restricts the long-term

TABLE 1. *Summary of studies using multivariate analysis techniques to find variables with increased risk for restenosis*

References	Patients	Angiographic follow-up[a] (%)	Definition of restenosis	Restenosis	Risk factors Patient	Risk factors Lesion	Risk factors Procedural
Holmes (17)	665	84%	NHLBI I or IV	34% of pts	Male Severity of angina No history of MI	Bypass graft	—
Mata[b] (19)	63	96%	↑ DS > 30% or DS >70%	23% of lesions	—	LAD or LCX > RCA Calcified stenosis % DS post-PTCA (40% vs 20%)	bar 0.9 vs. bar 1.1
Leimgruber (20)	1758	57%	>50% DS	30% of pts	Unstable angina	LAD ↑ %DS post-PTCA	Absence of intimal dissection gradient >15 mmhg
Myler[c] (21)	286	57%	>50% DS	57% of pts 43% of lesions	Diabetes Hypercholesterolemia New onset angina Current smoking	>95% DS pre-PTCA	↑ max pressure
Guiteras Val (22)	181	98%	↑ ≥30% DS	28% of pts 25% of lesions	Variant angina Multivessel disease	↑ % DS post-PTCA low Δ %DS pre-post	
Vandormael[c] (23)	209	62%	>50% DS	50% of pts	Male Diabetes	Proximal LAD Longer lesions	—
de Feyter[d] (24)	179	88%	>50% DS	32% of pts	Worsening AP or post-MI AP	—	—
Fleck (25)	110	86%	Δ MLCA >1 mm² (QCA)	44% of lesions	—	—	—
Halon[d] (26)	84	56%	>70% DS	25%	—	Multiple irregularities Decrease in coronary perfusion	—
Quigley[e] (27)	114	88%	>50% DS	32% of pts	Unstable angina Hypertension Diabetes	—	—
Renkin (28)	278	47%[c]	>50% DS	—	—	MLD post-PTCA	—
Rupprecht (29)	676	70%	>50% DS or loss of >50% of gain	29% of pts	Unstable angina	↑ %DS pre-PTCA ↑ %DS post-PTCA	long single inflation
Bourassa (30)	376	66%	≥50% DS + Δ 10% ↑ post-Fup	36% of pts 35% of lesions	Severity of angina	Length >10 mm %DS post-PTCA	
Hirshfeld (32)	694	74%	≥50% DS	40% of lesions	—	Length >10 mm Vein graft LAD % DS pre-PTCA % DS post-PTCA	bar 1.1–1.3

[a] Percentage of successfully dilated patients with angiographic follow-up.
[b] Multivessel dilatation.
[c] Multilesion dilatation.
[d] Unstable angina.
[e] For restenosis.
*****) = review of patients with clinical recurrence; **) = angiography + exercise thallium scintigraphy.

AP, angina pectoris; bar, balloon artery ratio; DS, diameter stenosis; Fup, follow-up; LAD, left anterior descending artery; LC, left circumflex; MI, myocardial infarction; Δ MLCA, change in minimal cross-sectional area; MLD, minimal luminal diameter; NHLBI, National Heart Lung Blood Institute classification; pts, patients; RCA, right coronary artery; ↑, increase; ↓, decrease; max, maximal; Δ, change; QCA, quantitative coronary analysis.

benefit of the procedure. Restenosis occurs in 17% to 40% of all dilated lesions, this variability being mainly a consequence of the completeness of angiographic follow-up, as well as of the criterion by which restenosis is defined (angiographic, clinical, physiologic). The patho-logical process of restenosis is usually completed within 2 to 5 months after the procedure, and rarely continues after 6 months (15–32). In the last 10 years, attempts to retard the rate of this late complication of PTCA have failed. Although many risk factors for restenosis have

TABLE 2. *Proposed primary success criteria*

Author (ref.)	YEAR	Angiographic criteria		Other criteria
		Diameter gain at PTCA (%)	Residual diameter post-PTCA (%)	
Grüentzig (51)	1983	≥20	—	Elimination of symptoms
Holmes (17)	1984	≥20	—	No in-hospital CABG
Kent (52)	1984	≥20	—	Absence of MI, death, CABG during hospitalization
Faxon (53)	1984	≥20	—	
Faxon (53)	1984	≥40	—	
O'Neill (54)	1984			Increase in CFR ≥ 1.2 gradient ≤ 25% of MAP
Meier (55)	1984	≥20	—	Functional improvement
Corcos (56)	1985	≥20	≤60%	
Levine (57)	1985	≥20	—	No complications (unspecified)
Mata (19)	1985	≥20	≤60%	
Kaltenbach (18)	1985	≥20		
Wijns (58)	1985	—	≤50%,	With good run-off and filling of the distal vessel
Serruys (59)	1985		≤50%	Elimination of symptoms
				Mean pressure gradient across the stenosis, normalized for MAP ≤ 0.2
Leimgruber (20)	1986	≥20	—	Absence of MI, CABG, in-hospital death
Bertrand (60)	1986	≥20	—	No complications (unspecified)
Vandormael (23)	1987	≥30	<50%	No in-hospital complications and functional improvement
Myler (21)	1987	≥35	<50%	Gradient less than 15 mmHg + absence of major in-hospital complications
Guiteras Val (22)	1987	≥20	—	Without procedure-related complications
de Feyter (24)	1988	—	<50%	Or transstenotic gradient index reduced to <0.30 +
				Relieve of acute ischemic symptoms, no death or CABG
Halon (26)	1989	≥20	<50%	—
Quigley (27)	1989	—	<50%	
Renkin (28)	1990	≥20	<50%	No major in-hospital complications
Rupprecht (29)	1990	≥20	<50%	—
				No major in-hospital complications

CABG, coronary artery bypass graft; CFR, coronary flow reserve; MAP, mean aortic pressure; MI, myocardial infarction.

been identified (Table I), most are difficult to influence and it seems to be impossible to reliably predict which patients or vessel segments will develop restenosis. Despite many well-designed and well-executed clinical trials of antithrombotic, antiproliferative, antiinflammatory, antispastic and lipid-lowering agents in the last 8 years (Table 2) (33–38), a pharmacological solution has not been reached. In addition, none of the new devices which have been developed to combat restenosis, including directional atherectomy (39–42), excimer laser (43,44), endoluminal prothesis of various design and content (45–47) or rotational angioplasty (48,49) have succeeded in achieving this goal. At present, it appears that although these devices will not replace "good old balloon angioplasty," each could find a niche and become the treatment of choice in specific circumstances. They include:

1. Any stent: for diseased saphenous veins, or for abrupt vessel closure following balloon angioplasty, or for lesions refractory to other devices.
2. Excimer laser in type C lesions or abrupt closure.
3. Directional atherectomy in complex, ulcerated lesions, particularly in large vessels not suitable for balloon angioplasty.

4. Rotational angioplasty for calcified or tortuous vessels not amenable to angioplasty or other techniques, or for a chronic total occlusion with a guidewire across lesion but a balloon will not advance.
5. Transluminal extraction catheter for degenerated saphenous vein grafts (50).

The ultimate answer as to whether these devices have a place in the treatment of coronary lesions, depends on the outcome of currently ongoing randomized trials comparing the various devices with balloon angioplasty with regard to acute and late outcome.

This chapter deals with the problem of how to assess early and late outcome after percutaneous transluminal coronary balloon angioplasty (and of any other interventional device). In theory, success may be defined according to four different approaches:

1. Symptomatic: subjective appraisal of the frequency and severity of ischemic episodes.
2. Functional: noninvasive diagnostic tests of myocardial perfusion using exercise or pharmacological stressors to develop and detect ischemia, using electrocardiogram echocardiographic or cardiac nuclear techniques.

3. Hemodynamic: coronary flow reserve, pressure-flow characteristics in the affected vessel.
4. Anatomic: degree of luminal narrowing, coronary angiography, intravascular ultrasound.

ASSESSMENT OF EARLY SUCCESS AFTER PTCA

The criteria for primary success after PTCA are reported in Table 2 and depicted in chronological sequence of their adoption into clinical practice (17–29,51–60). In the early years of PTCA, the majority of these cite the percent diameter of stenosis before PTCA in evaluating the outcome of the procedure, considering a reduction in diameter stenosis by 20% or more [>30% Vandormael (23), >40% Faxon (53)] sufficient to declare success. Several authors use the previous definition in combination with a second angiographic definition in evaluating the short-term efficacy of PTCA, namely a residual stenosis diameter of either less than 50% or less than 60% immediately after dilatation.

In addition to the above, most of the quoted authors require that no major complications become evident during the procedure itself or the convalescence period (such as in-hospital death, myocardial infarction, or need for emergency bypass surgery).

In the last 3 years, several restenosis prevention trials have defined the PTCA procedure as successful if the dilated lesion had a stenosis diameter of less than 50% (irrespective of the diameter gain) on visual assessment of the post-PTCA angiogram, without major procedural complications (death, nonfatal myocardial infarction, and emergency CABG) (35,36,61,62). Where these complications occurred during the in-hospital stay, the outcome of the PTCA was still defined as successful.

Symptomatic Criteria

Although the subjective improvement of symptoms (clinical status) after PTCA is probably the most desirable end point, it is also the least objective method of evaluation of success (63). The frequency of symptomatic improvement appears to be lower than that of angiographic success; only 80% to 85% of the patients with satisfactory angiographic result immediately post-PTCA exhibit such an improvement (64). Incomplete revascularizations or noncardiac chest pain, are two possible explanations for not having relief of symptoms in all patients having angiographically successful angioplasty.

Functional Criteria

In the immediate post-PTCA period, 7% of the patients continue to show an abnormal exercise ECG test or thallium scintigram after an angiographically successful PTCA. On the other hand, 52% of patients still have an abnormal ECG-gated radionuclide ventriculography after successful PTCA (65,66). This apparent inconsistency may be related to the mechanism of angioplasty, the time interval between PTCA and noninvasive diagnostic testing, and/or the test's sensitivity. As a general rule, there is an inverse relation between sensitivity and specificity for most indirect noninvasive tests, thereby limiting their clinical reliability (67,68). Although coronary luminal diameter is increased angiographically and symptoms of coronary insufficiency may be relieved by PTCA, a residual stenosis is always present as the atherosclerotic plaque itself is not totally obliterated (Fig. 1). Therefore, sensitive diagnostic tests in the immediate post-PTCA period, such as exercise radionuclide ventriculography, might still show minor abnormalities of left ventricular function during stress in areas with minimally compromised coronary blood flow.

Hemodynamic Criteria
Transstenotic Pressure Drop

Before low-profile balloon catheter shafts (<4F) and large-lumen guiding catheters became available for use in daily practice, adequate visualization of the post-PTCA result was at times difficult, and the early operators depended heavily on the reduction of translesional gradient to assess their result. Fluid dynamics models suggest that the translesional gradient should be inversely proportional to the fourth power of the stenosis diameter and directly proportional to the square of the rate of blood flow through the stenosis (69). However, the value of these measurements in assessing the physiologic significance of coronary stenoses, even those obtained with the smallest catheters, must be questioned.

First of all, the arterial translesional pressure gradient is affected by phasic changes in blood flow (Fig. 2): the maximal pressure gradient across a coronary stenosis occurs in early diastole (70,71), which is consistent with the finding that the pressure drop increases in a curvilinear fashion with increasing flow (72,73). Thus, within a narrowed segment, blood velocity increases and pressure decreases in accordance with Bernoulli's law.

Second, progressive miniaturization of the balloon catheter has facilitated the angioplasty procedure but precluded a reliable measurement of distal pressure.

Third, because of the physical presence of the dilation catheter across the stenotic cross section, the remaining vessel luminal area is further reduced and as a result blood flow through the obstruction is impeded (70,74). In fact, the measured pressure drop overestimates the true pressure difference across the stenosis in a predictable manner, which is dependant on the ratio of the diameter of the angioplasty catheter over the stenosis diam-

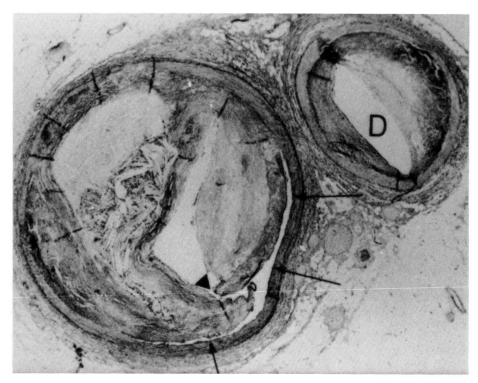

FIG. 1. Cross section through the proximal part of the left anterior descending artery and adjacent diagonal branch (D), of a 65-year-old woman who died accidentally immediately after PTCA. The atherosclerotic plaque shows disruption and splitting (*arrowhead*), and is dissected and lifted from the media (*arrows*). A hemorrhagic area within the plaque opposite the split has an appearance which suggests that its occurrence predates PTCA. Apart from an atherosclerotic narrowing of the lumen, the diagonal branch (D) does not show other changes. From Soward et al. (97), with permission.

eter (70,74,75). Comparison of balloon catheter measurements with a high-fidelity (HiFi) miniaturized tip transducer, showed that the HiFi transstenotic pressure drop measurements were markedly lower both before and after angioplasty than the corresponding measurements through the fluid-filled catheter lumen. Essentially, this difference is the result of using a catheter with a smaller shaft diameter (0.7 mm as opposed to about 1.0 to 1.2 mm for conventional balloon catheters).

Whereas the pressure distal to a coronary artery obstruction is dependent mainly on the severity of the stenosis and the amount of collateral flow to the corresponding myocardial region, it is entirely determined by the extent of this collateral circulation if antegrade flow is eliminated by an angioplasty catheter which totally obstructs the native vessel (76). The systolic translesional gradient defined as the difference between the proximal systolic pressure (measured through the guiding cath-

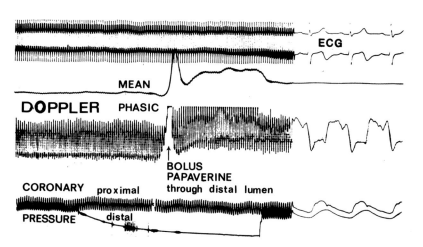

FIG. 2. Relationships of the translesional pressure gradient and the intracoronary Doppler blood flow velocity before and after 4 mg of intracoronary papaverine was administered distal to the stenotic lesion through the dilatation catheter lumen. It can be observed on the right-hand side of the tracing that the measured pressure gradient increases with increasing flow as a result of vasodilatation by papaverine. The changes in the tracings between the two arrows are artefactual, as a result of injection of papaverine.

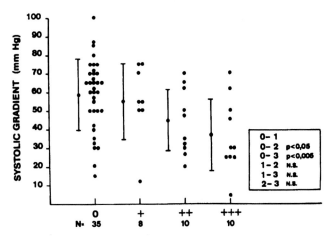

FIG. 3. Relation of the transstenotic pressure gradient to the extent of angiographically quantitated collateral circulation. The difference is significant, although there is a wide overlap. N, number of patients studied; O, no collaterals; +, just visible collaterals; ++, good visible collaterals; +++, contralateral vessel filled by collaterals; N.S., not statistically significant. From Probst (76), with permission.

eter) and the distal systolic pressure (measured by the dilation catheter) has a significant negative relation to the angiographically quantitated extent of the collateral circulation (Fig. 3); at the same time, patients with clearly visible collaterals before PTCA show a significantly higher recurrence rate relative to patients without angiographic evidence of collateral circulation (52% vs. 28%, $p < 0.05$) (76). Coronary artery wedge pressure, on the other hand, reflects not only visible but also potential (recruitable) collateral flow to the vessel segment distal to the inflated balloon (77). Data from Urban et al. show

that a high (≥ 30 mmHg) coronary wedge pressure during angioplasty is significantly associated with an increased incidence of restenosis (52% vs. 23%) as compared to a wedge pressure of less than 30 mmHg (78).

To summarize, current data suggest that the absolute value of the transstenotic pressure difference measured with a balloon catheter during catheterization does not accurately reflect the true pressure-flow-resistance characteristics across coronary lesions (74). However, recent technical developments (pressure guidewires) might reintroduce the practice of translesional pressure measurement.

Emanuellson et al. evaluated a newly constructed pressure sensor with a diameter of 0.45 mm in 15 patients undergoing balloon angioplasty (79). The sensor and an optic fiber were mounted on a 0.018-in guidewire, which was used in the angioplasty balloon catheter. The basic principle is that the sensor element modulates an optical reflection by pressure-induced elastic movements. The sensor is a relative pressure sensor, comparing the recorded pressure with the atmospheric pressure. Pressure gradients were recorded before and after PTCA. All pressure tracings were of satisfactory quality (Fig. 4). It can be used with every system over-the-wire (e.g., excimer laser and atherectomy), and in combination with a Doppler or intravascular ultrasound catheter it could be of great help for the evaluation of intravascular interventions. However, data correlating pressure gradients with the severity of lesions have to be awaited.

De Bruyne et al. tested *in vitro* and *in vivo* a new 0.015-in fluid-filled guidewire for distal pressure monitoring during PTCA. This new fluid-filled guidewire permits the measurements of the mean pressure and pressure

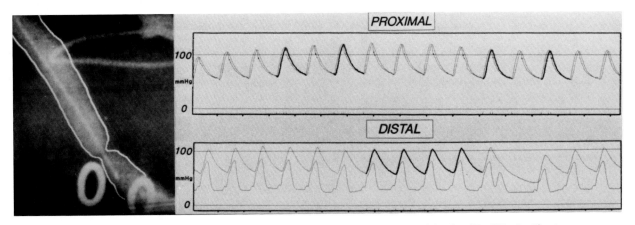

FIG. 4. A: The radiopaque, soft distal part of a 0.018-in pressure guidewire (RadiMedicalSystems, Uppsala, Sweden) is shown across a coronary stenosis. Note the relatively small dimension of the guidewire in comparison with the stenosis minimal lumen diameter, as measured using a computer-assisted automated edge detection technique (CAAS system, Pie Data, Maastricht, The Netherlands) (The minimal lumen diameter is 0.46 mm versus 1.30 mm, and the minimal cross-sectional area is 0.17 mm² versus 1.33 mm²). **B:** Coronary pressures recorded at baseline conditions through the guiding catheter and the micromachined optical sensor, positioned proximal (*upper tracing*) and distal to the stenosis (*lower tracing*). Note the large transtenotic gradient (mean gradient = 37 mmHg) with a prevalent diastolic component.

gradients across coronary stenoses and could aid in increasing the accuracy of angiographic assessment of coronary stenosis (80).

Blood Flow Velocity

With the recent invention and validation of a Doppler-tipped angioplasty guidewire (Cardiometrics, Inc, Mountain View, CA), selective measurement of blood flow velocity at the tip of a guidewire deep within a coronary artery and distal to the coronary stenosis became possible during coronary interventions.

Using this Doppler-tipped guidewire, Ofili et al. showed reversal of coronary blood flow velocity resulting from collateral flow development during angioplasty despite the absence of angiographically visible collaterals (Fig. 5) (81).

Using a Doppler probe mounted on the tip of an PTCA catheter, the effects of successive balloon inflations could be immediately evaluated by comparing the blood flow velocity recorded during peak reactive hyperemia (82). This approach, however, was limited by the persistence of the partially obstructive Doppler balloon catheter (cross-sectional area deflated = 0.68 mm²) at the site of the dilatation. Using a Doppler guidewire and a monorail technique, the balloon catheter can be withdrawn immediately after the inflation, as soon as the reappearance of antegrade flow is detected by the Doppler probe, as shown in Fig. 6. The peak increase in blood flow velocity during reactive hyperemia can be recorded with only the Doppler guidewire (CSA = 0.17 mm²) across the stenosis, and the increase in blood flow velocity after successive dilatations provides a direct functional assessment of the results of the procedure independent of angiography and immediately after inflation. The presence of the Doppler guidewire in the dilated artery distal to the lesion throughout the entire procedure makes it possible to monitor the development of flow-limiting complications (thrombus, intimal dissections, etc.).

Coronary Flow Reserve

The concept of coronary flow reserve as a functional measure of stenosis severity was initially proposed by Gould et al. (73). Two methodological approaches have

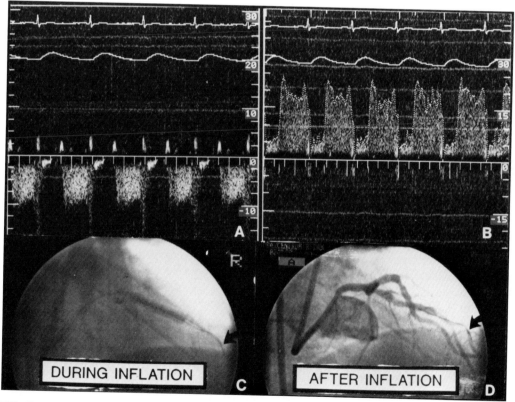

FIG. 5. A: Doppler recording distal to a severe stenosis of the left anterior descending artery during balloon inflation. The tip of the Doppler guidewire is indicated in the simultaneous fluoroscopy (**C**) by a curved arrow. Note the negative velocities observed before balloon dilatation, due to the presence of a well-developed collateral circulation from the right coronary artery. **B:** Reversal of flow, with a normal pattern of prevalent diastolic components, occurred after successful balloon dilatation and was subsequently confirmed with angiography (**D**).

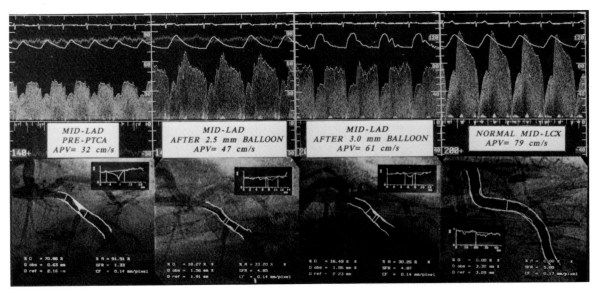

FIG. 6. Immediate assessment of the effects of balloon dilatation with a Doppler guidewire. The time-averaged maximal blood flow velocity (APV) is measured under conditions of peak reactive hyperemia immediately after balloon inflation and withdrawal of the balloon catheter (monorail technique) to avoid residual obstruction at the site of the dilatation. Note that the blood flow velocity recorded in the same position [middle segment of the left anterior descending artery distal to the stenosis (MID-LAD)] during pharmacologically induced maximal vasodilatation (PRE-PTCA, *left*) is half of the maximal flow after the final inflation with a 3-mm balloon. The blood velocity at peak reactive hyperemia is higher after the use of the 3-mm balloon than after the dilatation with a 2.5-mm balloon, in accordance with the further gain in minimal luminal diameter (from 1.56 mm to 1.86 mm) measured with quantitative coronary arteriography (ACA-DCI Philips). The peak effect of a pharmacologically induced (papaverine, 12.5 mg) maximal vaso-dilation in the angiographically normal left circumflex artery (LCX) is also shown for comparison on the right.

been developed to assess the flow reserve of individual coronary arteries in the clinical setting, and the definition of coronary flow reserve is therefore method-dependant.

The first approach uses quantitative coronary angiography to determine the pressure flow characteristics of coronary stenoses. Young et al. developed fluid dynamics equations that describe the relationship between the pressure distal to a stenosis and the flow (83,84). When coronary flow increases, the coronary perfusion pressure distal to the stenosis decreases in a nonlinear fashion. Kirkeeide et al. calculated a coronary flow reserve from the quantitative data (85). The major advantage of this approach is that it integrates multiple angiographically defined anatomical characteristics of a coronary stenosis into a single parameter. However, the effect of a coronary stenosis on blood flow is a response of an anatomic hemodynamic system in which the stenosis is but one component.

The second approach uses the ratio of maximal to resting coronary blood flow as a measure of coronary flow reserve (CFR). Temporary occlusion of a coronary artery, or potent pharmacological agents, can produce maximal coronary vasodilatation. This results in a hyperemic response characterized by a marked increase in

flow which gradually subsides (86,87,88). However, the pressure flow relationship during maximal vasodilatation varies substantially due to changes in other, unavoidable and unquantifiable variables, such as ventricular hypertrophy, heart rate, contractility, blood viscosity, and left ventricular end-diastolic pressure (89,90). This uncertainty limits the widespread clinical application of CFR, derived by current methods, in the description of coronary artery narrowing. We found this to be particularly true in the context of evaluation of the immediate effect of angiographically successful PTCA. In a recent study in unselected patients, the CFR values post-PTCA and at 24 hr, failed to reflect the changes in luminal diameter observed by quantitative angiography (91). These shortcomings do not decry the undoubted value of CFR measurements in selected patient, with single-vessel coronary artery disease and not in the setting of acute interventions, as previously shown in carefully selected patient subgroup (92,93).

Also for the assessment of restenosis post-PTCA, CFR has the attractive theoretical potential to provide a single measure of stenosis severity, taking into account the complete geometry of the stenosis.

A promising new technique measures the mean transit time of an injected contrast agent during maximum vasodilation, using videodensitometry, so that the variability of baseline blood flow is excluded, and an absolute physiological value is obtained (94). This method now needs to be objectively assessed in humans.

Anatomic Criteria

In view of the above, and with better coronary artery visualization provided by improvements in catheter design and radiographic imaging technology, coronary angiography has emerged as the most reliable method of judging the immediate (and late) results of intervention. However, there is the possibility of inaccuracy in luminal diameter measurements immediately after angioplasty because of the frequent inhomogeneous arterial opacification at the dilatation site, as a result of the passage of contrast material into split areas (Fig. 1) of the atherosclerotic plaque (3,7,95–99). In particularly, the presence of subintimal dissection can result in irregular angiographic vessel wall boundaries.

Visual Qualitative Assessment of Angiograms

Visual assessment of percentage diameter stenosis of a diseased coronary artery still remains the gold standard in more than 99% of centers performing coronary angiography (100,101). In addition, attempts to correlate closely the anatomy of a coronary stenosis and its physiologic significance by visual interpretation of cineangiograms are hampered by several serious shortcomings. The large intra- and interobserver variation (102–105), and lack of correlation with pathologic (106) and intraoperative (107) findings are well recognized. Furthermore, the reproducibility of visual lesion assessment is influenced by the severity of the coronary stenosis. In general, lesions with between 20% and 80% diameter obstruction (moderate lesions) have a wider range of intra- and interobserver variabilities than stenoses less than 20% or more than 80% (108). A recent report indicates that this variability may not be related to observer experience (108).

The accuracy of visual lesion assessment of coronary cineangiograms is limited in the range of the intermediate severity, where minor luminal changes in moderate lesions have major hemodynamic consequences. While resting coronary blood flow is not dramatically altered until an obstruction of at least 85% of the diameter is present, maximal coronary flow is already diminished by obstructions as small as 30%, and marked impairment of coronary flow reserve (CFR) occurs with the progression of diameter stenosis from 65% to 95% (109).

A recent report, where visual interpretation of coronary arteriograms was compared with quantitative coronary arteriographic assessment, confirmed earlier findings that (i) visual estimates of moderately severe stenosis were 30% higher than quantitatively measured actual percent diameter stenosis, (ii) visual estimates diagnosed significantly more three-vessel disease, and (iii) visual interpretation significantly overestimated initial lesion severity and underestimated stenosis severity after angioplasty (110,111).

Accurate determination of the degree of stenosis at this time can only be achieved *after* radiographic processing of cineangiograms; this prevents use of this information during interventional catheterization. However, practical semiautomated methods have been described (112,113) for measuring luminal dimensions from digital angiograms that allow immediate (on-line) quantitative analysis and assessment of results of intervention during catheterization. These software packages will soon be available for installation in all catheterization rooms.

Quantitative Coronary Angiography

Since visual interpretation of the coronary angiogram is a poor means of predicting the physiological importance of obstructive coronary artery disease (111), automatic quantification systems have been introduced in recent years to enhance objectivity and reproducibility in the assessment of coronary artery dimensions. These computer programs analyze the coronary lesion either by (i) automated border detection of the segment of interest (edge detection), or (ii) densitometric analysis of the radiographic image (using the concept that the density across an artery in a radiographic image is proportional to the cross-sectional area at that point) (114–116).

The Coronary Angiographic Analysis System (CAAS) has been in operation at the Thoraxcenter since 1982 and has been rigorously and extensively validated (117,118). An example of an analysis is shown in Fig. 7. Essentially, the boundaries of a selected coronary segment are detected automatically (so-called edge detection) from optically magnified and videodigitized regions of interest (512 × 512 pixels) of an end-diastolic cineframe. This step may soon be rendered unnecessary by the rapid development of on-line digital angiographic systems. Absolute diameter values are determined in millimeters, using the guiding catheter (each individual catheter tip is retained and measured by micrometer) as a scaling device. A correction factor is then introduced for the so-called pincushion distortion introduced by the image intensifier.

The problem of selecting a reference diameter is solved by using a computer-derived or interpolated reference diameter. By this technique the computer generates the original disease-free dimension of the segment of interest. From these absolute measurements (minimal luminal diameter-MLD, maximal luminal diameter, mean luminal diameter, and extent of obstruction) and

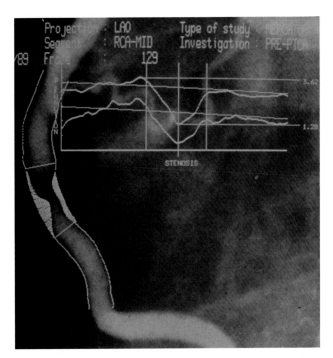

FIG. 7. The detected contours, together with the proximal and distal obstruction boundaries, for a mid lesion in the right coronary artery. The minimal lumen diameter is 1.28 mm, and the interpolated reference diameter is 3.23 (value not shown); these values correspond to a computed percentage diameter stenosis of 61% (value not shown). The difference in area (mm²) between the estimated outer contours and the detected luminal contours at the site of the obstruction, is a measure for the atherosclerotic plaque (*shaded area*).

the interpolated measurements obtained by the computer (symmetry, curvature, inflow-outflow angle, plaque area, roughness) many others may be derived, e.g., percent diameter stenosis, percent area stenosis, theoretical transstenotic pressure gradient, calculated poiseuille resistance and calculated turbulence resistance (Table 3) (119–122). The validity of the fluid dynamics equations used to describe the hemodynamics of a coronary stenosis based on quantitative arteriography has also been confirmed in the clinical setting (123). These derived hemodynamic parameters have been shown to correlate with the transstenotic pressure difference, and with exercise thallium 201 perfusion scintigraphy (124,125). In fact, as has been shown by Zijlstra, the calculated pressure drop over a stenosis as an integrated measurement of multiple angiographic dimensions, is a better anatomic predictor of the functional importance of a coronary stenosis than is percent diameter stenosis or obstruction area (126,127).

Although quantitative, computer-based analysis methods have enhanced objectivity, some pitfalls still exist. For one, the presence of overlapping branches interferes with the quantitative analysis of lesion severity from coronary angiograms. Also, a number of sources of variation in the angiographic data acquisition and analysis at different stages can be distinguished:

1. Pincushion distortion of image intensifier.
2. Differences in angles and height levels of x-ray systems.
3. Differences in vasomotor tone.
4. Variation in quality of mixing of contrast agent with blood.
5. The catheter used as scaling device (angiographic quality, influence of contrast in catheter tip on the calibration factor, size of catheter).
6. Deviations in the size of catheter as listed by the manufacturer from its actual size.
7. Variation in data analysis (reference diameter, length of analyzed segment, frame selection) (128,129).

Furthermore, assessment of the percentage area of stenosis from diameter measurements obtained from a single angiographic view assumes a symmetric circular cross section, an assumption which will not always be true. In a previous study in which 120 lesions were analyzed in several orthogonal projections, asymmetric lesions were seen in more than half of the cases (130). So, atherosclerotic disease does not always involve the entire circumference of the vessel, but instead frequently results in an asymmetrical or eccentric lesion. In fact, it has been estimated that approximately 70% of coronary artery stenoses are eccentric rather than concentric in nature (131). In addition, a previous study by our group has suggested that changes in the luminal area of an artery that are produced by the mechanical disruption of its internal wall as a result of angioplasty cannot be assessed accurately from the detected contours of the vessel from a single plane angiographic view (124). The diagnostic

TABLE 3. *Formulas for computation of various hemodynamic parameters following quantitative analysis of a coronary stenosis*

$$R_p = C_1 \cdot \frac{\text{obstruction length}}{\text{obstruction area}^2}$$

where $C_1 = 8 \cdot \pi \cdot$ (blood viscosity)

Blood viscosity = 0.03 g/cm · s

$$R_t = C_2 \cdot \left(\frac{1}{\text{obstruction area}} - \frac{1}{\text{normal distal area}} \right)^2$$

where $C_2 = \dfrac{\text{blood density}}{0.266}$

Blood density = 1.0 [g/cm³]

$$P_{grad} = Q \cdot (R_p + Q \cdot R_t)$$

where Q = mean coronary blood flow (ml/s)

P_{grad} = theoretical pressure gradient; R_p = Poiseuille resistance; R_t = turbulent resistance.

value of this type of measurement is restricted by the fact that dilatation frequently results in irregular angiographic vascular wall outlines, so that the cross-sectional area derived from the detected contours of the vessel will overestimate the true luminal cross-sectional area. To overcome this limitation, the use of videodensitometry to compute cross-sectional areas is advocated.

Videodensitometry assesses the relative area of a stenosis by comparing the density of contrast in the diseased and normal segments. The advantage here is that only a single view is required; this, however, must be perfectly perpendicular to the long axis of the vessel and there must be no overlapping or closely parallel sidebranches or other disturbing radiopaque structures. Only relative measurements are provided, so that edge detection data are also necessary to provide absolute measurements. A further drawback of this otherwise promising technique is its high sensitivity (more than that of edge detection) to x-ray scatter, veiling glare, beam hardening, and suboptimal contrast filling of the vessels.

Intravascular Imaging Techniques

Although contrast angiography remains the method of choice for quantitative assessment of atherosclerotic disease, it is a less than ideal reference standard because of limitations in

1. Detection of early or minimal atherosclerotic disease.
2. Differentiation of eccentric from concentric plaques.
3. Identification of plaque composition.
4. Detection of plaque ulceration or dissection.
5. Identification of thrombus.

Fiberoptic angioscopy is nonquantitative and difficult to use, but appears to be highly accurate in identifying intravascular thrombus and intimal disruption (132). Intravascular ultrasound has the potential for precisely quantitating the severity of atherosclerosis, assessing lesion composition, and identifying lesion disruption and dissection after coronary interventions (133–139). When comparing angiography, angioscopy, and ultrasound imaging after angioplasty, intimal tears, subintimal hemorrhage, intimal flaps, and arterial dissection were found at the angioplasty site by angioscopy and intravascular ultrasound, but were not detected by angiography (134). It is clear that the type of information derived from the three imaging techniques is quite different and that each may have a specific role in intravascular diagnosis and assessment of intracoronary interventions. An example of large dissection flap detected with intravascular ultrasound but not with angiography is shown in Fig. 8.

Although there is a great promise for intravascular ultrasound, limitations such as loss of image quality in severely diseased or heavily calcified vessels, as well as technical drawbacks with respect to size of the devices, hinder its general applicability (140).

Summary

On-line assessment of coronary flow reserve and digital angiographic analysis will emerge as the assessment

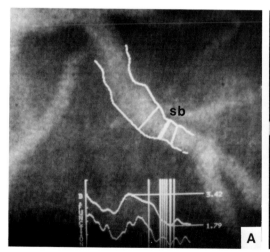 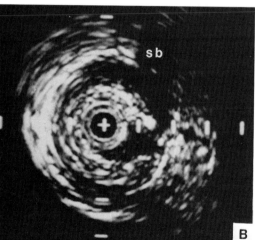

FIG. 8. A: Cineangiogram of a left circumflex artery after balloon dilatation. The contours of the vessel lumen are automatically detected and displayed in the diameter function in the lower part of the cineangiogram. The thick line indicates the position of the echographic catheter, and the large side branch (sb) visible in the echographic image is indicated. Note that no angiographic evidence of arterial dissection can be observed. **B:** Echographic intravascular cross section of a left circumflex artery after balloon dilatation. The presence of a dissection flap surrounded by a crescent-shaped false lumen is evident from seven o'clock to three o'clock in the image on the right. At eleven o'clock, a large side branch (sb) opens in the false lumen.

tools for any intervention in the near future, so that eye-balling of the stenosis will disappear. New angiographic guidelines will emerge from quantitative angiographic studies.

ASSESSMENT OF LATE SUCCESS AFTER PTCA

Before going into detail on how to assess the long-term effect of a successful coronary angioplasty, we first have to address the issue of restenosis. We believe that the word restenosis refers to the process by which a blood vessel tends to renarrow following the mechanical injury imparted by a balloon (or other device). This process of response to injury appears to consist of three components: elastic recoil, fibrocellular neointimal hyperplasia, and platelet deposition and mural thrombus formation.

Elastic Recoil

This refers to the ability of intact blood vessels to respond to mechanical stretch and has only recently been recognized by quantitative angiography (12–14,141, 142) and intravascular ultrasound (IVUS) (143). Objective data are scanty and conflicting but suggest that recoil occurs immediately following balloon deflation and has a doubtful contribution to the process of early and late restenosis (14,141,142). Recently, in a group of 70 patients, who underwent angiography 24 hr after PTCA, no significant differences were detected in minimal luminal diameter, minimal cross-sectional area, or reference diameter when comparing values immediately after dilatation and 24 hr later (unpublished observation).

Fibrocellular Neointimal Hyperplasia

Intimal hyperplasia is still regarded as the main pathological process by which progressive luminal renarrowing develops in the months following PTCA (144–160). Forrester et al. hypothesized that restenosis is a manifestation of the general wound healing process expressed specifically in vascular tissue (161). The temporal response to injury occurs in three characteristic phases: inflammation, granulation, and extracellular matrix remodeling. The major milestones in the temporal sequence of restenosis are platelet aggregation, inflammatory cell infiltration, release of growth factors, medial smooth muscle cell modulation and proliferation, protoglycan deposition, and extracellular matrix remodeling. Migration and replication of medial smooth muscle cells into a developing neointima is the cornerstone of

restenosis. Several growth factors have been described which appear to have a role in the restenosis process. However, the identity of the key factors and their exact actions are unknown.

Platelet Deposition and Mural Thrombus Formation

It has been accepted for some time that platelet deposition and mural thrombus formation are responsible—in combination with dissection—for the early restenosis seen shortly after coronary angioplasty. However, Schwartz et al. have recently put forward a new restenosis model, where platelets and thrombus play a central role and in which platelets are the main factor responsible for late restenosis (162). They observed in a porcine coronary injury model the universal presence of mural thrombus, which undergones endothelialization, then infiltration by mononuclear cells from the luminal aspect outward. Following this, cells staining positive for alpha actin (smooth muscle cells or myofibroblasts) appear on the luminal side of the degenerating surface (indicating that their origin in this model is apparently not the media at the site of damaged artery), and begin to migrate. They concluded that the magnitude of the luminal narrowing process may derive more from the volume of local mural thrombus at the site of arterial injury than from uncontrolled cellular proliferation.

Problems in Defining Restenosis

It is clear that the restenosis process is not well understood at the present time. This is the reason why there have been at least 13 different definitions, based on coronary angiographic findings applied by various clinical investigators attempting to address the problem of restenosis. These clinical studies in recent years have reported restenosis rates ranging between 25% and 55% (Table 1). This variation can be explained by the fact that

1. Angiographic follow-up ranges between 57% and 100%.
2. Time to follow-up ranges between 1 and 9 months.
3. Thirteen different criteria of restenosis have been applied (Table 5).
4. Visual assessment of the coronary angiogram is used in most studies (163).

Approaches to the Detection of Restenosis

As with the determination of early success of PTCA, maintained success or its counterpart, restenosis, may be evaluated by symptomatic criteria, functional criteria, and anatomic criteria.

Symptomatic Criteria

Maintained improvement in quality of life is the goal of any therapeutic treatment modality, but, as previously mentioned, it is also the least objective evaluation of success. The reappearance of angina as the criterion of restenosis underestimates the angiographic rate of restenosis, since the reported incidence of silent restenosis may be as high as 31% (164). Recently Califf et al. described that in studies with a high rate of angiographic follow-up, the probability that patients with symptoms had restenosis (positive predictive value) ranged from 48% to 92%, whereas the probability that patients without symptoms were free of restenosis (negative predictive value) ranged from 70% to 98% (165). The low positive predictive value found in many of these studies may be explained by the presence of other mechanisms of angina, such as incomplete revascularization or progression of disease in other vessels. In view of the above considerations, the usefulness of symptomatic criteria for the detection of restenosis is, at best, limited.

The paradox of angiographic recurrent stenosis in the absence of clinical symptoms can be explained, in part, by looking more closely at the definition of restenosis used. If restenosis is said to be present when there is a loss of at least 50% of the initial diameter gain, a 60% diameter stenosis that is reduced to 10% by angioplasty assumes recurrence with a diameter stenosis of 35% at follow-up. It is not surprising that such a patient is likely to be asymptomatic, since a diameter stenosis of 35% is usually not hemodynamically significant.

Functional Criteria

As far as detection of restenosis by noninvasive diagnostic tests is concerned, it can be said that in general an abnormal exercise ECG response or myocardial perfusion defect(s) on a thallium 201 (^{201}Tl) scintigram is either associated with an angiographically demonstrable restenosis of the dilated segment or is the result of the presence of additional disease (166–169). However, coronary collaterals to the myocardial region supplied by the dilated but restenosed vessel may provide adequate circulation to prevent exercise-induced thallium perfusion defects (170–174).

ECG Exercise Testing

Several studies have examined the ability of the exercise test to detect restenosis after coronary angioplasty. These studies have generally found that the presence of exercise-induced ST-segment depression, angina on exercise, or both are not highly predictive of restenosis,

whether the test is performed early or late after angioplasty. The positive predictive value of early exercise testing ranges from 29% to 60%, and the corresponding value for late exercise testing ranges from 39% to 64% (165,175). These low values are most likely a consequence of incomplete revascularization. It is, however, also possible that the noninvasive test accurately demonstrates a functionally inadequate dilatation, despite the appearance of angiographic success.

Thallium Scintigraphy

The positive predictive value of thallium scintigraphy for detection of restenosis, in series with a variable angiographic follow-up, ranged from 37% to 100% (165). Since coronary angiography is the gold standard for detection of restenosis in these studies, the reported value of a noninvasive test is determined not only by the actual accuracy of the test but also by the completeness of angiographic follow-up. In studies with a high angiographic follow-up rate, the negative predictive value of thallium scintigraphy varies between 42% and 100%. Tomographic imaging of nuclear scintigrams may prove superior to planar imaging for the detection of restenosis (176).

Of practical interest in this regard, a recent study (177), albeit in a small series of patients, suggests that exercise ^{201}Tl tomoscintigraphy with rest reinjection may be a useful means of detecting restenosis and would appear to be worthy of larger, more detailed, prospective studies along similar lines of design.

Anatomic Criteria

Although contrast angiography is still the gold standard, intracoronary biopsies and intravascular ultrasound imaging emerge as two new modalities of investigation in the early and late assessment of any intervention.

Intravascular Ultrasound

As stated earlier, intravascular ultrasound (IVUS) has the potential to offer new insights into the mechanisms, complications, and long-term results of coronary interventions. However, before IVUS can be accepted as an alternative to arteriography, several significant limitations need to be overcome. In particular, the size and relative inflexibility of the current devices prevent their routine use. In addition, the safety and accuracy of IVUS has yet to be demonstrated in clinical studies (143).

Histology

On-line in vivo histological assessment of biopsies taken with the atherectomy catheter is currently the only approach which can discriminate between classic atherosclerosis and fibrocellular hyperplasia. However, to what extent single biopsy samples represent the lesion as a whole is still undetermined. Although this technique is only applicable in a subset of patients with a lesion suitable for atherectomy treatment, it does offer an additional perspective. Some authors have suggested that there may be a relationship between the cellular density of the atherectomy specimen or the growth rate and migratory rate of these cells in culture and the later development of restenosis (178–182).

Coronary Angiography

In view of the above, coronary angiography is still the most objective and reliable means of assessing the long-term outcome of coronary interventions. As explained earlier, a quantitative computer-based analysis technique enhances objectivity, while it reduces the problem of high inter- and intraobserver variability inherent to visual interpretation of the coronary cineangiogram.

What Has Been Learned from Studies Using Quantitative Coronary Analysis?

Two virtually simultaneous studies addressing the issue of luminal changes in the months following PTCA, using coronary angiography at different preselected follow-up intervals, gave remarkably similar results (Fig. 9) (15,16). In the study carried out at the Thoraxcenter, the (mean) minimal lumen diameter increased slightly from

TABLE 4. *Criteria for angiographic restenosis in current use*

1. Loss of >30% diameter stenosis from post-PTCA to follow-up (NHLBI I).
2. An immediate post-PTCA diameter stenosis <50% and a diameter stenosis >70% at follow-up (NHLBI II).
3. A return to within 10% of the pre-PTCA diameter stenosis (NHLBI III).
4. Loss at follow-up of at least 50% of the initial gain after PTCA (NHLBI IV).
5. Loss of >20% diameter stenosis from post-PTCA to follow-up.
6. An immediate post-PTCA diameter stenosis <50% that increases to >50% at follow-up.
7. A diameter stenosis >50% at follow-up.
8. A diameter stenosis >70% at follow-up.
9. Area stenosis >85% at follow-up.
10. Loss of >1 mm² in stenosis area from post-PTCA to follow-up (25).
11. A change of ≥0.72 mm in minimal luminal diameter from post-PTCA to follow-up (15).
12. A change of ≥0.50 mm in minimal luminal diameter from post-PTCA to follow-up (16).
13. Diameter stenosis >50% at follow-up of a successfully dilated lesion (defined as diameter stenosis <50%, and a gain of >10% in luminal diameter, immediately after PTCA), excluding lesions with a <10% deterioration in diameter stenosis since PTCA (30).

2.06 mm directly after angioplasty to 2.11 mm at 30 days; it then decreased steadily to 1.93, 1.77, 1.69, and 1.82 mm at subsequent follow-up times (2, 3, 4, 5 months). Nobuyoshi et al. restudied 229 patients at 24 hr, and 1, 3, 6, and 12 months. Their findings were very similar to those from the Thoraxcenter. In addition, Nobuyshi found that lesion progression after 6 months was unusual. These data demonstrate a striking resemblance to the pattern of intimal hyperplasia after vascular injury in animals, which reaches a peak at 4 to 12 weeks (144–146).

A Continuous Approach to the Assessment of Restenosis

There have been recent claims that luminal renarrowing following PTCA follows a bimodal distribution. If this is true it would rationalize a categorical approach to the definition of restenosis. The angiographic studies of Serruys et al. and Nobuyshi et al. suggest the contrary: that restenosis is a continuous phenomenon affecting all dilated lesion to some degree and some more than others. Postmortem studies, although limited to small numbers, are consistent with these angiographic findings. The issue has recently been resolved by the clear demonstration, in a series of 1,445 lesions treated by PTCA with angiographic follow-up in 91%, that the change in minimal luminal diameter during follow-up and the percent diameter stenosis at follow-up follow a Gaussian or normal distribution (183). This study con-

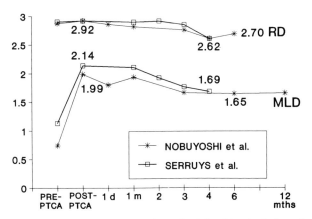

FIG. 9. Graphic representation of minimal luminal diameter (MLD) and reference diameter (RD) values as reported in the studies of Nobuyoshi et al. and Seruys et al. Virtually identical time trends are seen during 6-month follow-up.

clusively illustrates that the use of categorical criteria to define restenosis is misleading, even if these are derived from quantitative techniques. In the light of this evidence, the existence of more than 13 different categorical criteria (Table 4) can also be understood, since any arbitrary cutoff point may be selected and justified as necessary in attempts to divide patients, after PTCA, into two distinct groups, when in reality they form one group and must be described as such. We believe that results of intervention trials may now be much more elegantly presented in graphic form, with cumulative distribution curves displaying change in minimal luminal diameter (MLD) during follow-up for treated versus placebo populations (35) or indeed for PTCA versus stent, atherectomy, or laser.

Clinical Application of Minimal Lumen Diameter

A strong correlation between the threshold for exercise-induced myocardial ischemia (using thallium 201 tomoscintigraphy) and an absolute value for minimal luminal diameter of 1.4 mm has been suggested (184). In an ancillary study of the CARPORT trial, 350 patients who underwent successful PTCA for single-vessel disease and had exercise testing and repeat coronary angiography at follow-up, we found that an MLD of 1.45 mm correlates with the threshold for recurrence of angina pectoris (72%). Exercise-induced ST-segment depression was a less reliable predictor of luminal renarrowing, although the point of greatest diagnostic accuracy for a

positive exercise test also corresponded with a measured MLD of 1.45 mm (Fig. 10). This preliminary information suggests that, as the ultimate measure of long-term success of PTCA, the absolute value of MLD at follow-up may prove to be an even more useful clinical parameter than change in MLD during follow-up (185).

Summary

Coronary angiography is still the gold standard for evaluation of the long-term outcome of PTCA. Carefully controlled angiographic techniques and a quantitative assessment system must now be considered a prerequisite for any clinical study of coronary interventions.

ACKNOWLEDGMENT

The authors gratefully acknowledge the statistical advice of Jan GP Tijssen, PH.D. and the secretarial assistance of Hanneke Roerade.

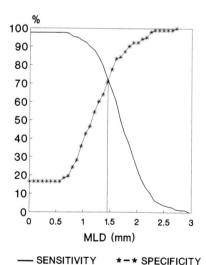

FIG. 10. Percentage correct classification of recurrence of angina (sensitivity) and percentage correct classification of absence of angina at follow-up (specificity) as a function of cutoff points for the different quantitative angiographic parameters. The point of intersection of the two curves denotes the cutoff point with the highest diagnostic accuracy.

REFERENCES

1. Gruentzig AR, Senning A, Siegenthaler WE. Nonoperative dilatation of coronary-artery stenosis. Percutaneous transluminal coronary angioplasty. *New Engl J Med* 1979;301:61–68.
2. Detre K, Holubkov R, Kelsy S, Cowley M, Kent K, Williams D, Myler R, Faxon D, Holmes D Jr, Bourassa M, Block P, Gosselin A, Bentivoglio L, Leatherman L, Dorros G, King S III, Galichia J, Al-Bassam M, Leon M, Robertson T, Passamani E, Co-Investigators of the NHLBI PTCA Registry. Percutaneous transluminal coronary angioplasty in 1985–1986 and 1977–1981. The National Heart Lung Blood Institute Registry. *N Engl J Med* 1988;318:265–270.
3. Block PC, Myler RK, Stertzer S, Fallon JT. Morphology after transluminal angioplasty in human beings. *N Engl J Med* 1981;305:382–385.
4. Castaneda-Zuniga WR, Formanek A, Tadavarthy M, Vlodaver Z, Edwards JE, Zollikofer C, Amplatz K. The mechanism of balloon angioplasty. *Radiology* 1980;135:565–571.
5. Sanborn TA, Faxon DP, Haudenschild C, Gottsman SB, Ryan TJ. The mechanism of transluminal angioplasty: evidence for formation of aneurysms in experimental atherosclerosis. *Circulation* 1983;5:1136–1140.
6. McBride W, Lange RA, Hillis LD. Restenosis after successful coronary angioplasty. Pathophysiology and prevention. *N Engl J Med* 1988;318:1734–1737.
7. Waller BF. "Crackers, breakers, stretchers, drillers, scrapers, shavers, burners, welders and melters." The future treatment of atherosclerotic coronary artery disease? A clinical-morphologic assessment. *J Am Coll Cardiol* 1989;13:969–987.
8. Ellis SG, Roubin GS, King SB III, Douglas JS, Weintraub WS, Thomas RG, Cox WR. Angiographic and clinical predictors of acute closure after native vessel coronary angioplasty. *Circulation* 1988;322:372–379.
9. Detre KM, Holmes DR, Holubkov R, Cowley MJ, Bourassa MG, Faxon DP, Dorros GP, Bentivoglio LB, Kent KM, Myler RK, Coinvestigators of the NHLBI PTCA Registry. Incidence and consequences of periprocedural occlusion: the 1985–1986 NHLBI PTCA Registry. *Circulation* 1990;82:739–750.
10. de Feyter PJ, van den Brand M, Laarman GJ, van Domburg R, Serruys PW, Suryapranata H. Acute coronary artery occlusion during and after percutaneous transluminal coronary angio-

plasty. Frequency, prediction, clinical course, management and follow-up. *Circulation* 1991;83:927–936.

11. Fischell TA, Derby G, Tse TM, Stadius ML. Coronary artery vasoconstriction routinely occurs after percutaneous transluminal coronary angioplasty. A quantitative arteriographic analysis. *Circulation* 1988;78:1323–1334.

12. Rensing BJ, Hermans WRM, Beatt KJ, Laarman GJ, Suryapranata H, van der Brand M, de Feyter PJ, Serruys PW. Quantitative angiographic assessment of elastic recoil after percutaneous transluminal coronary angioplasty. *Am J Cardiol* 1990;66:1039–1044.

13. Rensing BJ, Hermans WR, Strauss BH, Serruys PW. Regional differences in elastic recoil after percutaneous transluminal coronary angioplasty: a quantitative angiographic study. *J Am Coll Cardiol* 1991;17:34B–38B.

14. Rensing BJ, Hermans WR, Vos J, et al. Quantitative angiographic risk factors of luminal narrowing after coronary balloon angioplasty using balloon measurements to reflect stretch and elastic recoil at the dilatation site. *Am J Cardiol* 1992;69:584–591.

15. Serruys PW, Luijten HE, Beatt KJ, Geuskens R, de Feyter PJ, van den Brand M, Reiber JH, ten Katen HJ, van Es GA, Hugenholtz PG. Incidence of restenosis after successful coronary angioplasty: a time-related phenomenon. A quantitative angiographic study in 342 consecutive patients at 1, 2, 3 and 4 months. *Circulation* 1988;77:361–371.

16. Nobuyoshi M, Kimura T, Nosaka H, Mioka S, Ueno K, Hamasaki N, Horiuchi H, Oshishi H. Restenosis after successful percutaneous transluminal coronary angioplasty: serial angiographic follow-up of 299 patients. *J Am Coll Cardiol* 1988;12:616–623.

17. Holmes DR, Vlietstra RE, Smith HC, Vetrovec GW, Kent KM, Cowley MJ, Faxon DP, Gruentzig AR, Kelsey SF, Detre KM, van Raden MJ, Mock MB. Restenosis after percutaneous transluminal coronary angioplasty (PTCA): a report from the PTCA Registry of the National Heart, Lung, and Blood Institute. *Am J Cardiol* 1984;53:77C–81C.

18. Kaltenbach M, Kober G, Scherer D, Vallbracht C. Recurrence rate after successful coronary angioplasty. *Eur Heart J* 1985;6:276–281.

19. Mata LA, Bosch X, David PR, Rapold HJ, Corcos T, Bourassa MG. Clinical and angiographic assessment 6 months after double vessel percutaneous coronary angioplasty. *J Am Coll Cardiol* 1985;6:1239–1244.

20. Leimgruber PP, Roubin GS, Hollman J, Cotsonis GA, Meier B, Douglas JS, King SB III, Gruentzig AR. Restenosis after successful coronary angioplasty in patients with single-vessel disease. *Circulation* 1986;73:710–717.

21. Myler RK, Topol EJ, Shaw RE, Stertzer SH, Clark DA, Fishman J, Murphy MC. Multiple vessel coronary angioplasty: classification, results, and patterns of restenosis in 494 consecutive patients. *Cathet Cardiovasc Diagn* 1987;13(1):1–15.

22. Guiteras Val P, Bourassa MG, David PR, Bonan R, Crepeau J, Dyrda I, L'Espérance J. Restenosis after successful percutaneous transluminal coronary angioplasty: the Montreal Heart Institute experience. *Am J Cardiol* 1987;60(3):50B–55B.

23. Vandormael MG, Deligonul U, Kern MJ, Harper M, Presant S, Gibson P, Galan K, Chaitman BR. Multilesion coronary angioplasty: clinical and angiographic follow-up. *J Am Coll Cardiol* 1987;10(2):246–252.

24. de Feyter PJ, Suryapranata H, Serruys PW, Beatt K, van Domburg R, van den Brand M, Tijssen JJ, Azar A, Hugenholtz PG. Coronary angioplasty for unstable angina: immediate and late results in 200 consecutive patients with identification of risk factors for unfavorable early and late outcome. *J Am Coll Cardiol* 1988;12:324–333.

25. Fleck E, Regitz V, Lehnert A, Dacian S, Dirschinger J, Rudolph W. Restenosis after balloon dilatation of coronary stenosis: multivariate analysis of potential risk factors. *Eur Heart J* 1988;9:15–18.

26. Halon DA, Merdler A, Shefer A, Flugelman MY, Lewis BS. Identifying patients at high risk for restenosis after percutaneous transluminal coronary angioplasty for unstable angina pectoris. *Am J Cardiol* 1989;64:289–293.

27. Quigley PJ, Hlatky MA, Hinohara T, Rendall DS, Perez JA, Phillips HR, Califf RM, Stack RS. Repeat percutaneous transluminal coronary angioplasty and predictors of recurrent restenosis. *Am J Cardiol* 1989;63:409–413.

28. Renkin J, Melin J, Robert A, Richelle F, Bachy JL, Col J, Detry JMR, Wijns W. Detection of restenosis after successful coronary angioplasty: improved clinical decision making with use of a logistic model combining procedural and follow-up variables. *J Am Coll Cardiol* 1990;16:6:1333–1340.

29. Rupprecht HJ, Brennecke R, Bernhard G, Erber R, Pop T, Meyer J. Analysis of risk factors for restenosis after PTCA. *Cathet Cardiovasc Diagn* 1990;19:151–159.

30. Bourassa MG, Lespérance J, Eastwood C, et al. Clinical, physiologic, anatomic, and procedural factors predictive of restenosis after percutaneous transluminal coronary angioplasty. *J Am Coll Cardiol* 1991;18:368–376.

31. MacDonald RG, Henderson MA, Hirschfeld JW Jr, Goldberg SH, Bass T, Vetrovec G, Cowley M, Taussig A, Whitworth H, Margolis JR, Hill JA, Jugo R, Pepine CJ, for the M-Heart Group. Patient related variables and restenosis after percutaneous transluminal coronary angioplasty: a report from the M-Heart group. *Am J Cardiol* 1990;66:926–931.

32. Hirshfeld JW, Schwartz SS, Jugo R, Macdonald RG, Goldberg S, Savage MP, Bass TA, Vetrovec G, Cowley M, Taussig AS, Withworth HB, Margolis JR, Hill JA, Pepine CJ, and the M-Heart Investigators. Restenosis after coronary angioplasty: a multivariate statistical model to relate lesion and procedural variables to restenosis. *J Am Coll Cardiol* 1991;18:647–656.

33. Hermans WRM, Rensing BJ, Strauss BH, Serruys PW. Prevention of restenosis after percutaneous transluminal coronary angioplasty (PTCA): the search for a "magic bullet". *Am Heart J* 1991;122:1:171–187.

34. Sahni R, Maniet AR, Voci G, Banka VS. Prevention of restenosis by lovastatin after successful angioplasty. *Am Heart J* 1991;121:1600–1608.

35. Serruys PW, Rutsch W, Heyndrikx GR, Danchin N, Mast EG, Wijns W, Rensing BJ, Vos J, Stibbe J. Prevention of restenosis after percutaneous transluminal coronary angioplasty with thromboxane A2 receptor blockade. A randomized, double blind, placebo controlled trial. *Circulation* 1991;84:1568–1580.

36. MERCATOR study group. Does the new angiotensin converting enzyme inhibitor cilazapril prevent restenosis after percutaneous transluminal coronary angioplasty? The results of the MERCATOR-study: a multicenter randomized double-blind placebo-controlled trial. *Circulation* 1992;86:100–110.

37. Popma J, Califf RM, Topol EJ. Clinical trials of restenosis following coronary angioplasty. *Circulation* 1991;84:3:1426–1436.

38. White CW, Chaitman B, Knudtson ML, Chrisholm RJ, and the Ticlopidine Study Group. Antiplatelet agents are effective in reducing the acute ischemic complications of angioplasty but do not prevent restenosis: results from the ticlopidine trial. *Coronary Artery Res* 1991;2:757–767.

39. Safain RD, Gelbfish JS, Erny RE, Schnitt SJ, Schmidt D, Baim DS. Coronary atherectomy: clinical angiographic and histologic findings and observations regarding potential mechanisms. *Circulation* 1990;82:69–79.

40. Ellis SG, DeCasare NB, Pinkerton CA, Whitlow P, King SB, Ghazzal ZMB, Kereikes DJ, Popma JJ, Menke KK, Topol EJ, Holmes DR. Relation of stenosis morphology and clinical presentation to the procedural results of directional coronary atherectomy. *Circulation* 1991;84:644–653.

41. Popma JJ, De Ceasare NB, Ellis SG, Holmes DR, Pinkerton CA, Whitlow P, Ling SB, Ghazzal ZMB, Topol EJ, Garett KKN, Kereiakes DJ. Clinical, angiographic and procedural correlates of quantitative coronary dimensions after directional coronary atherectomy. *J Am Coll Cardiol* 1991;18:1183–1191.

42. Selmon MR, Hinohara T, Vetter JW, Robertson GC, Bartzokis TC, McAuley BJ, Sheehan DJ, Braden LJ, Simpson JB. Experience of directional coronary atherectomy: 848 procedures in 4 years. *Circulation* 1991;84:4:320 (abst).

43. Karsch KR, Haase KK, Voelker W, Bauambach A, Mauser M, Seipel L. Percutaneous coronary excimer laser angioplasty in patients with stable and unstable anginal pectoris: acute results and incidence of restenosis during 6 month follow-up. *Circulation* 1990;81:1849–1859.

44. Schwartz L, Andrus S, Sinclair IN, Plokker T, Dear WE, Spears RJ. Restenosis following laser balloon coronary angioplasty: results of a randomized pilot multicentre trial. *Circulation* 1991;84:4:1437 (abst).

45. Serruys PW, Strauss BH, Beatt KJ, Bertrand ME, Puel J, Rickards AF, Meier B, Goy JJ, Vogt P, Kappenberger L, Sigwart U. Angiographic follow-up after placement of a self-expanding coronary artery stent. *N Engl J Med* 1991;324:13–17.

46. Schatz RA, Baim DS, Leon M, Ellis SG, Goldberg S, Hirshfeld JW, Cleman MW, Cabin HS, Walker C, Stagg J, Buchbinder M, Teirstein PS, Topol EJ, Savage M, Perez JA, Curry RS, Whitworth H, Sousa JE, Tio F, Almagor Y, Ponder R, Penn IM, Leonard B, Levine SL, Fish D, Palmaz JC. Clinical experience with the Palmaz-Schatz coronary stent. Initial results of a multicenter study. *Circulation* 1991;83:148–161.

47. Serruys PW, Strauss BH, van Beusekom HM, van der Giessen WJ. Stenting of coronary arteries: has a modern Pandora's Box been opened? *J Am Coll Cardiol* 1991;17:143B–154B.

48. Bertrand ME, Lablanche JM, Leroy F, Bauters C, DeJargere P, Serruys PW, Meyer J, Dietz U, Erbel R. Percutaneous transluminal rotary ablation with the rotablator. The European experience. *Am J Cardiol* 1992;69:470–474.

49. Warth D, Bertrand M, Buchbinder M, Dietz U, Fourrier JL, Zacca N. Percutaneous transluminal coronary rotational ablation: six month restenosis rate. *Circulation* 1991;84:4:328 (abst).

50. Topol EJ. Promises and pitfalls of new devices for coronary artery diseases [Editorial]. *Circulation* 1991;83:689–694.

51. Gruentzig AR, Meier B. Percutaneous transluminal coronary angioplasty. The first five years and the future. *Int J Cardiol* 1983;2:319–323.

52. Kent KM, Bentivoglio LG, Block PC, Bourassa MG, Cowley MJ, Dorros G, Detre KM, Gosselin AJ, Gruentzig AR, Kelsey SF, Mock MB, Mullin SM, Passamani ER, Myler RK, Simpson J, Stertzer SH, van Raden MJ, Williams DO. Long-term efficacy of percutaneous transluminal coronary angioplasty [PTCA]: report from the National Heart, Lung, and Blood Institute PTCA Registry. *Am J Cardiol* 1984;53:27C–31C.

53. Faxon DP, Kelsey SF, Ryan TJ, McCabe CH, Detre K. Determinants of successful percutaneous transluminal coronary angioplasty: report from the National Heart, Lung, and Blood Institute Registry. *Am Heart J* 1984;108:1019–1023.

54. O'Neill WW, Walton JA, Bates ER, Colfer HT, Aueron FM, Le Free MT, Pitt B, Vogel RA. Criteria for successful coronary angioplasty as assessed by alterations in coronary vasodilatory reserve. *J Am Coll Cardiol* 1984;3:1382–1390.

55. Meier B, King III SB, Gruentzig AR, Douglas JS, Hollman J, Ischinger T, Galan K, Tankersley R. Repeat coronary angioplasty. *J Am Coll Cardiol* 1984;4:463–466.

56. Corcos T, David PR, Val PG, Renkin J, Dangoisse V, Rapold HG, Bourassa MG. Failure of diltiazem to prevent restenosis after percutaneous transluminal coronary angioplasty. *Am Heart J* 1985;109:926–931.

57. Levine S, Ewels CJ, Rosing DR, Kent KM. Coronary angioplasty: clinical and angiographic follow-up. *Am J Cardiol* 1985;55:673–676.

58. Wijns W, Serruys PW, Reiber JHC, de Feyter PJ, van den Brand M, Simoons ML, Hugenholtz PG. Early detection of restenosis after successful percutaneous transluminal coronary angioplasty by exercise-redistribution thallium scintigraphy. *Am J Cardiol* 1985;55:357–361.

59. Serruys PW, Umans V, Heyndrickx GR, van den Brand M, de Feyter PJ, Wijns W, Jaski B, Hugenholtz PG. Elective PTCA of totally occluded coronary arteries not associated with acute myocardial infarction; short-term and long-term results. *Eur Heart J* 1985;6:2–12.

60. Bertrand ME, LaBlanche JM, Thieuleux FA, Fourrier JL, Traisnel G, Asseman P. Comparative results of percutaneous transluminal coronary angioplasty in patients with dynamic versus fixed coronary stenosis. *J Am Coll Cardiol* 1986;8:504–508.

61. Schwartz L, Bourassa MG, Lesperance J, Aldridge HE, Kazim F, Salvatori VA, Henderson M, Bonan R, David PR. Aspirin and dipyridamole in the prevention of restenosis after percutaneous transluminal coronary angioplasty. *N Engl J Med* 1988;318:1714–1719.

62. Pepine CJ, Hirshfeld JW, MacDonald RG, Henderson MA, Bass TA, Goldberg S, Savage MP, Vetrovec G, Cowley M, Taussig AS, Withworth HB, Margolis JR, Hill JA, Bove AA, Jugo R. A controlled trial of corticosteroids to prevent restenosis after coronary angioplasty. *Circulation* 1991;81:1751–1753.

63. Holmes DR Jr, Schwartz RS, Webster MWI. Coronary restenosis: what have we learned from angiography. *J Am Coll Cardiol* 1991;17:14B–22B.

64. Kent KM, Bonow RO, Rosing DR, Ewels CJ, Lipson LC, Mc Intosh CL, Bacharach S, Green M, Epstein SE. Improved myocardial function during exercise after successful percutaneous transluminal coronary angioplasty. *N Engl J Med* 1982;306:441–446.

65. Rosing DR, Raden MJ, van Mincemoyer RM, Bonow RO, Bourassa MG, David PR, Ewels CJ, Detre KM, Kent KM. Exercise, electrocardiographic and functional responses after percutaneous transluminal coronary angioplasty. *Am J Cardiol* 1984;53:36C–41C.

66. Detrano R, Froelicher VF. Exercise testing: uses and limitations considering recent studies. *Prog Vardiovasc Disease* 1988;31:173–204.

67. Gould KL. Quantitative imaging in nuclear cardiology. *Circulation* 1982;66:1141–1146.

68. Hamilton GW, Trobaugh GB, Ritchie JL, Gould KL, DeRouen TA, Williams DL. Myocardial imaging with 201-thallium: an analysis of clinical usefulness based on Bayes' theorem. *Semin Nucl Med* 1978;8:358–364.

69. Mates RE, Gupta RL, Bell AC, Klocke FJ. Fluid dynamics of coronary artery stenosis. *Circ Res* 1978;42:152–162.

70. Ganz P, Harrington DP, Gaspar J, Barry WH. Phasic pressure gradients across coronary and renal artery stenoses in humans. *Am Heart J* 1983;106:1399–1406.

71. Wright CB, Doty DB, Eastham CL, Marcus ML. Measurements of coronary reactive hyperemia with a Doppler probe: Intraoperative guide to hemodynamically significant lesions. *J Thorac Cardiovasc Surg* 1980;80:888–897.

72. Epstein SE, Cannon RO III, Talbot TL. Hemodynamic principles in the control of coronary blood flow. *Am J Cardiol* 1985;56:4E–10E.

73. Gould KL, Lipscomb K. Effects of coronary stenoses on coronary flow reserve and resistance. *Am J Cardiol* 1974;34:48–55.

74. Serruys PW, Wijns W, Reiber JHC, de Feyter P, van den Brand M, Piscione F, Hugenholtz PG. Values and limitations of transstenotic pressure gradients measured during percutaneous coronary angioplasty. *Herz* 1985;10:337–342.

75. Leiboff R, Bren G, Katz R, Korkegi R, Katzen B, Ross A. Determinants of transstenotic gradients observed during angioplasty: an experimental model. *Am J Cardiol* 1983;52:1311–1317.

76. Probst P, Zangl W, Pachinger O. Relation of coronary arterial occlusion pressure during percutaneous transluminal coronary angioplasty to presence of collaterals. *Am J Cardiol* 1985;55:1264–1269.

77. Meier B, Luethy P, Finci L, Steffeninno GP, Rutishauer W. Coronary wedge pressure in relation to spontaneously visible and recruitable collaterals. *Circulation* 1987;75:906–913.

78. Urban P, Meier B, Finci L, deBruyne B, Steffenino G, Rutishauser W: Coronary wedge pressure: a predictor of restenosis after coronary balloon angioplasty. *J Am Coll Cardiol* 1987;10:504–509.

79. Emanuellsson H, Dohnal M, Lamm C, Tenerz L. Initial experience with a miniaturized pressure transducer during coronary angioplasty. *Cathet Cardiovasc Diagn* 1991;24:137–143.

80. De Bruyne B, Pijls NHJ, Paulus WJ, Vantrimpont PJ, Stockbroeckx J, de Moor D, Nelis O, Heyndrickx GR. In vitro and in vivo evaluation of a new 0.015 fluid filled guide wire for distal pressure monitoring during PTCA. *Circulation* 1991;84:II-1198 (abst).

81. Ofili E, Kern MJ, Tatineni S, Deligonul U, Aguirre F, Serota H, Labovitz AJ. Detection of coronary collateral flow by a Doppler-tipped guide wire during angioplasty. *Am Heart J* 1991;122:1:221–225.

82. Serruys PW, Juilliere Y, Zijlstra F, Beatt KJ, de Feyter PJ, Suryapranata H, van den Brand M, Roelandt J. Coronary blood flow velocity during percutaneous transluminal coronary angioplasty

as a guide for assessment of the functional result. *Am J Cardiol* 1988;61:253–259.

83. Young DF, Cholvin NR, Roth AC. Pressure drop across artificially induced stenoses in the femoral arteries of dogs. *Circ Res* 1975;36:735.

84. Young DF, Cholvin NR, Kirkeeide RL, Roth AC. Hemodynamics of arterial stenoses at elevated flow rates. *Circ Res* 1977;41:99.

85. Kirkeeide RL, Gould KL, Parsel L. Assessment of coronary stenoses by myocardial perfusion imaging during pharmacologic coronary vasodilation. Validation of coronary flow reserve as a single integrated functional measure of stenosis severity reflecting all its geometric dimentions. *J Am Coll Cardiol* 1986;7:103–113.

86. Hoffman JIE. Maximal coronary flow and the concept of coronary vascular reserve. *Circulation* 1984;70:153–159.

87. Bookstein JJ, Higgins CB. Comparative efficacy of coronary vasodilatory methods. *Invest Radiol* 1984;12:121–127.

88. Marcus M, Wright C, Doty D, Easthan C, Laughlin D, Krumm P, Fastenow C, Brody M. Measurements of coronary velocity and reactive hyperemia in the coronary circulation of humans. *Circ Res* 1981;49:877.

89. Klocke FJ. Measurements of coronary blood flow and degree of stenosis. Current clinical implications and continuing uncertainties. *J Am Coll Cardiol* 1983;1:31–41.

90. Serruys PW, Zijlstra F, Laarman GJ, Reiber JHC, Beatt K, Roelandt J. A comparison of two methods to measure coronary flow reserve in the setting of coronary angioplasty: intracoronary bloodflow velocity measurements with a Doppler catheter and digital subtraction cineangiography. *Eur Heart J* 1989;10:725.

91. Laarman GJ, Serruys PW, Suryapranata H, van den Brand M, Jonkers PR, de Feyter PJ, Roelandt JRTC. Inability of coronary blood flow reserve measurements to assess the efficacy of coronary angioplasty in the first 24 hours in unselected patients. *Am Heart J* 1991;122:631–638.

92. Zijlstra F, den Boer A, Reiber JHC, Van Es GA, Lubsen J, Serruys PW. The assessment of immediate and long-term functional results of percutaneous transluminal coronary angioplasty. *Circulation* 1988;1:15–24.

93. Hodgson JM, Riley RS, Most AS, Williams DO. Assessment of coronary flow reserve using digital angiography before and after successful percutaneous transluminal coronary angioplasty. *Am J Cardiol* 1987;60:61–65.

94. Pijls NHJ, Uijen GJH, Hoevelaken A, et al. Mean transit time for the assessment of myocardial perfusion by videodensitometry. *Circulation* 1990;81:1331–1340.

95. Essed CE, van den Brand M, Becker AE. Transluminal coronary angioplasty and early restenosis: fibrocellular occlusion after wall laceration. *Br Heart J* 1983;49:393–396.

96. Mizuno K, Kurita A, Imazeki N. Pathological findings after percutaneous transluminal coronary angioplasty. *Br Heart J* 1984;52:588–590.

97. Soward AL, Essed CE, Serruys PW. Coronary arterial findings after accidental death immediately after successful percutaneous transluminal coronary angioplasty. *Am J Cardiol* 1985;56:794–795.

98. Düber C, Jungbluth A, Rumpelt HJ, Erbel R, Meyer J, Thoenes W. Morphology of the coronary arteries after combined thrombolysis and percutaneous transluminal coronary angioplasty for acute myocardial infarction. *Am J Cardiol* 1986;58:698–703.

99. LaDelia V, Rossi PA, Sommers G, Kreps E. Coronary histology after percutaneous transluminal coronary angioplasty. *Texas Heart Inst J* 1988;15:113–116.

100. Marcus LM, Harrison DG, White CW, McPherson DD, Wilson RF, Kerber RE. Assessing the physiologic significance of coaonary obstructions in patients: importance of diffuse undetected atherosclerosis. *Prog Cardiovasc Dis* 1988;31:39–56.

101. Marcus ML, Skorton DJ, Johnson MR, et al. Visual estimates of percent diameter coronary stenosis: "a battered gold standard." *J Am Coll Cardiol* 1988;11:882–885.

102. DeRouen TA, Murray JA, Owen W. Variability in the analysis of coronary arteriograms. *Circulation* 19;55:324–328.

103. Detre KM, Wright E, Murphy ML, Taharo T. Observer agreement in evaluating coronary angiograms. *Circulation* 1975;52:979–986.

104. Meier B, Gruentzig AR, Goebel N, Pyle R, von Gosslar W, Schlumpf M. Assessment of stenoses in coronary angioplasty: inter- and intraobserver variability. *Int J Cardiol* 1983;3:159–169.

105. Zir LM, Miller SW, Dinsmore RE, Gilbert JP, Harthorne JW. Interobserver variability in coronary angiography. *Circulation* 1976;53:627–632.

106. Arnett EN, Isner JM, Redwood DR, Kent KM, Baker WP, Ackerstein H, Roberts WC. Coronary artery narrowing in coronary heart disease: comparison of cineangiographic and necropsy findings. *Ann Intern Med* 1979;91:350–356.

107. Shub C, Vlietstra RE, Smith HC, Fulton RE, Elveback LR. The unpredictable progression of symptomatic coronary artery disease: a serial clinical-angiographic analysis. *Mayo Clin Proc* 1981;56:155–160.

108. Beaumann GJ, Vogel RA. Accuracy of individual and panel visual interpretations of coronary arteriograms: implications for clinical decisions. *J Am Coll Cardiol* 1990;16:108–113.

109. Demer L, Gould KI, Kirkeeide R. Assessing stenosis severity: coronary flow reserve, collateral function, quantitative coronary arteriography, positron imaging and digital substraction angiography. A review and analysis. *Prog Cardiovasc Dis* 1988;30:307–322.

110. Fleming RM, Kirkeeide RL, Smalling RW, Gould KL. Patterns in visual interpretation of coronary angiograms as detected by quantitative coronary angiography. *J Am Coll Cardiol* 1991;18:945–951.

111. White CW, Wright CB, Doty DB, Hiratza LF, Eastham CL, Harrison DG, Marcus ML. Does visual interpretation of the coronary arteriogram predict the physiologic importance of a coronary stenosis? *N Engl J Med* 1984;310:819–824.

112. Tobis J, Nalcioglu O, Iseri L, Johnston WD, Roeck W, Castleman E, Bauer B, Montelli S, Henry WL. Detection and quantitation of coronary artery stenoses from digital subtraction angiograms compared with 35-millimeter film cineangiograms. *Am J Cardiol* 1984;54:489–496.

113. Kruger RA. Estimation of the diameter of and iodine concentration within blood vessels using digital radiography devices. *Med Phys* 1981;8:652–658.

114. Reiber JHC. An overview of coronary quantitative techniques as of 1989. In: Reiber JHC, Serruys PW, eds. *Quantitative coronary arteriography.* Dordrecht: Kluwer Academic Publishers. 1991:55–132.

115. Brown GB, Bolson EL, Dodge HT. Quantitative computer techniques for analyzing coronary arteriograms. *Prog Cardiovasc Dis* 1986;28:403–418.

116. Doriot P, Rutishauser W. On the accuracy of densitometric measurements of coronary artery stenosis based on Lambert-Beer's absorption law. In: Reiber JC, Serruys PW, eds. *New developments in quantitative coronary arteriography.* Dordrecht: Kluwer Academic Publishers; 1988:115–124.

117. Reiber JHC, Serruys PW, Kooijman CJ, Wijns W, Slager CJ, Gerbrands JJ, Schuurbiers JCH, den Boer A, Hugenholtz PG. Assessment of short-, medium-, and long-term variations in arterial dimensions from computer-assisted quantitation of coronary cineangiograms. *Circulation* 1985;71:280–288.

118. Reiber JHC, Serruys PW. Quantitative coronary angiography. In: Marcus ML, Schelbert HR, Skorton JD, Wolf GI, eds. *Cardiac imaging: a companion to Braunwalds heart disease.* Philadelphia: WB Saunders; 1991:211–280.

119. Brown BG, Bolson EL, Dodge HT. Arteriographic assessment of coronary atherosclerosis. Review of current methods, their limitations, and clinical applications. *Arteriosclerosis* 1982;2:2–15.

120. McMahon MM, Brown BG, Cuhingnan R, Rolett EL, Bolson E, Frimer M, Dodge HT. Quantitative coronary angiography: measurement of the "critical" stenosis in patients with unstable angina and single-vessel disease without collaterals. *Circulation* 1979;60:106–113.

121. Reiber JHC, Serruys PW, Slager CJ. Quantitative coronary and left ventricular cineangiography. Methodology and clinical applications. Dordrecht: Martinus Nijhoff Publishers; 1986.

122. Siebes M, Lenzen H, Gottwik M, Schlepper M. Influence of geometric errors in quantitative angiography on the evaluation of stenotic hemodynamics. *Comp Cardiol* 1983;4:385–388.

123. Zijlstra F, Serruys PW. Intracoronary blood flow velocity and transstenotic pressure drop in an awake human being during coronary vasodilation. *J Interven Cardiol* 1988;1:43–48.

124. Serruys PW, Reiber JHC, Wijns W, van den Brand M, Kooijman CJ, ten Katen HJ, Hugenholtz PG. Assessment of percutaneous transluminal coronary angioplasty by quantitative coronary angiography: diameter versus densitometric area measurements. *Am J Cardiol* 1984;54:482–488.

125. Wijns W, Serruys PW, Reiber JHC, van den Brand M, Simoons ML, Kooijman CJ, Balakumaran K, Hugenholtz PG. Quantitative angiography of the left anterior descending coronary artery: correlations with pressure gradient and results of exercise thallium scintigraphy. *Circulation* 1985;71:273–279.

126. Zijlstra F, Fioretti P, Reiber JHC, Serruys PW. Which cineangiographically assessed anatomic variable correlates best with functional measurements of stenosis severity? A comparison of quantitative analysis of the coronary cineangiogram with measured coronary flow reserve and exercise/redistribution thallium-201 scintigraphy. *J Am Coll Cardiol* 1988;12:686–691.

127. Zijlstra F, Reiber JC, Juillieve Y, Serruys PW. Normalisation of coronary flow reserve by percutaneous transluminal coronary angioplasty. *Am J Cardiol* 1988;61:55–60.

128. Reiber JHC, Serruys PW, Kooijman CJ, Slager CJ, Schuurbiers JCH, den Boer A. Approaches towards standardization in acquisition and quantitation of arterial dimensions from cineangiograms. In: Reiber JHC, Serruys PW, eds. *State of the art in quantitative coronary arteriography.* Dordrecht: Martinus Nijhoff Publications; 1986:145–172.

129. Hermans WRM, Rensing BJ, Paameyer J, Serruys PW. Experiences of a quantitative coronary angiographic core laboratory in restenosis prevention trials. In: Reiber JHC, Serruys PW, eds. *Coronary arteriography 1991.* Dordrecht: Kluwer Academic Publishers; 1992 (in press).

130. Wijns W, Serruys PW, van den Brand M, Reiber JHC, Suryapranata H, Hugenholtz PG. Progression to complete coronary obstruction without myocardial infarction in patients who are candidates for percutaneous transluminal angioplasty. A 90-day angiographic follow-up. In: Roskamm H, ed. *Prognosis of coronary heart disease. Progression of coronary arteriosclerosis.* Berlin: Springer-Verlag; 1983:190–195.

131. Freudenberg H, Lichtlen P. Postmortale Koronarangiographie. In: Lichtlen PR, ed. *Koronarangiographie.* Erlangen: Verlag Dr Med D Straube; 1979:341–357.

132. Sherman CT, Litvack F, Grundfest W, et al. Demonstration of thrombus and complex atheroma by in vivo angioscopy in patients with unstable angina pectoris. *N Engl J Med* 1986;315:913–919.

133. Tobis JM, Mallery JA, Gessert J, Griffith J, Mahon D, Bessen M, Moriuchi M, McLeay, McRae M, Henry WL. Intravascular ultrasound cross-sectional arterial imaging before and after balloon angioplasty in vitro. *Circulation* 1989;80:873–882.

134. Siegel RJ, Chae J, Forrestor JS, Ruiz CE. Angiography, angioscopy, and ultrasound imaging before and after percutaneous balloon angioplasty. *Am Heart J* 1990;120:1086–1090.

135. Yock PG, Fitzgerald PJ, Linker DT, Angelsen BAJ. Intravascular ultrasound guidance for catheter-based coronary interventions. *J Am Coll Cardiol* 1991;17:39B–45B.

136. Tobis JM, Mallery J, Mahon D, Lehmann K, Zalesky P, Griffith J, Gessert J, Moriuchi M, McRae M, Dwyer ML, Greep N, Henry WL. Intravascular ultrasound imaging of human coronary arteries in vivo. *Circulation* 1991;83:913–926.

137. Coy KM, Maurer G, Siegel RJ. Intravascular ultrasound imaging: a current perspective. *J Am Coll Cardiol* 1991;18:1811–1823.

138. Rosenfield K, Losordo DW, Ramaswamy K, Pasore JÓ, Langevin RE, Razvi S, Kosowsky BD, Isner JM. Three-dimensional reconstruction of human coronary and peripheral arteries from images recorded during two-dimensional intravascular ultrasound examination. *Circulation* 1991;84:1938–1956.

139. Werner GS, Buchwald A, Kreuzer H, Wiegand V. Intravascular ultrasound imaging of human coronary arteries after percutaneous transluminal angioplasty: morphologic and quantitative assessment. *Am Heart J* 1991;122:212–220.

140. Di Mario C, Serruys PW, Roelandt JRTC, et al. Detection and characterization of vascular lesions by intravascular ultrasound.

An in vitro qualitative and quantitative correlation with histology. *J Am Soc Echocardiogr* (*in press*).

141. Hermans WR, Rensing BJ, Strauss BH, Serruys PW. Methodological problems related to the quantitative assessment of stretch, elastic recoil, and balloon-artery ratio. *Cathet Cardiovasc Diagn* (*in press*).

142. Hanet C, Wijns W, Michel X, Schroeder E. Influence of balloon size and stenosis morphology on immediate and delayed elastic recoil after percutaneous transluminal coronary angioplasty. *J Am Coll Cardiol* 1991;18:506–511.

143. Isner JM, Rosenfield K, Losordo DW, et al. Combination balloon-ultrasound imaging catheter for percutaneous transluminal angioplasty. Validation of imaging, analysis of recoil, and identification of plaque fracture. *Circulation* 1991;84:739–754.

144. Clowes AW, Reidy MA, Clowes MM. Mechanisms of stenosis after arterial injury. *Lab Invest* 1983;49:208–215.

145. Stemerman MB, Spaet TH, Pitlick F, Cintron J, Lejnieks I, Tiell ML. Intimal healing: the pattern of reendothelialization and intimal thickening. *Am J Pathol* 1986;123:220–230.

146. Schwartz SM, Campbell GR, Campbell JH. Replication of smooth muscle cells in vascular disease. *Circ Res* 1986;58:427–444.

147. Ross R. The pathogenesis of athersosclerosis. An update. *N Engl J Med* 1986;314:488–500.

148. Steele PM, Chesebro JH, Stanson AW, Holmes DR Jr, Dewanjee MK, Badimon L, Fuster V. Balloon angioplasty: natural history of the pathophysiological response to injury in the pig model. *Circ Res* 1985;57:105–112.

149. Wilentz JR, Sanborn TA, Haudenschild CC, Valeri CR, Ryan TJ, Faxon DP. Platelet accumulation in experimental angioplasty: time course and relation to vascular injury. *Circulation* 1987;75:636–642.

150. Lindner V, Reidy MA. Proliferation of smooth muscle cells after vascular injury is inhibited by an antibody against basic fibroblast growth factor. *Proc Natl Acad Sci USA* 1991;88:3739–3743.

151. Ip JH, Fuster V, Badimon L, Badimon J, Taubman MB, Chesebro JH. Syndromes of accelerated atherosclerosis: role of vascular injury and smooth muscle cell injury. *J Am Coll Cardiol* 1990;15:1667–1687.

152. Clowes AW. Pathologic intimal hyperplasia as a response to vascular injury and reconstruction. In. Rutherford RB, ed. *Vascular surgery.* Philadelphia: WB Saunders; 1989:266–275.

153. Liu MW, Roubin GS, King SB. Restenosis after coronary angioplasty. Potential biologic determinants and role of intimal hyperplasia. *Circulation* 1989;79:1374–1387.

154. Schwartz SM, Campbell GR, Campbell JH. Replication of smooth muscle cells in vascular disease. *Circ Res* 1986;58:427–444.

155. Fingerle J, Au YPT, Clowes AW, Reidy MA. Intimal lesion formation in rat carotid arteries after endothelial denudation in absence of medial injury. *Arteriosclerosis* 1990;10:1082–1087.

156. Fingerle J, Johnson R, Clowes AW, Majesky MW, Reidy MA. Role of platelets in smooth muscle cell proliferation and migration after vascular injury in rat carotid artery. *Proc Natl Acad Sci USA* 1989;86:8412–8416.

157. Lindner V, Lappi DA, Baird A, Majack RA, Reidy MA. Role of basic fibroblast growth factor in vascular lesion formation. *Circ Res* 1991;68:106–113.

158. Jawien A, Lindner V, Bowen-Pope DF, Schwartz SM, Reidy MA, Clowes AW. Platelet derived growth factor (PDGF) stimulates arterial smooth muscle cell proliferation in vivo. *FASEB J* 1990;4:342 (abst).

159. Hammacher A, Hellman U, Johnsson A, Östman A, Gunnarsson K, Westermark B, Wasteson Ä, Heldin CH. A major part of platelet-derived growth factor purified from human platelets is a heteromer of one A and one B chain. *J Biol Chem* 1988;263:16493–16498.

160. Majesky MW, Reidy MA, Bowen-Pope DF, Hart CE, Wilcox JN, Schwartz SM. PDGF ligand and receptor gene expression during repair ligand. *J Cell Biol* 1990;111:2149–2158.

161. Forrester JS, Fishbein M, Helfant R, Fagin J. Paradigm for restenosis based on cell biology: clues for the development of new preventive therapies. *J Am Coll Cardiol* 1991;17:758–769.

162. Schwartz RS, Huber KC, Edwards WD, Camrud AR, Jorgensen

M, Holmes DR. Coronary restenosis and the importance of mutal thrombus: results in a porcine coronary model. *Circulation* 1991;84:II–71 (abst).

163. Beatt KJ, Serruys PW, Hugenholtz PG. Restenosis after coronary angioplasty: new standards for clinical studies. *J Am Coll Cardiol* 1990;15:491–498.

164. Califf RM, Fortin DF, Frid DJ, Harlan WR III, Ohman EM, Bengtson JR, Nelson CL, Tcheng JE, Mark DB, Stack RS. Restenosis after coronary angioplasty. An overview. *J Am Coll Cardiol* 1991;17:2B–17B.

165. Califf RM, Ohman EM, Frid DJ, Fortin DF, Mark DB, Hlatky MA, Herndon JE, Bengtson JR. Restenosis: the clinical issue. In: Topol EJ, ed. *Textbook of interventional cardiology.* Philadelphia: WB Saunders; 1990:363–394.

166. Scholl JM, Chaitman BR, David PR, Dupras G, Brévers G, Val PG, Crépeau J, Lespérance J, Bourassa MG. Exercise electrocardiography and myocardial scintigraphy in the serial evaluation of the results of percutaneous transluminal coronary angioplasty. *Circulation* 1982;66:380–390.

167. Hirzel HO, Nuesch K, Gruentzig AR, Luetolf UM. Short- and long-term changes in myocardial perfusion after percutaneous transluminal coronary angioplasty assessed by thallium-201 exercise scintigraphy. *Circulation* 1981;63:1001–1007.

168. Legrand V, Aueron FM, Bates ER, O'Neill WW, Hodgson JM, Mancini GBJ, Vogel RA. Value of exercise radionuclide ventriculography and thallium 201 scintigraphy in evaluating successful coronary angioplasty: comparison with coronary flow reserve translesional gradient and percent diameter stenosis. *Eur Heart J* 1987;8:329–339.

169. O'Keefe H Jr, Lapeyre AC, Holmes DR Jr, Gibbons RJ. Usefulness of early radionuclide angiography for identifying low risk patients for late restenosis after percutaneous transluminal coronary angioplasty. *Am J Cardiol* 1988;61:51–54.

170. Eng C, Patterson RE, Horowitz SF, Halgash DA, Pichard AD, Midwall J, Herman MV, Gorlin R. Coronary collateral function during exercise. *Circulation* 1982;66:309–316.

171. Gregg DE, Patterson RE. Functional importance of the coronary collaterals. *N Engl J Med* 1980;303:1404–1406.

172. Rigo P, Becker LC, Griffith LSC, Alderson PO, Bailey IK, Pitt B, Burow RD, Wagner HN Jr. Influence of coronary collateral vessels on the results of thallium-201 myocardial stress imaging. *Am J Cardiol* 1979;44:452–458.

173. Smith SC Jr, Gorlin R, Herman MV, Taylor WJ, Collins JJ Jr. Myocardial blood flow in man: effects of coronary collateral circulation and coronary artery bypass surgery. *J Clin Invest* 1972;51:255–265.

174. Hansen JF. Coronary collateral circulation: clinical significance and influence on survival in patients with coronary artery occlusion. *Am Heart J* 1989;117:290–294.

175. Laarman GJ, Luijten HE, van Zeyl LG, et al. Assessment of "silent" restenosis and long-term follow-up after successful angioplasty in single vessel coronary artery disease: the value of quantitative exercise electrocardiography and quantitative coronary angiography. *J Am Coll Cardiol* 1990;16:578–585.

176. Jain A, Mahmarian JJ, Borges-Neto S, et al. Clinical significance of perfusion defects by thallium-201 single photon emission tomography following oral dipyridamole early after coronary angioplasty. *J Am Coll Cardiol* 1988;11:970–976.

177. Marie PY, Danchin N, Juilliere Y, Briancon S, Karcher G, Bertrand A, Aliot E, Cherrier F. Detection of quantitative coronary angiography-defined restenosis after PTCA by exercise TI-201 tomoscintigraphy with rest reinjection: a prospective study. *Eur Heart J* 1991;12[Suppl]:P1757 (abst).

178. Johnson D, Hinohara T, Selmon M, Robertson G, Braden L, Simpson J. Histologic predictors of restenosis after directional coronary atherectomy. *J Am Coll Cardiol* 1991;17:53A (abst).

179. Dartsch PC, Voisard R, Betz E. In vitro growth characteristics of human atherosclerotic plaque cells: comparison of cells from primary stenosing and restenosing lesions of peripheral and coronary arteries. *Res Exp Med* 1990;190:80–87.

180. Voisard R, Dartsch PD, Seitzer U, Hannelu MA, Kochs M, Hombach V. The effect of cytostatic agents on proliferative activity and cytoskeletal components of palque cells from human coronary arteries. *Eur Heart J* 1991;12:385 (abst).

181. Strauss BH, Verkerk A, van Suylen RJ, Umans V, de Feyter PJ, van der Giessen WJ, Jongkind JF, Serruys PW. Smooth muscle cell culture from human coronary lesions. *Circulation* 1990;82:III–496 (abst).

182. Bauriedel G, Windsetter U, Kandolf R, Hofling B. Increased migratory activity of human smooth muscle cells from peripheral and coronary restenosis plaques. *Eur Heart J* 1991;12:291 (abst).

183. Rensing BJ, Hermans WR, Deckers JW, de Feyter PJ, Tijssen JGP, Serruys PW. Luminal narrowing after percutaneous transluminal coronary balloon angioplasty follows a near Gaussian distribution. A quantitative angiographic study in 1445 successfully dilated lesions. *J Am Coll Cardiol* (in press).

184. Wijns W, Serruys PW, Simoons ML, van den Brand M, de Feyter PJ, Reiber JHC, Hugenholtz PG. Predictive value of early maximal exercise test and thallium scintigraphy after successful percutaneous transluminal coronary angioplasty. *Br Heart J* 1985;53:194–200.

185. Rensing BJ, Hermans WRM, Deckers JW, de Feyter PJ, Serruys PW. Which angiographic parameter best describes functional status 6 months after successful single vessel coronary balloon angioplasty? *J Am Coll Cardiol* (in press).

Practical Angioplasty,
edited by David P. Faxon.
Raven Press, Ltd., New York © 1993.

CHAPTER 14

The Management of Patients Following Successful Coronary Angioplasty

Jesse W. Currier and Mark L. Leitschuh

One of the most rewarding aspects of interventional cardiology is observing the improvement in functional capacity and quality of life in patients who have undergone successful coronary angioplasty. What one defines as success is dependent on the goals which one sets prior to undertaking the procedure. For the younger patient with single- or double-vessel coronary artery disease and normal left ventricular function, the goal is complete revascularization and immediate and long-term symptom-free status without the necessity of taking medication (1). In the very elderly patient with severe three-vessel disease and refractory angina who is felt to be a poor candidate for coronary artery bypass surgery, incomplete revascularization with some, but not total, improvement in symptoms might be a reasonable goal.

Another factor which will influence the management of patients both in hospital, and after discharge following coronary angioplasty, is the setting in which the procedure is performed. Patients undergoing a totally elective procedure will obviously be managed differently than those who undergo angioplasty in the setting of acute myocardial infarction or cardiogenic shock.

The following discussion on the management of patients after successful coronary angioplasty will consider these and other factors important in determining long-term success following the procedure. In-hospital management will be discussed first, with an emphasis on recognition of early complications and appropriate treatment strategies. This will be followed by out-of-hospital management over the first 6 months, including issues related to the timing of return to work and physical activity. Since this is also the time frame in which

restensois occurs, we will explore the various clinical manifestations of this difficult problem.

IN-HOSPITAL MANAGEMENT

Immediate Evaluation Following Coronary Angioplasty—The First 24 Hours

The first step following coronary angioplasty is the determination of the angiographic success of the procedure and the risk of abrupt closure of the vessel dilated. Assuming an adequate angiographic result has been obtained, close visual inspection with state-of-the-art imaging equipment is necessary to determine if there is evidence of major dissection or intracoronary thrombus present at the site of the dilatation. If the patient is stable and there is no evidence of major dissection or clot, he or she can be managed in a noncritical care unit equipped with hemodynamic and electrocardiographic monitoring units. Heparin is given at a dose of 100 U/kg at the beginning of the case and a drip of 1,000 U/hr is started. The activated clotting time (ACT) is followed, and the heparin dose is adjusted to keep the ACT over 300 seconds. If there are no complications, the heparin drip is discontinued after 2 hr and the vascular sheaths are removed at 4 hr after the procedure. The patient should remain at bedrest without bending at the hip for 8 hr, at which time he or she may sit up in bed and ambulate. Discharge from the hospital can be planned within 24 to 48 hr after admission, assuming the patient has ambulated without difficulty. Such an approach has been suggested for outpatient angioplasty and in one study has been found to be safe (2). This somewhat aggressive approach may, however, be unsuitable for elderly patients, even if no complications have occurred during the procedure.

JW Currier and ML Leitschuh: Division of Cardiology, Medical College of Wisconsin, Milwaukee, Wisconsin

A more cautious approach should be taken for those patients who have (i) experienced complications such as hypotension, serious arrhythmias, or vascular access problems during the angioplasty, (ii) developed in-laboratory abrupt closure from major coronary dissection or intracoronary thrombus, or (iii) undergone urgent or emergent angioplasty in the setting of unstable angina or acute myocardial infarction. These patients should be monitored in a coronary care or step-down unit and maintained on intravenous heparin for 12 to 24 hr with the vascular sheaths in place. Close attention should be given to the possibility of out-of-laboratory abrupt closure. Sheaths are removed the following day if the patient is stable. If heparinization is deemed necessary for more than 24 hr, it can generally be safely restarted within 2 to 4 hr after sheath removal.

This generalized approach to the management of patients is outlined in Fig. 1. The specific issues that will be discussed below include (i) the evaluation of postcoronary angioplasty chest pain, (ii) physical activity prior to hospital discharge, (iii) recommendations regarding medications, and (iv) the need for noninvasive testing and its interpretation prior to hospital discharge.

Evaluation of Chest Pain Following Coronary Angioplasty

The development of chest pain within the first 24 hr after angioplasty is common, of multiple etiologies, and should always be completely and comprehensively evaluated. The most serious source is that of abrupt closure of the vessel dilated, which can occur in 4.9% of patients in the cardiac catheterization laboratory and 1.9% of patients outside of the laboratory (3). Most abrupt closures

TABLE 1. *Evaluation of chest pain following successful coronary angioplasty*

1. Detailed history to determine if pain consistent with angina.
2. 12-lead ECG to evaluate for evidence of ischemia.
3. Assure adequate anticoagulation by checking ACT (should be >300 sec). Give extra heparin as necessary.
4. Treat possible spasm with nitrates and calcium channel blockers.
5. Optimize rate-pressure product (BP × HR).
6. Repeat coronary angiography to rule out abrupt closure if pain is not relieved by above measures and evidence exists for ischemia.

ECG, electrocardiogram; ACT, activated clotting time; BP, blood pressure; HR, heart.

occur in the first 24 hr, with rare cases occurring up to 1 to 2 weeks after the procedure (4). Ellis et al. found several procedural and angiographic predictive factors, including lesion length, stenosis at a bend of 45 degrees or more, stenosis at a branch point, stenosis-associated thrombus or filling defect, intimal tear, or other stenosis located in the same vessel. The NHLBI Registry 1985–1986 found both patient and lesion characteristics to be independent predictors of acute closure (5). The patient factors were triple-vessel disease, acute coronary insufficiency, or a subjective assessment that the patient was at high risk for bypass surgery. The lesion characteristics included a stenosis greater than 90%, diffuse or multiple discrete morphology, thrombus, and collateral flow from the vessel with the stenosis. As mentioned above, patients at high risk for abrupt closure warrant more vigilant monitoring during the first 24 hr following the procedure.

Other possible etiologies for chest pain shortly after angioplasty include the presence of thrombus at the site without total vessel occlusion, coronary vasospasm, or pericarditis, especially in patients with recent myocardial infarction. In addition, in the patient without complete revascularization, residual coronary artery disease with myocardial ischemia may produce chest pain.

The evaluation and treatment of chest pain following angioplasty will be somewhat dependent on the presumed etiology and the clinical suspicion for the presence of true ischemia. A general approach is outlined in Table 1. All patients with chest pain should have a 12-lead electrocardiogram (ECG) performed to determine if significant changes are present which are consistent with ischemia. The patient is then treated for possible coronary vasospasm or thrombus with an intensification of anticoagulation, nitroglycerin, or calcium channel blocker regimen. An ACT of less than 300 seconds should be promptly treated with heparin. If the patient was felt to be completely revascularized at the completion of the procedure and there is clear-cut evidence for transmural ischemia which does not respond to the above measures, he or she should be returned to the cath-

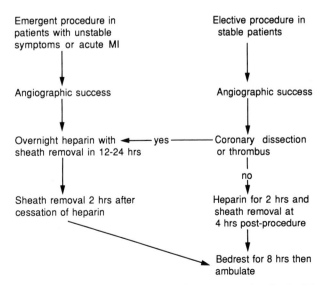

FIG. 1. Immediate evaluation and treatment of patients following successful coronary angioplasty.

eterization laboratory for angiography to determine if abrupt closure is present. If abrupt closure is present, repeat angioplasty should be performed. If the patient is not completely revascularized and responds to intensification of the medical regimen outlined above, it may be possible to observe the patient over the next 24 hr. It is often our practice to treat such patients with 3 to 5 days of systemic heparin following sheath removal, especially if angiographic evidence of dissection was present. Recurrent chest pain despite adequate anticoagulation and calcium channel blockade is an indication for returning to the cardiac catheterization laboratory.

In-Hospital Physical Activity Following Coronary Angioplasty

The level of physical activity and the timing at which the activity takes place is again dependent on the setting and the results of the procedure. As noted above, if the procedure is done electively and is without immediate complications, the vascular sheaths can be removed within 3 to 4 hr after the procedure is completed, and the patient can sit up and ambulate within 6 to 8 hr after sheath removal. If the patient continues to do well, he or she may be discharged the following morning with instructions to avoid heavy lifting or strenuous activity for the following 2 to 3 days. If the patient is elderly or otherwise debilitated, a longer period of in-hospital rehabilitation may be warranted.

If the patient has suffered an acute or recent or myocardial infarction prior to the angioplasty, the patient should undergo routine cardiac rehabilitation both in hospital and following discharge. A more aggressive approach to return to work and other activities may be indicated if the patient benefited from myocardial salvage with thrombolytic therapy or direct angioplasty and is completely revascularized (6).

Medications

Medical therapy following coronary angioplasty is directed toward (i) preventing abrupt closure or coronary vasospasm, (ii) treating possible myocardial ischemia in patients left incompletely revascularized, and (iii) possibly interrupting the process of restenosis. Since aspirin therapy has been shown to significantly reduce the incidence of abrupt closure (7), all patients are routinely started on aspirin at a dose of 325 mg daily the day prior to angioplasty and are continued on it indefinitely after the procedure in order to take advantage of its possible role in the secondary prevention of acute ischemic syndromes (8). Heparin is given intravenously at the start of angioplasty at a dose of 100 U/kg as a bolus and the patient is started on a heparin drip of 1,000 U/hr. The ACT is monitored and additional heparin is given in

order to keep the level at or greater than 300. The drip is maintained for 2 hr after the angioplasty, and then the heparin is discontinued. The sheaths are removed in approximately 2 to 3 hr after stopping the heparin, when the ACT is less than 200. If there is concern regarding the risk of abrupt closure, the heparin is continued until the following morning with close monitoring of the ACT. Heparin is occasionally continued for 3 to 5 days in patients with a large clot burden, or when very major dissections occur. In this case, heparin is decreased to half-dose for 2 to 3 hr, the sheaths are removed, and full anticoagulation therapy is continued in 2 hr.

Nitroglycerin is administered intravenously if there is concern that coronary spasm may occur, but is not routinely given at our institution. Other antianginal medications postprocedure can be tapered over the next 3 to 5 days if the patient is completely revascularized. Calcium channel blockers are given before the angioplasty and for 1 wk to 1 month after the procedure, for treatment of possible coronary vasospasm.

The treatment of restenosis is discussed below, but it should be noted that at this point no therapy has been unequivocally shown to prevent restenosis. If such therapy becomes available, it may be necessary to administer the drug before starting the procedure in order to interrupt the complex biochemical and cellular processes involved in restenosis.

In-Hospital Noninvasive Testing

The use of noninvasive testing, such as exercise stress tests with or without thallium scanning, prior to hospital discharge must be individualized and is not recommended as a routine. If the angioplasty was done electively and is without complications, there is generally no need to perform exercise testing at this time. Indeed, evidence exists that thallium scanning may be falsely positive and only revert to normal after an extended period of time (9). One area where exercise testing may be helpful for stable, uncomplicated patients is in attempts to improve the level of confidence regarding return to work or other activity. We have shown that patients who undergo exercise testing have an increase level of confidence in undertaking a number of activities, including return to work (10).

Other situations exist where the use of exercise testing may be helpful prior to discharge. In those patients who experience atypical chest pain, especially when left incompletely revascularized, exercise testing may be helpful in determining if objective evidence of myocardial ischemia exists. In addition, if the final angiographic result is less than optimal, exercise testing may be helpful in determining if ischemia develops at high work loads in the area of myocardium which is served by the dilated vessel. Although some concern has been raised regarding the safety of predischarge exercise testing, especially in those patients with unstable angina or myocardial infarction prior to the procedure, we have shown that exercise testing within 24 to 48 hr is safe in stable, uncomplicated, elective angioplasty (10).

Some studies have suggested that early abnormal thallium scans are predictive for the development of restenosis (11), but most studies report that exercise testing, with or without thallium scanning, lacks sufficient sensitivity and specificity to be of clinical usefulness in asymptomatic patients in predicting restenosis (12). The specific strategy for evaluation and treatment of restenosis is discussed in a later section.

Predischarge Patient Counseling

Although both the patient and the cardiologist are pleased and relieved by a successful outcome following coronary angioplasty, one should not minimize the seriousness of the situation to the patient. In addition to warning of recurrent symptoms of angina due to restenosis, time should be spent with the patient discussing risk factor modification in hopes of slowing the progression of the existing coronary artery disease. Out-of-hospital cardiac rehabilitation should be considered for all patients following coronary angioplasty, for both the physiological and psychological benefit which it offers. Continued smoking has been shown to be associated with a higher rate of restenosis (13), and smoking cessation should be strongly suggested to all patients. Studies from our institution have shown that elevated cholesterol levels are also associated with a higher rate of restenosis, but further studies are needed to determine if modification of lipid levels will limit restenosis (14).

OUT-OF-HOSPITAL MANAGEMENT

Physical Activity and Return to Work

One of the areas of angioplasty which is least well studied relates to the issues involved in return to work and other activities following a successful procedure. Many of the recommendations given to a patient are based on the personal management styles of the various physicians caring for the patients. In a recent study at our institution, managing physicians were surveyed regarding when they would allow their patients to return to work, and to physical and recreational activities following a successful, uncomplicated coronary angioplasty. Although most patients were discharged within 2 days following the procedure, there was a wide variation regarding when the managing physician would allow a return to work or other activities, especially those viewed as being physically strenuous (10). It is difficult to make specific recommendations in this area due to variabilities such as age, extent of residual coronary disease, and the

type of work which the patient does. However, the following general recommendations may apply to the majority of patients.

If the patient was working prior to the angioplasty and has not suffered a myocardial infarction, he or she may return to work shortly after the angioplasty. If the work does not require strenuous physical activity, as few as 2 to 3 days of rehabilitation may be sufficient. In jobs which require more physical activity, one must be assured that vascular complications at the site of sheath placement do not occur, and therefore heavy lifting should be avoided for 3 to 4 days. Some individuals advocate exercise testing before returning to strenuous physical activity, but little prognostic information is available to support this approach and the cost is not inconsequential. One interesting study recently reported that a longer lag time exists in return to work than would have been predicted (15). The best predictor of early return to work was the self-efficacy score, a psychosocial concept which reflects the degree of self-confidence to perform the job they previously held. This result would support in-depth patient counseling in order to improve patient confidence about performing their job at the earliest date possible. In regards to specific physical activities, these patients may return to activities requiring low levels of exertion (i.e. driving, cooking, light household cleaning) within 1 to 2 days. For more strenuous activity such as tennis, skiing, or yard work, a wait of 1 to 2 weeks is generally indicated.

For those patients who have suffered a recent or acute myocardial infarction, a more prolonged period of cardiac rehabilitation is indicated. This is generally best done in the outpatient, supervised programs which are available in most medical centers. The guidelines for return to work and other activities are generally determined by the functional capacity of the patient and the extent of myocardial damage, not the angioplasty procedure itself. Most patients return to work at some level within 4 to 8 weeks of hospital discharge, and specific recreational and activities of daily living can be resumed as dictated by the postmyocardial infarction time frame.

Management of Recurrent Chest Pain Following Angioplasty

The development of recurrent chest pain after hospital discharge but within the first 6 months following coronary angioplasty is usually due to incomplete revascularization or the presence of restenosis at the site of the angioplasty (16). In patients with incomplete revascularization, a decision should be made regarding the ability to obtain more complete revascularization with angioplasty. If this is felt to be possible, the patient should have angioplasty of any remaining significant stenosis. If, on the other hand, it is felt that no further revascularization is possible with angioplasty due to technical, angiographic, or clinical reasons, aggressive medical therapy or coronary artery bypass surgery are the only remaining options. Since it is often difficult to determine the etiology of the chest pain, it is our practice to perform cardiac catheterization on most of these patients. For those with incomplete revascularization who are being considered for coronary artery bypass surgery, a graft should be placed distal to the area dilated, even if the artery is patent in patients who are within the time frame of restenosis.

In patients who develop chest pain within the first 6 months following the angioplasty, especially when revascularization is complete, strong consideration should be given to the possibility of restenosis. In spite of extensive attempts to prevent it, approximately 20% to 40% of patients suffer renarrowing at the site of the dilatation. No medical therapy is currently available to prevent this process, despite numerous trials with various agents. We are, therefore, left with detecting and treating the process when it occurs.

Studies by ourselves and others (17) have shown that the majority of patients with restenosis present with exertional angina, with only a small percentage presenting with acute myocardial infarction (see Table 2). Patients often progress in symptoms from a lower to a higher class of angina if intervention is not undertaken, but few progress to unstable angina or acute infarction within the time frame of scheduling an elective angioplasty (2 to 3 weeks). There is a correlation between the presenting symptom prior to the initial angioplasty and the presentation at the time of restenosis, such that patients initially presenting with acute myocardial infarction or unstable angina are more likely to present with similar symptoms at the time of restenosis. Therefore, it is reasonable to consider urgent catheterization and angioplasty in patients whose original procedure was performed for the treatment of unstable angina or acute myocardial infarction.

Chest pain which occurs outside the window of restenosis, especially after 1 year, is more likely to represent progression of coronary artery disease rather than restenosis (16). Appropriate therapy at this time is based on the extent of disease and other clinical factors.

Noninvasive Testing

Much has been written regarding the use of exercise testing following discharge in patients with a successful angioplasty. Such testing is of potential use in determining the extent of residual myocardial ischemia which results from a less than optimal angiographic result or from incomplete revascularization. A more controversial area is the use of exercise testing to predict or detect restenosis. As noted earlier, exercise testing appears to lack the sensitivity and specificity needed to accurately predict restenosis (12). In regards to the ability to detect restenosis, Califf reports that a positive test result is only moderately accurate in identifying patients with angiographically defined restenosis, but a negative result provides a high level of assurance that restenosis is absent (18). In the patient with symptoms very suggestive of angina, we favor repeat angiography rather than exercise testing to confirm the presence of restenosis. In patients with atypical symptoms, it is reasonable to obtain more objective evidence of ischemia with the use of exercise testing, with or without thallium.

Long-term Outcome Following Successful Angioplasty

There are now a series of patients reported in the literature with long-term follow-up after coronary angioplasty. The group from Emory found that at 5 years, the risk of death was 3.7% and of myocardial infarction 6%. Twenty percent of patients had had a second angioplasty and 16% had undergone coronary artery bypass grafting (CABG). Ninety percent of the patients were symptomatic at the time of initial angioplasty, but only 15% were symptomatic at the time of follow-up (1).

In a smaller series of 46 patients, 3-year results showed an excellent functional capacity. Exercise time increased from 9.8 min preangioplasty to 18.3 min after angioplasty, and this was maintained over 3 years. Angiographic restenosis occurred in 29% of patients at 6 months, and in only 1 patient over the ensuing 2.5 years (19).

These data have been since confirmed in a serial angiographic study from the Montreal Heart Institute (20). At 5 months, 38% of patients had restenosis following angioplasty. Repeat angiography, at an average of 34 months, showed late restenosis in only 1%. Progression of disease at 34 months was seen in 34% of patients.

These results confirm the generally excellent long-term results in patients with successful angioplasty and reinforce the need for risk factor modification and close clinical follow-up in the hope of preventing and detecting the progression of disease.

CONCLUSIONS

In order to successfully manage patients following angioplasty, one must individualize treatment strategies based on the circumstances surrounding the procedure and the desired goal of the therapy. Close attention should be paid to the presence of chest pain at any time

TABLE 2. *Clinical presentation at the time of restenosis*

Symptom	Occurrence (%)
Exertional angina	85.5
Average CHA class	2.6 + 1.0
Unstable angina	11.3
Acute myocardial infarction	1.6
Asymptomatic with + ETT	1.6

ETT, exercise tolerance test.

after the procedure and it should be evaluated completely as outlined above. Of equal importance should be counseling of the patient regarding the possibility of restenosis and the need for risk factor modification. In order to accomplish these goals it is important for the patient to have close clinical follow-up, either by the cardiologist or the patient's primary care provider. In the later case, good communication is necessary between the referring physician and the interventional cardiologist in order to assure that the patient has adequate follow-up. If such measures are taken, the majority of patients undergoing successful angioplasty can obtain excellent long-term results from the procedure.

REFERENCES

1. Talley JD, Hurst JW, King SB, Douglas JS, Roubin GS, Gruentzig AR, Anderson HV, Weintraub WS. Clinical outcome 5 years after attempted percutaneous transluminal coronary angioplasty in 427 patients. *Circulation* 1988;77:820–829.

2. Cragg DR, Friedman HZ, Almany SL, Gangadharan V, Ramos RG, Levine AB, LeBeau TA, O'Neil WO. Early hospital discharge after percutaneous transluminal coronary angioplasty. *Am J Cardiol* 1989;64:1270–1274.

3. Cowley MJ, Dorros G, Kelsey SF, Van Raden M, Detre KM. Acute coronary events associated with percutaneous transluminal angioplasty. *Am J Cardiol* 1984;53:12C–16C.

4. Sinclair IN, McCabe CH, Sipperly ME, Baim DS. Predictors, therapeutic options and long-term outcome of abrupt reclosure. *Am J Cardiol* 1988;61:61G–66G.

5. Ellis SG, Roubin GS, King SB, Douglas JS, Weintraub WS, Thomas RG, Cox WR. Angiographic and clinical predictors of acute closure after native vessel coronary angioplasty. *Circulation* 77;1988:372–379.

6. Topol EJ, Burek K, O'Neil WW, Kewman DG, Kander NH, Shea MJ, Schork MA, Kirschit J, Juni JE, Pitt BP. A randomized controlled trial of hospital discharge three days after myocardial infarction in the era of reperfusion. *N Engl J Med* 1988;318:1083–1088.

7. Schwartz L, Bourassa MG, Lespérance J, et al. Aspirin and dipyridamole in the prevention of restenosis after percutaneous transluminal angioplasty. *N Engl J Med* 1988;318:1714–1719.

8. Antiplatelet Trialists' Collaboration. Secondary prevention of vascular disease by prolonged antiplatelet treatment. *BMJ* 1988;296:320.

9. Manyari DE, Knudtson M, Kloiber R, Roth D. Sequential thallium-201 myocardial perfusion studies after successful percutaneous transluminal coronary artery angioplasty: delayed resolution of exercise-induced scintigraphic abnormalities. *Circulation* 1988;77:86–95.

10. Leitschuh ML, Balady GJ, Jacobs AK, Weiner DA, Ryan TJ. Safety and utility of early exercise testing after PTCA: results of a randomized trial. *J Am Coll Cardiol* 1991;17:237A.

11. Breisblatt WM, Weiland FL, Spaccavento LJ. Stress thallium-201 imaging after coronary angioplasty predicts restenosis and recurrent symptoms. *J Am Coll Cardiol* 1988;12:1199–1204.

12. Califf RM, Ohman EM, Frid DJ, Fortin DF, Mark DB, Hlatky MA, Herndon JE, Bengtson JR. Restenosis: the clinical issues. In: Topol E, ed. *Textbook of interventional cardiology.* Philadelphia: WB Saunders; 1990:199–223.

13. Galan KM, Deligonul V, Kern MJ, Chaitman BR, Vandermael MG. Increased frequency of restenosis in patients continuing to smoke after percutaneous transluminal coronary angioplasty. *Am J Cardiol* 1988;61:260–263.

14. Jacobs AK, Folan DJ, McSweeney SM, Faxon DP, Kellet MA, Sandborn TA, Ryan TJ. Effect of plasma lipids on restenosis following coronary angioplasty. *J Am Coll Cardiol* 1987;9:183A.

15. Fitzgerald ST, Becker DM, Celentano DD, Swank R, Brinker J. Return to work after percutaneous transluminal coronary angioplasty. *Am J Cardiol* 1989;64:1108–1112.

16. Joelson JM, Most AS, Williams DO. Angiographic findings when chest pain recurs after successful percutaneous transluminal coronary angioplasty. *Am J Cardiol* 1987;60:792–795.

17. Joelson JM, Becker DJ, Most AS, Williams DO. Initial presentation predicts clinical manifestation of restenosis after successful coronary angioplasty. *Circulation* 1988;78(Suppl II):633.

18. Califf RM, Fortin DF, Frid DJ, Harlan WR, Ohman EM, Bengtson JR, Nelson CL, Tcheng JE, Mark DG, Stack RS. Restenosis after coronary angioplasty: an overview. *J Am Coll Cardiol* 1991;17:2B–13B.

19. Rosing DR, Cannon RO, Watson RM, Bonnow RO, Mincemayer R, Ewels C, Leon M, La Katos E, Epstein SE, Kent KM. Three year anatomic, functional, and clinical followup after successful PTCA. *J Am Coll Cardiol* 1987;9:1–7.

20. Cequior A, Bonan R, Crepeau J, Cote G, De Guise P, Joly P, Lespérance J, Waters PD. Restenosis and progression of coronary atherosclerosis after coronary angioplasty. *J Am Coll Cardiol* 1988;12:49–55.

CHAPTER 15

Coronary Atherectomy

Robert F. Fishman and Donald S. Baim

The equipment and techniques of conventional angioplasty have improved markedly since its development in 1977 (1–3). Despite broader application, improved success rate, and lower complication rate, however, conventional angioplasty continues to be plagued by several limitations. These include (i) failure to cross a stenosis or occlusion, (ii) failure to dilate a rigid or eccentric lesion, (iii) the development of abrupt closure, and (iv) restenosis (4). Coronary atherectomy has been developed in an effort to overcome some of these limitations (5–7).

Several different atherectomy devices have been introduced for use in native coronary arteries and saphenous vein bypass grafts (SVG). All use cutting surfaces rotated at high speeds to reduce coronary stenoses by either removing the obstructing tissue from the body, or pulverizing it into minute particles safe for distal embolization. Devices which remove plaque include (i) the Simpson AtheroCath (Devices for Vascular Intervention, Redwood City, CA), (ii) the transluminal extraction catheter (TEC) (Interventional Vascular Technologies, Inc., San Diego, CA), (iii) the rotational atherectomy system (C. R. Bard, Inc., Billerica, MA), and (iv) the Fischell pullback atherectomy catheter (Arrow/MedInnovations, Inc., Reading, PA). Devices which rely on plaque abrasion and pulverization include (i) the Auth Rotoblator (Heart Technology, Inc., Seattle, WA), (ii) the Kensey catheter (Theratek International, Miami, FL), (iii) the atherolytic reperfusion guidewire (Medrad, Pittsburgh, PA) and (iv) the low-speed rotational angioplasty catheter (ROTAC). To date, the technique of directional coronary atherectomy (DCA) using the Simpson AtheroCath has received the most widespread investigational and clinical use in the coronary system, and will be the major focus of this chapter.

RF Fishman and DS Baim: Harvard-Thorndike Laboratory, Cardiovascular Division, Beth Israel Hospital, Boston, Massachusetts

It was hypothesized that the controlled method of excision and retrieval of tissue by DCA would (i) reduce the incidence of abrupt vessel closure by limiting the incidence of dissection, flaps, and thrombus; (ii) reduce the incidence of restenosis by removing the obstructing lesion and leaving a smoother surface, thereby decreasing platelet aggregation and limiting intimal hyperplasia; and (iii) expand the treatment of lesions currently considered unfavorable for conventional balloon angioplasty due to calcified, ulcerated, eccentric, lengthy, ostial, or bifurcation morphology (8).

Directional coronary atherectomy was developed and refined by Dr. John B. Simpson at Sequoia Hospital, Redwood City, CA, using cadaveric peripheral arteries (9). The procedure was first applied clinically in the peripheral arterial system in 1985 (5) and in the coronary circulation in 1987 (6). As of January, 1991, more than 2000 patients have undergone DCA using the Simpson AtheroCath.

INDICATIONS

The indications for DCA are continually changing as the technology improves and physicians gain more experience. Because of differences in technique, even experienced conventional angioplasty operators require further training before attempting to perform DCA.

Clinical Indications

Patients referred for DCA should have symptoms and exercise test evidence of myocardial ischemia in association with a significant obstructing lesion suitable for DCA. Patients ideally should be free of significant peripheral vascular disease, and they should be considered suitable for coronary artery bypass surgery in the event of an atherectomy complication.

Angiographic Criteria

Angiographic indications for DCA are listed in Tables 1 and 2. The technique is most easily and safely performed in 3.0 to 4.0-mm diameter proximal and mid left anterior descending (LAD) arteries with focal, eccentric, de novo, or restenosis lesions. However, DCA is also quite effective in treating LAD origin, aorta-ostial, ulcerated, SVG, or bifurcation lesions, in which the efficacy of conventional angioplasty remains limited (10). Certain lesion features, however, still contraindicate DCA. These include

1. Diffusely diseased vessels.
2. Total occlusions (unless first successfully recanalized by conventional angioplasty).
3. Lesions with significant angulation (>45°).

TABLE 1. *Angiographic indications of DCA difficulty*

Highly favorable lesions

Proximal/mid or ostial LAD
Proximal LCX with a short left main and shallow takeoff
3.0–3.5-mm diameter vessel
Restenosis lesion
Eccentric
Focal
Saphenous vein graft without thrombus or calcification

Favorable lesions

Proximal/mid RCA
Accessible mid LCX
2.5–4.0-mm diameter vessel
De novo lesions
Concentric
Tubular
Ulcerated
Aortoostial

Challenging

Distal LAD/RCA >2.5 mm in diameter
Protected left main
Moderate angulation
Moderate tortuosity of proximal vessel
Mild diffuse length
Moderate calcification
Adajacent distal lesion
Presence of thrombus

Not recommended

Unprotected left main
Highly angulated segment
Excessive turtuosity of proximal segment
Vessels <2.5 mm in diameter
Degenerated saphenous vein grafts
Long/spiral dissections
Heavy calcifications
Moderate disease in left main
Total occlusion unless successfully recanalized by
  conventional angioplasty

TABLE 2. *Definitions of lesion characteristics*

Discrete:	Lesion length of ≤10 mm
Tubular:	Lesion length of 11–20 mm
Diffuse:	Lesion length of >20 mm
Eccentric:	A stenosis with asymmetry in any angiographic projection
Calcification:	Radioopaque density at the lesion or in the target vessel as seen on cineangiogram
Ostial involvement:	A stenosis involving the ostium of the left main, RCA or saphenous vein graft (aorta-ostial) or LAD or diagonal (non-aorta-ostial)
Ulceration:	A lesion with a contrast-filled crater
Bifurcation lesion:	Involvment of a moderate to large sized branch that contains a stenosis of >50% at its origin

4. Severe tortuosity proximal to or immediately distal to the lesion.
5. Severe vascular calcification, especially calcified ostial lesions.
6. A lesion in a circumflex artery whose origin is steeply angulated from the left main.
7. Vessels <2.5 mm in diameter.
8. Lesions lying beyond a moderately diseased left main trunk.

While DCA for abrupt closure after attempted angioplasty has been effective in selected cases (8,11), some investigators advise caution in the application of DCA to angioplasty-induced dissections, given the increased risk of vessel perforation (12,13).

TECHNICAL ASPECTS

The Simpson AtheroCath is a multilumen catheter which terminates in a windowed cylindrical housing unit that encloses a cup-shaped cutter (Figs. 1 and 2). A balloon is mounted to the housing opposite the window and is used to press the window up against the diseased vessel wall. The cutter is connected to a hollow torque cable, through whose central lumen a steerable 0.014-in guidewire can be passed. A battery powered motor drive unit rotates this cable and the attached cutter at 2,000 rpm, as it is advanced using the cutter advancement control lever. The flexible nose cone at the distal tip facilitates atraumatic catheter passage, and serves as a specimen collection chamber.

Device Selection

The currently available sizes of device housings for the coronary circulation are 5 French (F), 6F, and 7F (Table 3). The working diameter of each device is based on the combined size of the housing plus the inflated balloon. The working diameter of the 6F device is 3.5 mm. There

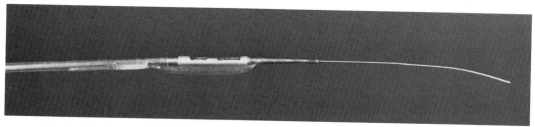

FIG. 1. The Simpson AtheroCath (Devices for Vascular Intervention). See text for details.

are two 7F devices: one for native arteries with a 4.0-mm working diameter, and one for vein grafts with a 4.5-mm working diameter (the larger diameter is due to a larger attached balloon). Device size is selected by estimating the size of the normal vessel adjacent to the stenosis (the reference segment). In general, one should choose a device whose working diameter is no more than 0.5 mm larger than the reference segment. We thus generally use a 6F device when the reference diameter is less than 3.0 mm and a 7F device when the reference diameter is greater than 3.0 mm, or when there is significant residual stenosis after use of the 6F device with balloon inflation pressures up to 40 psi. Only rarely (i.e., subtotal occlusions in calcified or moderately tortuous vessels) is the 5F device used to partially debulk the plaque and facilitate subsequent passage of a definitive larger device.

Preparing the Catheter

The balloon is filled with 60% contrast (full-strength Renografin-60 or Angiovist-282) after aspirating lumen air for approximately 3 sec. Contrast is then slowly infused into the balloon lumen under a positive pressure no greater than 60 psi (4 atm). Any residual luminal air is purged out of the self-vent at the tip of the balloon during this process. Make sure no visible air remains within the balloon, and do not apply negative pressure to the balloon while the device is outside the body, since this could result in aspiration of air back into the balloon. Flush the proximal port with sterile physiologic saline. A 0.014-in wire can be backloaded from the distal tip if the cutter is positioned in the middle of the housing window so the wire can be seen to enter the cutter lumen. If the wire is front loaded from the proximal end of the catheter, the cutter should be fully advanced to its distal stop. Make the appropriate bend on the distal tip of the wire, and make sure that it moves freely within the catheter. Do not use an ACS DOC wire, as the atherectomy catheter may not easily pass over the connection. Attach the motor drive unit and check for proper cutter movement and rotation.

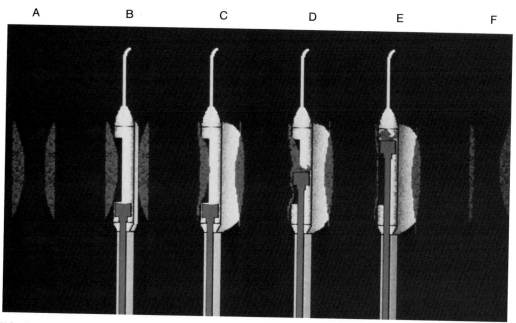

FIG. 2. Schematic representation of atherectomy device and procedure. **A:** Coronary artery segment with stenotic lesion before atherectomy. **B:** Atherectomy device in place across the lesion. **C:** Atherectomy device with balloon inflated. **D, E:** As rotating cup-shaped cutter is advanced, material is shaved from stenotic lesion. **F:** Coronary artery segment after atherectomy.

TABLE 3. *Catheter sizes*

Catheter size	Housing diameter (mm)	Inflated balloon diameter (mm)	Working diameter (mm)	Equivalent PTCA catheter size (mm)
5 French	1.7	1.3	3.0	2.5
6 French	2.0	1.5	3.5	3.0
7 French	2.3	1.7	4.0	3.5
7 French Graft	2.3	2.2	4.5	4.0

Initial Procedure

Patients have been pretreated with aspirin 325 mg daily and dypyridamole 50 mg four times daily, starting at least 24 hr prior to the procedure, and continuing indefinitely after discharge. After insertion of a 9F arterial sheath, 10,000 U of heparin are given, and additional heparin is given throughout the procedure (2,500 U approximately every 30 min) to maintain an activated clotting time of more than 300 sec. We generally perform baseline coronary angiography using standard 9F angioplasty guiding catheters. Once angiography confirms the presence of a critical lesion amenable to atherectomy, the 9F arterial sheath is exchanged for an 11F sheath. When the iliac artery is tortuous we recommend using a long 11F arterial sheath.

Guiding Catheter

Conventional angioplasty guiding catheters are *not* suitable for atherectomy due to their acute angulation and relatively small lumens. Special 11F guiding catheters have been developed by Devices for Vascular Interventions (DVI) that have gentle curves rather than the sharp angles of conventional guiding catheters so as to facilitate the passage of the rigid atherectomy housing. The 11F guides have an inner diameter of 9F (3 mm) (Fig. 3). These guides are available in shapes equivalent to left Judkins (JCL3.5 and JCL4.0) and right Judkins (JCR4) catheters. Guides for the downward-pointing right coronary artery (RCA) or grafts (JRinf), and upward pointing grafts (JRG, JLG) are also available. The guide is inserted over an 8F introducing catheter and an 0.038-in guidewire. When inserting the introducing catheter into the guide, the guide should be momentarily straightened in order to minimize the potential of damage to the side holes in the guide. Once the guide–introducing catheter combination has been advanced into the ascending aorta, the inner introducing catheter and wire are then removed and the guide is flushed and filled with contrast. The guide is connected to the coronary manifold using a large bore rotating hemostatic valve (DVI). Modification of the O-ring fitting to include a self-closing disc valve helps reduce blood loss during catheter manipulation. The 11F guide has excellent torque control, but is quite stiff. It should be engaged gently, and

not deeply seated in the vessel ostium. Overmanipulation can lead to ostial dissections, especially in the right coronary artery. If contrast load will be a clinical limitation, diluted contrast can be used for the procedure, reserving full-strength contrast for the pre- and postprocedure angiography.

Positioning the Device

Introduce the device into the guide carefully, with the wire withdrawn just inside the distal tip of the atherectomy device, before trying to insert it into the rotating hemostatic valve. Once the device is in the ascending aorta just proximal to the side holes of the guide, advance the 0.014-in wire so that it exits the main lumen of the guide rather than a side hole, and position it in the main vessel beyond the target lesion (rather than a distal branch vessel). The maneuvers necessary to advance the atherectomy device across the target lesion are different from those used to advance a conventional angioplasty balloon. With the cutter advanced to its distal position, gently advance the device by combining gentle forward pressure with continuous rotation, until the nose cone enters into the proximal portion of the vessel. Gently lifting or rotating the guiding catheter in order to align

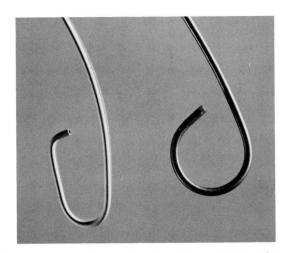

FIG. 3. Guiding catheters for directional coronary atherectomy (Devices for Vascular Intervention) are constructed with gentle curves rather than sharp angles. **Left:** A 9F JL4 guiding catheter for conventional angioplasty. **Right:** An 11F JCL3.5 guiding catheter for coronary atherectomy (4).

the device with the long axis of the vessel will ease insertion. Continue to apply forward pressure and rotate the device, but do not attempt to force it into a lesion or around curves, as excessive force might cause trauma to the vessel wall. If the device will not cross the lesion, consider using a smaller device, or predilating the lesion with a small (2.0–2.5 mm) conventional angioplasty balloon. It is not generally advisable to routinely predilate the lesion prior to atherectomy because balloon dilatation may make subsequent tissue removal more difficult. Atherectomy of ostial lesions should not be attempted unless the device is coaxially aligned with the artery, so that DCA of aorta-ostial lesions require significant experience in manipulating the guide and device. A portion of the rigid cutter window must remain in the aorta, depriving the cutter of full support.

Once across the lesion, the device is rotated under fluoroscopy until the cutting window is seen in profile, oriented toward the greatest bulk of eccentric plaque. An initial balloon inflation pressure of 10 to 20 psi is used to press the cutting window against the plaque, while the motor-driven cutter is advanced slowly across the window over a period 5 sec. Low inflation pressures help minimize concominant angioplasty effect and maximize tissue retrieval. The assistant takes charge of balloon inflation and holds the guidewire in place during cutter advancement, to avoid excessive guidewire motion. After each cut, the balloon is deflated and the device is rotated 90 degrees to reorient the window within the lesion. The balloon is then inflated partially (to 10 psi) as the cutter is retracted in preparation for the next cuts. This prevents distal embolization of debris and/or retrieved tissue from the nose cone. The balloon is then inflated fully as the cut is made. Cuts should be made only in orientations where there is angiographic (or ultrasonic) evidence of disease, to avoid damage to normal vessel walls. The cutter should be advanced to its distal stop with each cut, in order to make sure that the cut is complete and the strip of plaque is parted off from the vessel wall. If the cutter fails to advance completely to the distal stop, the collection chamber may be full. The device and guidewire should be withdrawn every four to six cuts to empty the collection chamber by backflushing from the device tip. The cutter lumen should also be flushed and balloon integrity checked. If there is a residual stenosis but no additional tissue can be removed with balloon inflation pressure up to 60 psi (4 atm), consider switching to a larger device. Calcified lesions often require higher inflation pressures (40–60 psi) and slower advancement of the cutter. The number of passes and final device size will be determined by the size of the reference segment and the presence of residual disease. Recrossing the stenosis with the guidewire and atherectomy device after the initial series of cuts is generally quite easy. Success is defined as tissue removal with a residual stenosis of less than 50%, without having to use a postatherectomy balloon dilatation, and the absence of a major complication (Q-wave myocardial infarction, emergency bypass surgery, or death).

Supplemental Conventional Balloon Angioplasty

As previously discussed, conventional angioplasty balloon dilatation should not be done routinely prior to atherectomy unless it is necessary to pass the atherectomy device across the lesion, since predilatation can potentially decrease the amount of tissue retrieved by atherectomy. If predilatation is necessary prior to atherectomy, only a small (2.0–2.5 mm) balloon should be used. Restenotic lesions are generally easier to cross, given the softer nature of intimal hyperplasia compared to de novo lesions, and rarely need predilatation. Postatherectomy dilatation with conventional angioplasty balloons should be reserved for lesions which cannot be crossed with the atherectomy device, or for those in which significant residual stenosis can no longer be debulked using the appropriately sized device. Conventional angioplasty can also be used to tack up small to moderate dissections, and to rescue side branches compromised by the atherectomy.

Potential Difficulties

Failure to Cross

This is the most common problem with the current bulky and rigid atherectomy device. If the initial combination of continuous rotation and forward advancement fails, consider switching to a smaller device, or predilating the lesion with a small conventional angioplasty balloon at low pressure. If still unable to cross, conventional angioplasty is required.

Difficult Movement of the Guidewire

Hold the wire while advancing the cutter. Do not allow the wire to enter a distal branch as the guidewire may become trapped and fracture as torque is applied by high speed rotation of the cutter.

Cutter Will Not Advance

Try to straighten the catheter to relieve binding on the cutter torque cable. Consider deflating the balloon to allow completion of the cut, and parting off of the specimen from the vessel wall. Check the motor drive unit for proper function. If the cutter still will not advance, gently remove the device while maintaining forward pressure on the advancement control lever in order to retain any collected specimens.

Loss of Side Branch

If the cutter window must be positioned across a side branch, there is a chance of branch closure. Consider whether side branch loss would be clinically tolerated prior to device insertion. Such side branches can usually be rescued by either DCA or conventional angioplasty.

Thrombus

If there is a significant thrombus burden, consider using intracoronary urokinase, before or after DCA, although this may increase the risk of bleeding at the femoral artery insertion site, given the 11F puncture.

Femoral Vascular Damage

Patients are at increased risk due to the large sheath required for vascular access. We recommend performing iliac angiography with half-strength contrast at the end of the procedure to document good distal flow. If there is iliac disease, or distal flow is impeded, the sheath should be removed as soon as possible. For routine sheath removal, we have found a reduced incidence of vascular complications if the sheath removal is delayed until the activated clotting time is less than 180 sec. Heparin may be reinstituted 2 hr after sheath removal.

CURRENT STATUS OF DIRECTIONAL CORONARY ATHERECTOMY

Acute Angiographic Results

More than 2,000 coronary atherectomy procedures have been performed with the Simpson AtheroCath, as of January, 1991. Success has been achieved in 83% to 90% of lesions, despite the fact that the procedure was attempted in many lesions generally considered to be unfavorable for conventional angioplasty. The DVI Multicenter Registry analyzed 1,020 DCA procedures performed in 1,140 lesions at 14 clinical centers between October 1, 1986 and December 31, 1989 (14). This study included patients with clinical or exercise-induced ischemia, and focal proximal stenoses or stenoses with marked eccentricity or irregularities, in arteries with a reference diameter greater than or equal to 2.5 mm. Patients with ongoing myocardial ischemia, an acute myocardial infarction (MI) within 14 days, severe congestive heart failure, excessive coronary calcifications, unprotected left main lesions, or severe peripheral vascular disease were excluded. Lesion distribution included: LAD (53%), RCA (22%), circumflex (CX) (6%), left main (3%), and SVG (17%). Lesion location was ostial (10%),

proximal (50%), mid (33%), and distal (7%). The majority (54%) of lesions were focal, but 35% were tubular (10–20 mm) and 11% were larger than 20 mm. Sixty-three percent of lesions were eccentric and 15% were calcified. Conventional angioplasty was required prior to DCA in 21% and after DCA in 14% of lesions. The overall success rate was 83%.

At the Beth Israel Hospital between August, 1988 and June, 1991, we performed DCA on more than 200 lesions comprising approximately 9% of all interventional procedures. We recently reported our experience in the first 76 lesions (7): DCA success was achieved in 67 (88%) of lesions. Eight additional patients underwent successful angioplasty after failed DCA (7 patients for failure to cross with the atherectomy device and one for aorta-ostial graft lesion that had a poor DCA result). Diameter stenosis was reduced from 80 ± 11% to 5 ± 15% after atherectomy (Fig. 4). There was no difference in the residual stenosis when the device size (6F or 7F) was compared, but the 7F device yielded a larger postprocedure lumen diameter (3.7 ± 0.6 mm versus 2.6 ± 0.4 mm for the 6F device). The improvement in diameter stenosis after DCA is thus generally superior to that seen after conventional angioplasty (15).

Hinohara and colleagues reported the experience at Sequoia Hospital (10) in 382 procedures involving 447

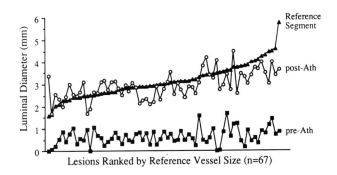

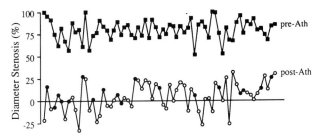

FIG. 4. Plots of quantitative angiographic results before and after successful coronary atherectomy in 67 lesions. **Top:** Absolute luminal diameter (mm) before and after atherectomy compared with the reference segment. **Bottom:** Percent diameter stenosis before and after atherectomy. Each lesion is represented by a single point along the horizontal axis, ranked in order of increasing reference segment diameter. Lesions that later developed restenosis are indicated in bottom panel by closed instead of open circles (7).

lesions. Atherectomy was successful in 89.5% of lesions with a procedural success rate (subsequent balloon angioplasty) of 94.4%. De novo lesions had a lower success rate than restenosis lesions (84% versus 93%). Success rates varied with the involved vessel: LAD (92.6%), CX (93.3%), RCA (83.5%), left main (75%) and SVG (91.4%), but not lesion location (ostial, proximal and mid and/or distal). Success rates for non–aorta-ostial (LAD, diagonal) was 100% while that of aorta-ostial lesions was 71%. The atherectomy success rate for simple lesions was 97%, while that of complex lesions (eccentric, ≥10 mm in length, calcified, ostial, dissection ulceration, flap-like, angulated, tortuous, bifurcation, thrombus) was 87%. The success rate was lowest for calcified de novo lesions (52%, versus 83% for calcified restenosis lesions). Among angiographic complex lesions, the presence of calcium was the strongest predictor of failed atherectomy. Success rate was also lower (75%) for de novo lesions over 10 mm in length.

Thus, atherectomy can be performed successfully in a variety of lesions within native coronary arteries and SVGs. The acute angiographic results are excellent despite the presence of lesion characteristics generally considered to be unfavorable for conventional angioplasty (eccentric, ostial, and bifurcation lesions with abnormal

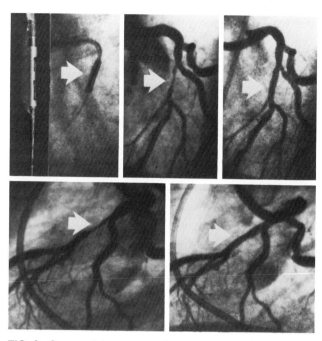

FIG. 6. Successful coronary atherectomy performed in a 53-year-old man with an eccentric mid LAD stenosis that was at the site of prior conventional angioplasty. **Top:** The 6F Athero-Cath outside the body and positioned in the mid LAD (LAO cranial view), pre- and postprocedure angiography. **Bottom:** Pre- and postprocedure angiography in the lateral view.

contour) (Figs. 5 and 6). With appropriate training on case selection and device use, the success and complication rates among new operators (those starting DCA since FDA approval in Fall, 1990) have been generally comparable to those of experienced operators during the investigational phase. While atherectomy now has its own Current Procedural Terminology (CPT) code, institution and professional reimbursements are provided at the conventional angioplasty level.

Complications

Based on the data of the DVI Multicenter Registry of 1,648 patients (1,774 lesions) the incidence of complications following DCA appears to be similar to that of conventional angioplasty (16). Major complications [death, emergency coronary artery bypass graft (CABG); or Q-wave MI] occurred in 5.7% of patients, of which 3.8% were directly attributable to the DCA procedure. Specifically, death occurred in 0.8%, emergency CABG in 3.8% and Q-wave MI in 0.7% of patients. Angiographic risk factors associated with a major complication included (i) RCA atherectomy, (ii) diffuse disease, (iii) eccentric stenosis, and (iv) de novo lesions (17). It should be noted that during the preapproval investigation the incidence of major complications decreased from 5.3% to 2.5% with increased operator experience, improved equip-

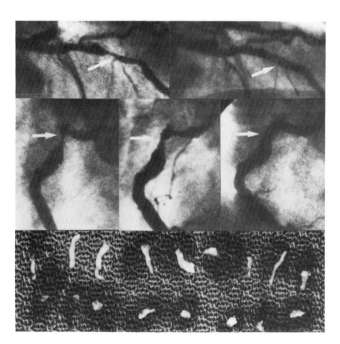

FIG. 5. Successful coronary atherectomy performed on an eccentric mid LAD stenosis (*top panels*) and a proximal-RCA stenosis (*middle panel*) in a 64-year-old man. A 6F atherectomy was used in the LAD and a 7F (4.0 mm working diameter) was used in the RCA. The bottom panel shows the retrieved tissue specimens. Histologic examination revealed atherosclerotic plaque and intimal hyperplasia in both the LAD and RCA lesions. There was evidence of thrombus in the RCA lesion.

ment design, and refined case selection. Reasons for urgent CABG included coronary obstruction at the site of atherectomy (1.8%), perforation (0.3%), dissection due to guidewire (0.2%), and ostial dissection due to the guide (0.4%). There was a trend toward higher rates of emergency CABG for lesions of 20 mm or more (18), de novo lesions (19), and complex morphology (13). Hinohara et al. (10) reported a 0% incidence of major complications for simple lesions, compared to a 3.8% incidence for complex lesions. The major complication rate was 5% for lesions over 10 mm or lesions with calcium or abnormal contour (ulceration, dissection, flap).

Popma reported an abrupt closure rate of 4.2% in 1,020 procedures for 1,140 lesions (14), with an increased risk of abrupt closure in de novo lesions, RCA atherectomy, and diffuse disease. There tended to be a lower incidence of abrupt closure in SVG atherectomy. Salvage angioplasty was effective in half (16/32) of the patients in whom it was attempted, but 24 patients underwent emergency CABG.

Less severe complications occurred in 7% to 11% of patients (16,20,21), a number which compares favorably with conventional angioplasty (22). Non–Q-wave MI occurred in 3.4% of patients in the DVI Registry (16), 4.5% in the Beth Israel series (7), and 3.8% in the Mayo Clinic cohort (21). Other clinical complications reported by the Registry include prolonged chest pain (5.5%), ventricular tachycardia (1.1%), ventricular fibrillation (0.5%), femoral vascular repair (1.7%), and hypotension (1.8%). We have noted that immediately following the procedure, some patients experience pleuritic discomfort not associated with objective evidence of ongoing ischemia, such as impaired coronary flow, ST-segment changes, or elevations in cardiac filling pressures (22). The incidence of femoral vascular complication requiring surgical repair appears to be somewhat higher than that of conventional angioplasty; this is likely due to the use of an 11F arterial sheath (23). Predictors of femoral vascular complications when using large sheaths include advanced age, female gender, presence of peripheral vascular disease, and diabetes (24). Reversible causes of hypotension include blood loss, tamponade, vasodilator medications, and vasovagal reactions.

Angiographic complications have also been reported by the DVI Registry including dissection (6.5%), loss of side branch (2.7%), coronary vasospasm (2.2%), distal embolization (1.9%), coronary perforation (0.5%), new lesion at a non-DCA site (0.3%), and coronary pseudoaneurysm (0.1%) (16). Rowe, in a nonrandomized study documented a decreased (11%) dissection rate for DCA compared to conventional angioplasty (37%) (25). Others have shown an increased risk of dissection with DCA in lesions larger than 20 mm (18,19), but not for procedures in which subintimal components (media, adventitia) were recovered (7,26,27). Side-branch occlusion is generally recognized before the patient leaves the

catheterization laboratory, and can be managed by conventional angioplasty. Other less frequent complications have included nose-cone separation, guidewire fracture, and intracoronary air embolism (16).

Late Follow-Up

The initial hope was that coronary atherectomy would lower the incidence of restenosis by providing larger, smoother arterial lumens compared to conventional angioplasty. Although follow-up data remains limited, it appears that the restenosis rate with DCA remains comparable to that for angioplasty (25–30%). We reported (7) a restenosis rate of 30% in 76 lesions according to a 6-month life-table analysis, with a trend of a lower rates of restenosis in de novo lesions compared to restenosis lesions (20% versus 40%). Although controlled trials have yet to be performed, this restenosis rate may be somewhat lower than might be expected for similar lesions dilated by conventional angioplasty (4).

Various lesion and patient characteristics appear to be associated with different rates of restenosis after DCA. The DCA Investigator Group reported on 6-month angiographic follow-up in 384 lesions (77% compliance) (28). The restenosis rate was higher in SVGs compared to native coronary arteries (50.3% vs. 40.3%). Within each category, de novo lesions had a significantly lower restenosis rate than restenosis lesions. Kaufman et al. reported that in spite of high success rates, restenosis remains high after DCA in SVGs (29). Holmes reported the follow-up data from the Mayo Clinic series of 124 patients (30). Restenosis rates were as follows: for de novo lesions in native coronary arteries 37%, and in SVGs 55%; for restenosis lesions in native coronary arteries 49%, and in SVGs 71%. Restenosis and recurrent symptoms have occurred within a similar time frame to that seen after conventional angioplasty. The severity of angina and incidence of death and infarction was highest in the patients undergoing DCA of SVGs. Selmon et al. reported angiographic follow-up for 52 lesions in SVGs (31). The overall restenosis rate was 59.6% (46.2% for de novo lesions, 73.1% for restenosis lesions). The authors concluded that although DCA can be performed effectively on SVGs, restenosis rates remain high, with a high (6.9%) risk of distal embolization.

Simpson et al. reported an overall restenosis rate of 24.2% for native, de novo lesions (32). The restenosis rates varied depending on the lesion location (ostial, 46.2%; proximal, 16.1%; mid and/or distal, 22.7%), and the reference vessel size (<3.0 mm, 33.3%; >3.0 mm, 18.4%), but not lesion length, or whether the lesion was in the LAD versus the RCA. Hinohara et al. (33) reported an overall restenosis rate of 36% (29% for de novo, 40% for restenosis lesions). They documented a significantly higher incidence of restenosis for lesions larger than 10 mm (51% vs. 30% for <10 mm), vessels smaller than 3.0 mm (44% vs. 29% for ≥3.0 mm), lesions with calcium absent (39% vs. 19% if present) and vessels with a postprocedure residual stenosis <−10% (57% versus 34% if >−10%). The authors conclude that restenosis following DCA is lower in shorter lesions, when vessel size is 3.0 mm or more, and without DCA overdilatation.

Schmidt et al. (34) reported that the risk of restenosis following DCA is higher with a smaller post-DCA luminal diameter, a cholesterol level over 200 mg%, and a lower NYHA class, but not with acute ischemic status, lesion eccentricity, native versus SVG lesions, prior angioplasty, reference artery size, pre- or post-DCA percent stenosis, or histologic depth of resection. Hinohara et al. (35) reported that recent (<4 months) previous angioplasty and lesions larger than 10 mm predicted recurrent restenosis following DCA of restenosis lesions.

DeCesare et al. caution against causing acute ectasia (final stenosis < 0%) because of a higher rate of restenosis with occasional aneurysm formation (36). There ap-

peared to be a higher incidence of coronary ectasia when there was associated thrombus.

Histologic Observations

Atherectomy provides a unique opportunity for detailed study of atherosclerosis and restenosis in human coronary arteries. At the Beth Israel Hospital, standard light microscopy revealed atherosclerotic plaque (95%), media (61%), and adventitia (31%) in 131 coronary atherectomy specimens from 116 patients (37) (Fig. 7). The incidence of recovering these components was higher for de novo than for restenosis lesions. This probably relates to the higher incidence of lesion eccentricity in the de novo as compared to the restenosis lesions. This would increase the likelihood of performing a cut directed at a relatively disease-free portion of the vessel. Intimal proliferation was seen in 45% of de novo lesions and 96% of restenosis lesions (Fig. 8). The intimal hyperplasia was immunophenotypically and histologically identical in

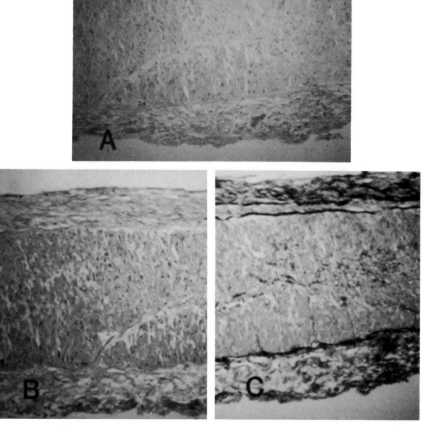

FIG. 7. Photomicrograph of retrieval of deep wall components during coronary atherectomy. Atherectomy sample taken from a 61-year-old man with class iv angina and a subtotal, eccentric, ulcerated stenosis in left anterior descending coronary artery. Intima (*top*), media, and adventitia (*bottom*) were identified (original magnification, × 6.3). **A:** Hematoxylin and eosin stain. **B:** Mason-trichrome stain. **C:** Van-Gieson stain for elastic tissue (7).

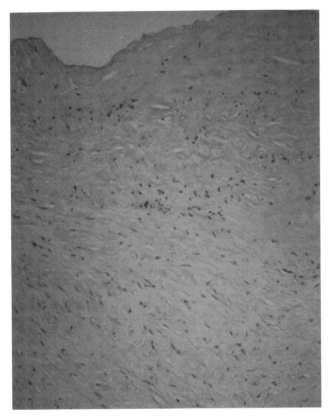

FIG. 8. Photomicrograph of intimal proliferation in a 42-year-old man with postinfarction angina after a recent anterior Q-wave myocardial infarction. There is marked intimal proliferation in association with atherosclerotic plaque (original magnification, × 6.3).

the de novo and restenosis lesions. These data confirm the association between restenosis and intimal hyperplasia regardless of the procedure performed (angioplasty, DCA, laser balloon angioplasty, or stent). Despite the recovery of deep wall components, there were no acute clinical sequelae.

At the Mayo Clinic (26) adventitial tissue was identified in 30% of lesions and media in 51%, also without clinical sequelae. The authors had expected that retrieval of deep wall components might lead to dissection, perforation, pseudoaneurysm formation, or secondary occlusive thrombus. In a follow-up study, (38) the authors suggest that the extent of intimal hyperplasia seen in a response to DCA may be related to the depth of tissue resection in vein graft lesions and coronary artery restenosis lesions (after angioplasty), but not in de novo atheromatous coronary artery lesions. The overall restenosis rate in their study was 50%: 42% when intima alone was resected, 50% when media was resected, and 63% when adventitia was resected. The authors suggested that the vascular injury associated with subintimal resection may be a more potent stimulus of smooth muscle cell proliferation than is the limited injury that occurs when the resection is confined to the atheromatous intima.

The Sequoia Hospital data revealed media from 40.8% of lesions and adventitia from 16.8% of lesions (39). Angiographic perforation or pseudoaneurysm formation was present in 1.7% of all lesions, but in 10.3% of the lesions with adventitial retrieval. Negative post-DCA residual stenoses (<0%) were associated with a higher incidence of retrieval of media (75% versus 36%) or adventitia (39% versus 11%) compared with positive residual stenoses. However, there was not a higher rate of dissection, haziness, or filling defects when media or adventitia was recovered. Analysis of Sequoia and Beth Israel data (40) suggest retrieval of deep wall components does not increase the risk of subsequent restenosis.

Mechanisms of Directional Coronary Atherectomy

Conventional angioplasty enlarges the coronary lumen by cracking and disrupting atherosclerotic plaque and separating the plaque from the media, in order to allow stretching of the vessel wall (41–43). Early studies using DCA suggested that the degree of improvement in luminal diameter appeared to be a function of the quantity of tissue excised, and that with multiple serial passes it was possible to nearly completely resect stenoses (44). However, subsequent studies (7,45,46) have suggested that at least a portion of the improvement seen with coronary atherectomy is due to mechanical dilatation rather than tissue removal. Safian reported that by geometric calculation, complete atherectomy of an occluded 3.0-mm vessel 10 mm in length should remove approximately 70 mg of tissue (assuming a plaque specific gravity of 1.0). The average weight of atherectomy specimens was 18.5 mg, suggesting that factors other than tissue removal alone may be playing a role in procedure success. Mechanical dilatation may occur either by the Dotter effect (47) during passage of the rigid atherectomy device, or stretching of weakened vessel wall components caused by low-pressure balloon inflations during subsequent cuts.

Sharaf and Williams showed that simply passing the atherectomy catheter across the lesion decreased the mean percent diameter stenosis from 77 ± 9% to 24 ± 8% (48). Atherectomy cuts further reduced the stenosis to 6 ± 9%. Smucker et al. evaluated the relative contribution of atherectomy and the angioplasty effect using intracoronary ultrasound (46). Coronary lesions were imaged after the first and final cuts. They reported that when the atherectomy protocol is designed to minimize vascular stretching, the first cut still increases the lumen size; however, most of the increase in lumen size occurs after the first cut. Some (10%) of this subsequent improvement in luminal area after atherectomy was due to angioplasty effects, although the predominant cause of increased lumen size remained plaque removal.

Garratt et al. studied the coronary arteries of three

patients who died at various intervals after DCA (49). It is of note that the vessel wall was not injured by plaque fracturing or medial dissection as would be seen with angioplasty. The authors suggest that remodeling of atheroma is of less importance in atherectomy than in conventional balloon angioplasty. Penny et al. have suggested that the improvement in vessel lumen diameter occurs via a combination of atherectomy and facilitated mechanical angioplasty (45). Excision of plaque and media during DCA may cause disruption of the internal elastic lamina and thinning of the vessel wall, increasing the radial compliance of the vessel. Subsequent balloon inflations may then cause focal stretching of the vessel wall in regions of increased radial compliance, further enlarging the lumen (Fig. 9). Further studies will be needed, possibly with the aid of intravascular ultrasound or angioscopy, to discern the true mechanism of DCA.

Future Directions

With the aid of intracoronary ultrasound devices it has been determined that angiography underestimates the residual plaque burden present after DCA (50). A catheter which combines ultrasound imaging and atherectomy has been developed and is in its early stage of testing (51). It is possible that more aggressive debulking, guided by intracoronary ultrasound may decrease the rate of restenosis without increasing the risk of damage to normal vessel walls. On-line three-dimensional reconstruction facilitates the analysis of stenoses without the use of contrast, and may extend the utility of intravascular ultrasound during interventional procedures (52).

Further refinements in catheter technology may decrease the incidence of restenosis by maximizing the ath-

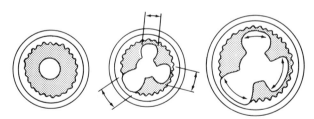

FIG. 9. Schematic of the proposed mechanism for improvement in vessel lumen by a combination of atherectomy and facilitated mechanical angioplasty. **Left:** Concentric stenosis in a coronary artery. The shaded area represents intimal plaque contained within the internal elastic lamina (wavy line). **Middle:** Excision of plaque and media at eight o'clock results in thinning of the vessel wall; subsequent cuts at one and four o'clock do not penetrate the media. **Right:** With disruption of the internal elastic lamina, radial compliance increases so that subsequent balloon inflations cause focal stretching of the vessel wall within the channels produced by previous atherectomy cuts (facilitated angioplasty). The resulting lumen appears smooth and free of residual stenosis in any angiographic projection, despite only partial atherectomy with the continued presence of residual intimal plaque (45).

erectomy effect and minimizing the angioplasty effect (8). The incidence of peripheral vascular complications and ostial dissections may decrease with the introduction of smaller guiding catheters. The change in balloon material from Surlyn to polyethylene tetraphthalate (PET) has reduced the size of the profile of the atherectomy device and has allowed the guiding catheter size to be decreased from 11F to 9.5F. Acute procedural success rate may improve with the introduction of a device with a more flexible distal housing.

Histologic analysis of atherectomy specimens is an exciting tool in the study of atherosclerosis and the mechanism of restenosis after interventional procedures. With the aid of newer molecular biologic techniques we may gain further insight into the underlying mechanisms such that appropriate pharmacologic agents may be directed toward reversing atherosclerosis and preventing restenosis.

Other Atherectomy Devices

Experience with other atherectomy devices in the coronary circulation remains limited in comparison with the Simpson AtheroCath. While all atherectomy catheters rely on high speed rotation to eliminate plaque, only the transluminal extraction catheter (TEC), the Bard rotational atherectomy system (BRAS), and the pullback atherectomy catheter (PAC), share with the Simpson AtheroCath the feature of actually removing atherosclerotic material from the body. The TEC device is a motorized stainless steel element with a conical cutting head that rotates at 750 rpm (Fig. 10). The device applies suction to the cutter head, aspirating pulverized atheroma fragments and collecting them in a hand-held bottle. The device is advanced over a 0.104-in steerable guidewire. The BRAS device is a flexible catheter (5–9F) with a special helical wire that serves as an auger device to retrieve debris, as a sharpened outer catheter is advanced across a lesion while rotating at 1200 rpm. This device is just entering clinical trials (53,54).

Clinical trials using the TEC device in the coronary circulation are currently underway. Sketch et al. reported multicenter data involving 147 patients with 155 lesions (55). The device was used alone in 67 patients and combined with conventional angioplasty in 88 patients. The overall success rate was 93%. The mean diameter stenosis decreased from 74 ± 11% to 35 ± 15%. Emergency CABG was required in 5% (3 dissections, 3 vessel disruptions, 1 thrombosis). Restenosis rates were 29% for RCA lesions, 33% for restenosis lesions, 38% if the postprocedure stenosis was less than 30%, and 52% for LAD lesions. It is of note that there were no reported distal embolizations (56,57). Leon et al. reported (58) that restenosis was independent of lesion length and recent MI, and that efficacy was slightly lower in eccentric

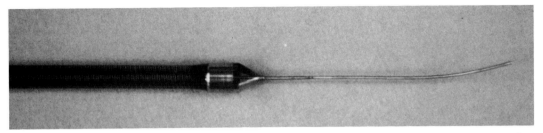

FIG. 10. The transluminal extraction catheter (TEC) (Interventional Vascular Technologies, Inc.). See text for details.

lesions. O'Neill et al. reported (59) the results of 125 lesions within SVGs (mean age 8.8 years), 30% of which had diffuse disease and/or thrombus, thus making them less than ideal candidates for conventional angioplasty. The success rate was 96%, but 76% of procedures required subsequent angioplasty. Again, there were no distal embolizations reported. Kramer et al. (60) reported the use of the TEC device in acute ischemic syndromes (acute MI, post-MI angina, and unstable angina). They noted thrombus frequently, and the presence of thrombus was associated with a better outcome. The TEC system appears to be useful for patients with high-grade de novo lesions and restenosis lesions, diffusely diseased vessels, and total occlusions (as long as they have been recanalized), and may have possibilities as a thrombectomy catheter (61).

The Fischell pullback atherectomy device (62) is an over-the-wire (0.014–0.018-in) system comprised of two separate catheters—a flexible outer closing catheter with an inner movable cut-collect catheter, which has a hollow collecting chamber. The distal end of the device is advanced through the lesion, the closing catheter is pulled back proximal to the lesion over the stationary cutter, and the cutting catheter is rotated (~2,000 rpm) and pulled back through the lesion until the blade contacts the closing catheter. The device is currently manufactured with blade sizes of 2.5, 3.0, and 3.5 mm diameter, and coronary devices with cutting blades of 1.7 mm or smaller are being developed. The current device has been tested in human cadaveric superficial femoral arteries. Fischell et al. reported (62) a reduction in the mean diameter stenosis from 95% to 21% using this device.

The device was very effective in cutting calcified plaque. Clinical testing of this device for the treatment of peripheral vascular disease is underway.

The Rotablator and the other rotational devices discussed below all rely on plaque abrasion and pulverization to treat atherosclerotic disease. These devices have been called athero-abrasion devices since tissue is not removed from the body (63). The Rotablator is a steerable, flexible, over-the-wire (0.009-in) system with a diamond studded elliptical-shaped burr powered by an air turbine (Fig. 11). During rotation (100,000–180,000 rpm) sterile saline is perfused around the drive shaft to lubricate and cool. The burrs come in various sizes ranging from 1.5 mm to 4.5 mm, with the larger sizes being reserved for peripheral vessels. The obvious concern is the potential clinical significance of distal embolization of particulate debris. While most particles are between 2 and 10 microns with the smaller burr sizes, some particles may be 15 to 20 microns or bigger using the larger burr size (63). When particulate matter retrieved after device use has been injected into the left coronary artery of pigs (64) or into canine femoral arteries (65) there were no local ischemic complications. A proposed advantage of this device is that it selectively ablates the inelastic atherosclerotic plaque, while sparing normal tissue (63). In order to avoid damage to normal tissue, it is recommended that the initial burr size be 0.5 mm smaller than the reference segment.

Buchbinder et al. (66) studied 140 lesions in 118 patients in a multicenter trial using the Rotoblator. Lesions were eccentric (58%), calcific (29%), within tortuous segments (34%), and at bifurcation points (25%). The acute

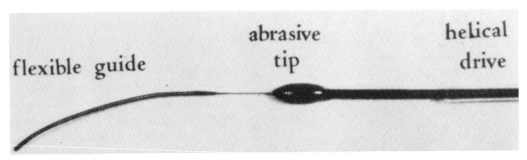

FIG. 11. The Rotablator (Heart Technology, Inc.). See text for details.

lesion success rate was 95%. The mean stenosis decreased from 86.5% to 40.4%. Subsequent angioplasty was required by 41.5% of the lesions, with a subsequent residual stenosis rate of 22.6%. Complications included coronary spasm (3.3%), non–Q-wave MI (2.5%), and emergency CABG (0.8%). Other investigators have reported similar results (67–70). Worrisome complications that have been reported when the device is used in the peripheral circulation include hemoglobinuria (63%), spasm (23%), and groin hematomas (23%) (71). O'Neill et al. reported that transient cessation of flow (no reflow phenomenon) in 20% of patients was managed successfully by intracoronary nitroglycerine and sublingual nifedipine (72). Cheirif et al. performed continuous two-dimensional ECHO during both conventional angioplasty and Rotablator procedures (73). They documented a low incidence of regional wall motion abnormalities during the Rotablator procedure, an observation that possibly implied a limited effect by distal embolization of particulate matter. Preliminary results of 6-month follow-up angiography suggest that restenosis rates remain on the order of 30% to 44% (72,73). Niazi et al. suggested that LAD lesions, ostial and proximal locations, and lesions in SVGs have a higher incidence of restenosis, while there was no difference in patients with unstable angina, de novo lesions, and those patients receiving adjunctive balloon angioplasty (74).

The disadvantages of the Rotablator include (i) an exposed cutting surface which may damage normal endothelium, (ii) the presence of microembolization of particulate matter, (iii) thermal and mechanical injury of formed blood elements (i.e., hemoglobinuria), (iv) vessel spasm, and (v) the need for large introducing sheaths (8F for 2.0–2.5-mm burrs, 9F for 3.0-mm, 11F for 3.5-mm, 12F for 4.0-mm, and 14F for 4.5-mm). Advances in technology (including expandable burrs) may further improve the utility of this device.

Three devices hold promise for treating the nemesis of conventional balloon angioplasty: the total occlusion. These devices, which have been tested in the peripheral circulation, include the atherolytic reperfusion guidewire, the Kensey catheter, and low-speed rotational angioplasty. The atherolytic reperfusion guidewire is a 0.035-in wire with a bullet-shaped tip attached to a handheld battery-driven power control unit which rotates the wire at 200 to 2000 rpm (61). This creates a channel through which a conventional angioplasty balloon or other device may pass. The problem with the system is that it is hard to maintain a coaxial alignment within the true lumen of an occluded vessel, thereby increasing the risk of perforation. Newer designs will use steerable 0.014-in wires. Clinical trials remain preliminary.

The Kensey catheter creates a fine jet spray that develops a vortex which is directed laterally against the vessel wall. This action dilates and also serves to maintain a coaxial alignment within the vessel. The device is a flexible polyurethane catheter (5–9F) with a rotating metal cam driven at 10,000 rpm. The irrigations fluid is pressurized by air cylinders and exits the catheter at the base of the cam. The atheromatous plaque is pulverized into 5- to 10-micron particles (61). Snyder reported the results in 20 patients with significant femoral occlusive disease (75). Significant improvements in luminal diameter were achieved in 10 of 13 patients with stenoses and 4 of 10 with total occlusions. Conventional angioplasty was used in 11 of 14 successful cases.

The low-speed rotational angioplasty catheter is a 2.2-mm device composed of four steel wires with a rounded tip covered in polyolefin or Teflon shrinking tube (4). The device spins at 200 rpm. The inner lumen allows passage of a 0.035-in wire.

Case Examples

Patient 1

A 53-year-old man with a history of cigarette smoking and a family history of early coronary artery disease presented with unstable angina. Diagnostic catheterization revealed an eccentric 95% stenosis in the mid left anterior descending artery (LAD) and normal left ventricular function. Directional coronary atherectomy was performed using a 6F AtheroCath through an 11F JCL3.5 guiding catheter. Two passes and seven cuts with a maximum balloon inflation pressure of 20 psi yielded 16 mg of tissue. There was no significant residual stenosis nor evidence of dissection (Fig. 12). Histologic examination of the retrieved specimens revealed evidence of atherosclerotic plaque and thrombus without evidence of deep wall components. The patient remained symptom-free with a negative exercise tolerance test, and follow-up catheterization performed at 6 months revealed a 10% residual stenosis at the atherectomy site.

Patient 2

An 80-year-old man with hypertension, diabetes mellitus, and a family history of early coronary disease had a 7-year history of stable exertional angina. He developed acute pulmonary edema and hypotension requiring placement of an intraaortic balloon, after prostate surgery. He subsequently had unstable angina. Diagnostic catheterization revealed a 90% proximal LAD stenosis and a 90% ramus stenosis, anterolateral and apical hypokinesis, and elevated right and left heart filling pressures. Directional coronary atherectomy was performed on the LAD using a 7F AtheroCath through an 11F JCL3.5 guiding catheter. Six cuts were made in a circumferential fashion, but no tissue fragments were recovered. Examination of the device revealed a defective balloon. A second device was used with a total of 10 cuts at a maxi-

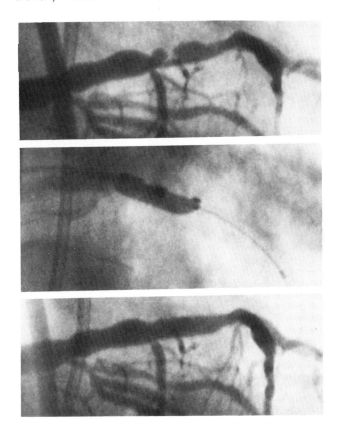

FIG. 12. Successful DCA of a lesion unsuitable for conventional angioplasty (patient 1). **Top:** A severe, eccentric, ulcerated lesion in the mid LAD is shown in the RAO cranial projection. **Middle:** The 6F AtheroCath with the balloon inflated, housing window pointed superiorly and the cutter in the middle of the window. **Bottom:** Following atherectomy the lumen is smooth with no significant residual stenosis.

mum balloon pressure of 40 psi with 7 tissue fragments obtained. There was a 0% residual stenosis without evidence of dissection. The ramus lesion was successfully dilated with conventional balloon angioplasty (Fig. 13). Histologic examination of the retrieved tissue revealed atherosclerotic plaque, media, and adventitia.

The patient presented $4\text{-}\frac{1}{2}$ months later with recurrent angina. Diagnostic catheterization revealed an 80% stenosis in the LAD at the site of prior atherectomy and a 50% ramus stenosis. The LAD lesion was again treated with atherectomy. A 7F AtheroCath was used to perform a total of 19 cuts and the retrieval of 12 specimens. There was no significant residual stenosis. Histologic examination of the retrieved tissue revealed atherosclerotic plaque, intimal hyperplasia, media, and adventitia. The patient subsequently did well, without return of his angina. At 6 months, follow-up catheterization revealed a 30% residual stenosis at the site of DCA.

Patient 3

A 75-year-old man with hypertension, hypercholesterolemia, a history of cigarette smoking, and a family his-

tory of early coronary artery disease developed exertional angina and had a positive exercise tolerance test (76). Diagnostic catheterization revealed severe three-vessel coronary artery disease and normal left ventricular function. The patient underwent successful coronary artery bypass surgery with placement of a left internal mammary artery (LIMA) to the LAD, a saphenous vein graft (SVG) to the second and third obtuse marginals, and a SVG to the posterior descending artery (PDA). Two months later he redeveloped angina. Diagnostic catheterization performed 4 months after surgery revealed 80% aortoostial stenosis of both SVGs. Additionally, there was a 90% stenosis of the distal LIMA to LAD anastamosis.

Ostial atherectomy was performed in both graft lesions using a 7F AtheroCath (4.5 mm working diameter). Treatment of the lesion in the SVG to the obtuse marginals required predilatation with a 5.0-mm conventional angioplasty balloon. Even though this only enlarged the lumen slightly, it allowed passage of the atherectomy catheter which resulted in a 4.0-mm lumen (Fig.

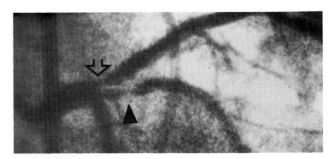

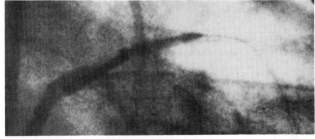

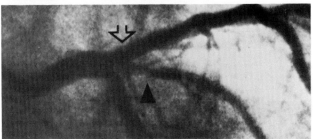

FIG. 13. Successful DCA of an ostial LAD stenosis (*open arrow*) and conventional angioplasty of a ramus stenosis (*closed arrow*) in an 80-year-old man (patient 2). **Top:** Preprocedure angiography. **Middle:** 7F AtheroCath positioned across the ostial LAD stenosis. **Bottom:** Post-procedure angiography revealing no significant residual stenosis and a smooth lumen in the LAD and a good result with conventional angioplasty in the ramus.

14). Primary atherectomy of the SVG to the PDA was successful without predilation. Histologic examination of the retrieved tissue revealed intimal hyperplasia. The stenotic distal LIMA to LAD anastamosis and a stenotic first diagonal branch were successfully treated with conventional angioplasty. The patient had no recurrent anginal symptoms at 6-month follow-up.

Conclusion

Interventional cardiologists now have a number of tools at their disposal to treat coronary artery disease. Although these new devices have appeared promising in their early clinical trials, the ultimate role (if any) for each of them remains to be settled. To date, the gold standard for comparison remains plain old balloon angioplasty (POBA). While each of the new devices attempts to improve on this technique, the results with directional coronary atherectomy suggest that it may be

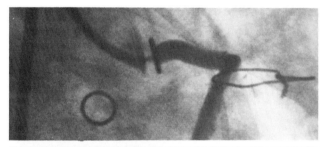

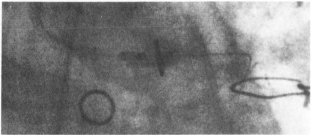

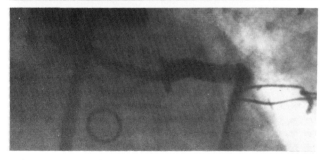

FIG. 14. Successful DCA of an ostial saphenous vein graft stenosis to the obtuse marginals (patient 3). **Top:** Saphenous graft en face demonstrates that the ostial stenosis is within the aortic wall. The aortic lumen is defined by angiographic dye reflux, and the adventitial side of the aorta is demarcated by the metallic ring marker. **Middle:** The 7F AtheroCath (4.5 mm working diameter) in position. **Bottom:** The result obtained following atherectomy, demonstrating an approximate 4.0-mm lumen (76).

used to safely provide excellent acute angiographic results. Because of its predictability, DCA may become the procedure of choice for certain lesions whose angiographic appearances make them unfavorable for conventional angioplasty: eccentric, ulcerated, ostial, or bifurcation lesions within native coronary arteries and saphenous vein bypass grafts. The role of DCA as a tool in the removal of angioplasty-induced dissections remains unclear. The TEC system may prove useful in diffusely diseased vessels and lesions with thrombus, while the Rotablator may be of value in diffusely diseased, calcified vessels. The Kensey catheter, low-speed rotational angioplasty, and, in particular, the atherolytic reperfusion guidewire may overcome the problem of crossing chronic total occlusions, provided that coronary perforation is avoided. Clearly, greater clinical experience with these new devices is necessary, particularly as regards restenosis rates, before advocating their widespread use in lieu of conventional angioplasty. A randomized trial of DCA versus conventional angioplasty in de novo lesions (CAVEAT) is now beginning. In the meantime, we continue to view the overall utility of these new devices with cautious optimism.

REFERENCES

1. Gruentzig AR, Senning A, Siegenthaler WE. Nonoperative dilatation of coronary artery stenoses—percutaneous transluminal coronary angioplasty. *N Eng J Med* 1979;301:61–68.
2. Kent KM, Bentivoglio LG, Block PC, et al. Percutaneous transluminal coronary angioplasty: report from the registry of the National Heart, Lung and Blood Institute. *Am J Cardiol* 1982;41:2001–2020.
3. Detre K, Holubkov R, Kelsey S, et al. Percutaneous transluminal coronary angioplasty in 1985–1986 and 1977–1981. *N Eng J Med* 1988;318:265–270.
4. Safian RD, Baim DS. New devices for coronary intervention: intravascular stents and coronary atherectomy catheters. In: Grossman W, Baim DS, eds. *Cardiac catheterization, angiography, and intervention.* Philadelphia: Lea & Febinger; 1991:467–491.
5. Simpson JB, Selmon MR, Robertson GC, et al. Transluminal atherectomy for occlusive peripheral vascular disease. *Am J Cardiol* 1988;61:96G–101G.
6. Hinohara T, Selmon MR, Robertson GC, et al. Directional coronary atherectomy: new approaches for treatment of obstructive coronary and peripheral vascular disease. *Circulation* 1990;81 [Suppl IV]:79–91.
7. Safian RD, Gelbfish JS, Erny RE, et al. Coronary atherectomy: clinical, angiographic, and histological findings and observations regarding potential mechanisms. *Circulation* 1990;82:69–79.
8. Robertson GC, Hinohara T, Selmon MR, et al. Directional coronary atherectomy. In: Topol EJ, ed. *Textbook of interventional cardiology.* Philadelphia: WB Saunders; 1990:563–579.
9. Simpson JB, Johnson DE, Thapliyal HV, et al. Transluminal atherectomy: a new approach to the treatment of atherosclerotic vascular disease. *Circulation* 1985;72[Suppl III]:146(abstract).
10. Hinohara T, Rowe MH, Robertson GC, et al. Effect of lesion characteristics on outcome of directional coronary atherectomy. *J Am Coll Cardiol* 1991;17:1112–1120.
11. Vetter JW, Simpson JB, Robertson GC, et al. Rescue directional coronary atherectomy for failed balloon angioplasty. *J Am Coll Cardiol* 1991;17:384A(abst).
12. Whitlow PL, Robertson GC, Rowe MH, et al. Directional coronary atherectomy for failed percutaneous transluminal coronary angioplasty. *Circulation* 1990;82[Suppl III]:1(abst).
13. Robertson GC, Rowe MH, Selmon MR, et al. Directional coro-

nary atherectomy for lesions with complex morphology. *Circulation* 1990;82[Suppl III]:312(abstract).

14. Popma JJ, Topol, EJ, Hinohara T, et al. Abrupt vessel closure after directional coronary atherectomy: clinical, angiographic, and procedural outcome. *J Am Cell Cardiol* 1992:19:1372–1379.

15. Muller DWM, Ellis SG, Debowey DC, Topol EJ. Quantitative angiographic comparison of the immediate success of coronary angioplasty, coronary atherectomy, and endoluminal stenting. *Am J Cardiol* 1990;66:938–942.

16. Hinohara T, Simpson JB. Multicenter experience of directional coronary atherectomy (*unpublished*).

17. U.S. Directional Coronary Atherectomy Investigator Group. Complications of directional coronary atherectomy in a multicenter experience. *Circulation* 1990;82[Suppl III]:311(abstract).

18. Robertson GC, Selmon MR, Hinohara T, et al. The effect of lesion length on outcome of directional atherectomy. *Circulation* 1990;82[Suppl III]:623(abst).

19. Hinohara T, Rowe MH, Robertson GC, et al. Comparison of outcome of directional coronary atherectomy in de novo and restenosed lesions. *Circulation* 1990;82[Suppl III]:624(abstract).

20. Robertson GC, Hinohara T, Selmon MR, et al. Complications: early experiences of percutaneous coronary atherectomy. *J Am Coll Cardiol* 1989;13:222A.

21. Kaufmann UP, Garratt KN, Vliestra RE, et al. Coronary atherectomy: First 50 patients at the Mayo Clinic. *Mayo Clin Proc* 1989;64:747–752.

22. Carrozza JP, Baim DS, Safian RD. Risks and complications of coronary atherectomy. In: Holmes DR, ed. *Atherectomy.* Cambridge, MA: Blackwell Scientific Publishing; 1992;132–148.

23. Bredlau CE, Roubin GS, Leimgruber PP, et al. In hospital morbidity and mortality in patients undergoing elective coronary angioplasty. *Circulation* 1985;72:1044–1052.

24. Alderman JD, Gabliani GI, McCabe CH, et al. Incidence and management of limb ischemia with percutaneous wire-guided balloon catheters. *J Am Coll Cardiol* 1987;9:524–530.

25. Rowe MH, Hinohara T, White NW, et al. Comparison of dissection rates and angiographic results following directional coronary atherectomy and coronary angioplasty. *Am J Cardiol* 1990;66:49–53.

26. Garratt KN, Kaufmann UP, Edwards WD, et al. Safety of percutaneous coronary atherectomy with deep arterial resection. *Am J Cardiol* 1989;64:538–540.

27. Selmon MR, Robertson GC, Simpson JB, et al. Retrieval of media and adventitia by directional coronary atherectomy and angiographic correlation. *Circulation* 1990;82[Suppl III]:624(abstract).

28. U.S. Directional Coronary Atherectomy Investigator Group. Restenosis following directional coronary atherectomy in a multicenter experience. *Circulation* 1990;82[Suppl III]:679(abst).

29. Kaufmann UP, Garratt KN, Vlietstra RE, Holmes DR. Transluminal atherectomy of saphenous vein aortocoronary bypass grafts. *Am J Cardiol* 1990;65:1430–1433.

30. Holmes DR, Garratt KN, Bell MR. Follow-up events after directional coronary atherectomy. *Circulation* 1990;82[Suppl III]:493(abst).

31. Selmon MR, Hinohara T, Robertson GC, et al. Directional coronary atherectomy for saphenous vein graft stenoses. *J Am Coll Cardiol* 1991;17:23A(abstract).

32. Simpson JB, Rowe MH, Selmon MR, et al. Restenosis following directional coronary atherectomy in de novo lesions of native coronary arteries. *Circulation* 1990;82[Suppl III]:313(abst).

33. Hinohara T, Selmon MR, Robertson GC, et al. Angiographic predictors of restenosis following directional coronary atherectomy. *J Am Coll Cardiol* 1991;17:385A(abstract).

34. Schmidt DA, Kuntz RE, Penny WF, et al. Predictors of angiographic restenosis following coronary atherectomy. *Circulation* 1990;82[Suppl III]:492(abstract).

35. Hinohara T, Rowe MH, Robertson GC, et al. Predictors of recurrent restenosis following directional coronary atherectomy for restenosed lesions. *Circulation* 1990;82[Suppl III]:624(abstract).

36. deCesare NB, Popma JJ, Whitlow PC, et al. Excision beyond the "normal" arterial wall with directional coronary atherectomy—acute and long term outcome. *J Am Coll Cardiol* 1991;17:384A(abstract).

37. Schnitt SJ, Safian RD, Kuntz RE, et al. Histologic findings in specimens obtained from percutaneous directional coronary atherectomy. *Hum Pathol,* 1992;23:415–420.

38. Garratt KN, Holmes DR, Bell MR, et al. Restenosis after directional coronary atherectomy: differences between primary atheromatous and restenosis lesions and influence of subintimal tissue resection. *J Am Coll Cardiol* 1990;16:1665–1671.

39. Selmon MR, Robertson GC, Simpson JB, et al. Retrieval of media and adventitia by directional coronary atherectomy and angiographic correlation. *Circulation* 1990;82[Suppl III]:624(abstract).

40. Kuntz RE, Selmon MR, Robertson GC, et al. Excision of deep wall components by directional coronary atherectomy does not increase restenosis *Circulation* 1991;84 [Suppl II]:81(abstract).

41. Block PC. Mechanism of transluminal angioplasty. *Am J Cardiol* 1984;53:69C–71C.

42. Block PC, Myler RK, Stertzer S, Fallon TJ. Morphology after transluminal angioplasty in human beings. *N Engl J Med* 1981;305:382–385.

43. Faxon DP, Weber VK, Haudenschild C, et al. Acute effects of transluminal angioplasty in three experimental models of atherosclerosis. *Arteriosclerosis* 1982;2:125–133.

44. Johnson DE, Braden L, Simpson JB. Mechanism of directional transluminal atherectomy. *Am J Cardiol* 1990;65:389–391.

45. Penny WF, Schmidt DA, Safian RD, Erny RE, Baim DS. Insights into the mechanism of luminal improvement after directional coronary atherectomy. *Am J Cardiol* 1991;67:435–437.

46. Smucker ML, Howard PF, Scherb DE, et al. Is intracoronary ultrasound a valid means to assess the mechanism of atherectomy. *J Am Coll Cardiol* 1991;17:126A(abstract).

47. Dotter CT, Judkins MP. Transluminal treatment of arteriosclerotic obstructions. *Circulation* 1964;30:654.

48. Sharaf BL, Williams DO. "Dotter effect" contributes to angiographic improvement following directional coronary atherectomy. *Circulation* 1990;82[Suppl III]:310(abstract).

49. Garratt KN, Edwards WD, Vliestra RE, et al. Coronary morphology after percutaneous directional coronary atherectomy in humans: autopsy analysis of three patients. *J Am Coll Cardiol* 1990;16:1432–1436.

50. White NW, Webb JG, Rowe MH, et al. Atherectomy guidance using intravascular ultrasound: quantitation of plaque burden. *J Am Coll Cardiol* 1989;80[Suppl II]:374(abstract).

51. Yock PG, Fitzgerald PJ, Jang YT, et al. Initial trials of a combined ultrasound imaging/mechanical atherectomy catheter. *J Am Coll Cardiol* 1990;15:105A(abstract).

52. Rosenfield K, Losordo DW, Palefski P, et al. On-line 3-D reconstruction of 2-D intravascular ultrasound images during balloon angioplasty: clinical application in patients undergoing percutaneous balloon angioplasty. *J Am Coll Cardiol* 1991;17:156A(abstract).

53. Smalling RW, Cassidy DB, Waldemar A, et al. Initial experience with a flexible rotational atherectomy system designed for removal of coronary and small peripheral atheromas. *J Am Coll Cardiol* 1989;13:223A(abstract).

54. Battler A, Scheinowitz M, Rath S, et al. Bard rotary atherectomy system (BRAS) in normal canine arteries. *J Am Coll Cardiol* 1989;13:223A(abstract).

55. Sketch MH, O'Neill WW, Tcheng JE, et al. Early and late outcome following coronary transluminal extraction-endarterectomy: a multicenter experience. *Circulation* 1990;82[Suppl III]:310(abst).

56. Stack RS, Quigley PJ, Sketch MH, et al. Treatment of coronary artery disease with the transluminal extraction-endarterectomy catheter: initial results of a multicenter study. *Circulation* 1989;80[Suppl II]:583(abstract).

57. Stack RS, Phillips HR, Quigley PJ, et al. Multicenter registry of coronary atherectomy using the transluminal extraction-endarterectomy catheter. *J Am Coll Cardiol* 1990;15:196A(abstract).

58. Leon MB, Pichard AD, Kramer BL, et al. Efficacious and safe transluminal extraction atherectomy in patients with unfavorable coronary lesions. *J Am Coll Cardiol* 1991;17:219A(abstract).

59. O'Neill WW, Meany TB, Kramer BL, et al. The role of atherectomy in the management of saphenous vein graft disease. *J Am Coll Cardiol* 1991;17:384A(abstract).

60. Kramer B, Larkin T, Niemyski P, Parker M. Coronary atherectomy in acute ischemic syndromes: implications of thrombus on treatment outcome. *J Am Coll Cardiol* 1991;17:385A(abstract).

61. Wholey MH. New reperfusion devices: the Kensey catheter, the atherolytic reperfusion wire device, and the transluminal extraction catheter. *Radiology* 1989;172:947–952.

62. Fischell TA, Fischell RE, White RI, Chapolini R. Ex-vivo results using a new pullback atherectomy catheter (PAC). *Cathet Cardiovasc Diagn* 1990;21:287–291.

63. Bertrand ME, Fourrier JL, Auth DC, et al. Percutaneous coronary rotational angioplasty. In: Topol EJ, ed. *Textbook of interventional cardiology.* Philadelphia: WB Saunders; 1990:580–589.

64. Zacca NM, Raizner AE, Noon GP, et al. Treatment of symptomatic peripheral atherosclerotic disease with a rotational atherectomy device. *Am J Cardiol* 1989;63:77–80.

65. Ahn SS, Auth DC, Marcus DR, Moore WS. Removal of focal atheromatous lesions by angioscopically guided high-speed rotary atherectomy. *J Vasc Surg* 1988;7:292–300.

66. Buchbinder M, O'Neill W, Warth D, et al. Percutaneous coronary rotational ablation using the Rotablator: results of a multicenter study. *Circulation* 1990;82[Suppl III]:309(abstract).

67. Scheiman G, McDaniel M, Fenner J, et al. Quantitative angiographic assessment of percutaneous transluminal rotational ablation. *Circulation* 1990;82[Suppl III]:493(abstract).

68. Bertrand ME, Fourrier JL, Dietz U, DeJaegere P. European experience with percutaneous transluminal coronary rotational ablation: immediate results. *Circulation* 1990;82[Suppl III]:310(abst).

69. Rodriguez AR, Zacca N, Heibig J, et al. Coronary rotary ablation using a single large burr and without balloon assistance. *Circulation* 1990;82[Suppl III]:310(abstract).

70. Fourrier JL, Bertrand ME, Auth DC, et al. Percutaneous coronary rotational angioplasty in humans: preliminary report. *J Am Coll Cardiol* 1989;14:1278–1282.

71. Dorross G, Iyer S, Zaitoun R, et al. Acute angiographic and clinical outcome of high-speed percutaneous rotational atherectomy (Rotablator). *Cathet Cardiovasc Diag* 1991;22:157–166.

72. O'Neill WW, Friedman HZ, Cragg D, et al. Initial clinical experience and early follow-up of patients undergoing mechanical rotary endarterectomy. *Circulation* 1989;80[Suppl II]:584(abstract).

73. Cheirif J, Heibig J, Harris S, et al. Rotational ablation is associated with less myocardial ischemia than PTCA. *Circulation* 1990;82[Suppl III]:493(abstract).

74. Niazi K, Cragg DR, Strzelecki M, et al. Angiographic risk factors for coronary restenosis following mechanical rotational atherectomy. *J Am Coll Cardiol* 1991;17:218A(abstract).

75. Snyder SO, Wheeler JR, Gregory RT, et al. The Kensey catheter: preliminary results with a transluminal atherectomy tool. *J Vasc Surg* 1988;8:541–543.

76. Kuntz RE, Piana R, Schnitt SJ, et al. Early ostial vein graft stenoses: management by atherectomy. *Cathet Cardiovasc Diagn* 1991;24:41–44.

CHAPTER 16

Excimer Laser Coronary Angioplasty

Bradley H. Evans, Neal Eigler, and Frank Litvack

BACKGROUND AND PHYSICS

Since the first human percutaneous transluminal angioplasty was performed 1977 (1,2), improvements in equipment and technique have increased the indications for balloon angioplasty. Concurrently, acute procedural success rates have increased (3). Despite this progress, several limitations remain which, if solved, may limit the number of coronary bypass surgeries performed (4–8). The most important limitation of balloon angioplasty is restenosis, the incidence of which has not decreased since the introduction of angioplasty (9,10). These limitations have stimulated the development of new devices, such as the excimer laser, that are capable of removing plaque from coronary arteries.

Excimer (an acronym for excited dimer) laser energy is produced by pulsing an electrical discharge across a mixture of an inert gas (helium, neon or argon), another inert gas (xenon or krypton) and a highly dilute halogen compound (such as 0.1% hydrogen chloride or fluorine). This results in emission of energy in the ultraviolet portion of the spectrum, between 193 and 351 nm, the wavelength depending on the gases used. The 308-nm xenon chloride (XeCl) excimer laser we currently use (Advanced Interventional Systems, Irvine, CA) emits 225 mJ per pulse at 200 to 300 nanoseconds. The pulse repetition rate can be varied from 2 Hz to 50 Hz.

Nanosecond pulsed energy from the XeCl excimer laser ablates tissue by photochemical mechanisms involving direct bond breakage and desorption of molecular products. Importantly, this ablation appears to occur with minimal thermal effect on adjacent tissue. Initial necropsy and animal studies have shown that excimer laser ablation of tissue occurs with great precision, in

contrast to the blast injury and carbonization that occurs with the continuous wave lasers (11,12). Excimer lasers are also unique in their ability to ablate calcified material such as calcified plaque (11,13). Preliminary data suggest that excimer-induced lesions heal more completely and with less damage to the arterial wall than those produced by other lasers (14).

The first successful excimer laser coronary angioplasty (ELCA) was performed at Cedars-Sinai Medical Center in August, 1988 (15). Subsequent clinical reports suggested that excimer laser angioplasty could be performed safely in the human coronary circulation (16–19). Shortly after this initial experience a nonrandomized multicenter trial was initiated which has currently enrolled more than 1,500 patients (with 1,810 lesions). Preliminary reports conclude that ELCA may be particularly suited for long diffuse lesions in native vessels, as well as saphenous vein grafts, calcified lesions, aortoostial lesions and total occlusions crossable by a guidewire (13,20–22).

What follows is an introduction to the practical aspects of excimer laser coronary angioplasty in the coronary arteries, including basic technical aspects, indications, complications and their management, and expected outcomes. For those physicians planning to perform ELCA this information should not be considered as a replacement of comprehensive training but an introduction to the selection of patients and the performance of the procedure.

EQUIPMENT

The system currently in use at Cedars-Sinai Medical Center consists of a magnetically switched Thyratron-driven 308 nm XeCl pulsed excimer laser. The device has a pulse width of 180 to 220 ns with an output of more than 200 mJ at 20 Hz. Laser energy is delivered through

BH Evans: The Thoracic Clinic, Portland, Oregon; N Eigler and F Litvack: Cedars-Sinai Medical Center, Los Angeles, California

multifiber catheters 1.3 (4.0F), 1.6 (4.7F), 2.0 (6.0F) or 2.2 mm (6.6F) in diameter. The currently available catheters have over 200 individual 50-micron silica fibers in a concentric array, arranged around a central lumen that accepts a 0.018-in guidewire. The shaft is composed of flexible polyethylene with a proximal Y-adaptor for introduction of the coronary guidewire into the central lumen and connection of the fiberoptics to the laser power source (Fig. 1).

Standard angioplasty guide catheters are used: 8 French (8F) catheters for ELCA with 1.3-mm and 1.6-mm laser catheters, and 9F for 2.0-mm and 2.2-mm-catheters. Guide catheters with large lumens (8F, 0.079 in; 9F, 0.092 in) offer adequate luminal size for hand injection and assessment of vessel patency and runoff while the laser catheter is within the guide catheter. Current generation laser catheters are not as trackable as the latest generation PTCA balloons. It is therefore more often necessary to solidly engage the guiding catheter. Efficient tissue ablation requires good contact with the lesion. If difficulty is encountered with the Judkins shape, an Amplatz of appropriate size is frequently a useful alternative.

It should be noted that the 2.0-mm and larger laser catheters do not fit through all commercially available Y-adaptors. It is best to confirm that all ancillary equipment is compatible prior to the procedure.

A coronary guidewire is selected from one of the following currently available: the 0.018 Hi-Torque Floppy "Xtra Support" [Advanced Cardiovascular Systems (ACS), Temecula, CA], a 0.016 Hyperflex (USCI, Inc., Billarica, MA), or a 0.018-in intermediate or standard wire. Guidewires with a diameter of 0.014 in have insufficient shaft column strength to maintain the laser catheter coaxial within the artery. This potentially increases intravascular trauma during passage of the laser fiber. The ACS 0.018-in high torque floppy wire is generally unacceptable for ELCA because this wire has a relatively long taper in the shaft that may allow for loss of coaxiality. The 0.018 Hi-Torque Floppy "Xtra Support" wire consists of a floppy tip design combined with the shaft taper of the High Torque Standard model. Excimer laser coronary angioplasty should always be performed over the solid mandrel portion of the wire to maintain catheter coaxiality and should never be continued over the platinum spring coil tip of the guide wire, as this may result in perforation.

Standard percutaneous transluminal coronary angioplasty (PTCA) balloons can be used for performing adjunctive balloon angioplasty following excimer laser cor-

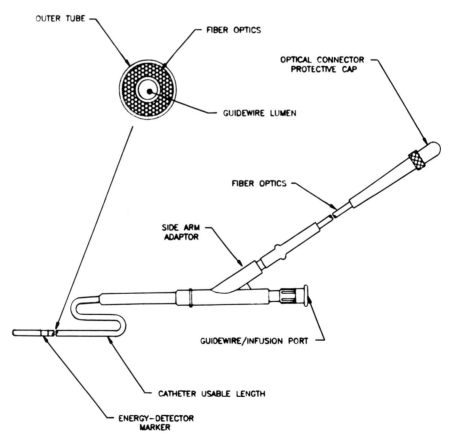

FIG. 1. ELCA catheter.

TABLE 1. *Characteristics of type A, B, and C lesions (23)*

Type A lesions (High success, 85%: low risk)	Type B lesions (Moderate success, 60–85%: moderate risk)	Type C lesions (Low success, 60%: high risk)
Discrete	Tubular (10–20 mm in length)	Diffuse (>2 cm length)
Concentric, less than totally occlusive	Eccentric	Excessive tortuosity of proximal segment
Readily accessible	Moderately angulated segment, >45° <90°	Extremely angulated segments > 90°
Nonangulated segment, <45°	Irregular contour	Total occlusion > 3 months old
Smooth contour	Moderate to heavy calcification	Inability to protect major side branches
Little or no calcification	Total occlusion < 3 months old	Degenerated vein grafts with friable lesions
Not ostial in location	Bifurcation lesions requiring double guidewires	
No major side-branch involvement	Some thrombus present	
Absence of thrombus		

B1 (one adverse characteristic).
B2 (≥ two adverse characteristics) (24).

onary angioplasty. It is advisable to have an adequate supply of balloons in various sizes that can be exchanged over a 0.018-in guidewire so that repetitive wire placement is avoided. Currently available balloons that will accept an 0.018-in guidewire include the ACS RX, Pinkerton and Stack Perfusion balloons (Advanced Cardiovascular Systems, Temecula, CA), the 0.018 Slider (Mansfield, Mansfield, MA), the 18K (Medtronic Inc., San Diego, CA), and the 0.018 MVP (Scimed, Minneapolis, MN).

It is helpful to work with a procedure table that is longer than the usual cardiac table (approximately 10 ft versus 7 ft). This facilitates the handling of 300-cm length wires which are more frequently used with ELCA than in balloon angioplasty.

The laboratory must be fully equipped to handle complex interventional cases in critically ill patients. There should be adequate floor space to accommodate sophisticated support and resuscitation equipment such as a volume cycled respirator, anesthesia machine, intraaortic balloon pump, and a percutaneous cardiopulmonary bypass device, in addition to the laser equipment.

POTENTIAL INDICATIONS AND CONTRAINDICATIONS

Patients suitable for excimer laser coronary angioplasty should have symptomatic coronary artery disease and/or objective evidence of myocardial ischemia sufficient to warrant either balloon angioplasty or bypass surgery. In addition the patient should have angiographically documented stenosis or occlusions of native coronary arteries or bypass grafts thought to be traversable by angioplasty guidewires. Currently, patients with evolving myocardial infarction or with resting ischemia unrelieved with medical therapy are excluded. Lesions best suited for excimer laser coronary angioplasty include certain types of B1, B2, or type C lesions (Table 1).

The initial ELCA experience (first 100 patients) at Cedars-Sinai Medical Center suggests that this procedure is an acutely effective and safe therapy for lesions identified as not well suited for balloon angioplasty (20).

Current potential indications for ELCA may include

1. Stenosis of native coronary arteries which are longer than 10 to 15 mm.
2. Stenosis or occlusions in saphenous vein grafts.
3. Rigid lesions not dilatable by conventional balloon angioplasty.
4. Aortoostial lesions.
5. Left anterior descending ostial lesions.
6. Diffusely diseased coronary segments (>20 mm).
7. Total occlusions that can be crossed by a coronary guidewire.

Current contraindications include

1. Unprotected left main stenosis.
2. Patient not a candidate for bypass surgery (unless no other clinical options are available.
3. Laser catheter diameter is greater than 60% to 70% of the diameter of the coronary segment being treated.
4. Inability to cross lesion with coronary guidewire.
5. True bifurcation lesions.
6. Acutely dissected lesions.

Potential relative contraindications include

1. Highly eccentric lesions.
2. Lesions on an acute bend (>45°).

TECHNICAL DETAILS

Because of the risk of coronary artery perforation and its sequelae, laser angioplasty is considered less forgiving than conventional balloon angioplasty. Excimer laser angioplasty should not be practiced by novice or occasional angioplasters. Operators should possess a high level of experience and skill before performing this procedure. This should include extensive experience with complex angioplasty cases.

Training in excimer angioplasty includes completion of a basic training course as well as hands-on experience under the supervision of an experienced operator. This hands-on training with experienced operators is crucial because there are substantive differences compared with PTCA.

Patients who meet the selection criteria noted above are treated with 324 mg of aspirin and a calcium channel antagonist, starting no later than the day prior to the procedure. Diagnostic and setup angiography are performed using standard techniques. Intravenous heparin boluses are administered (10,000–15,000 units) to raise the activated clotting time to greater than 350 sec and maintain it at this level for the duration of the procedure. Selective intracoronary nitroglycerin (200 mcg) is given prior to control angiography, and following laser angioplasty. The use of intracoronary nitroglycerin has been useful to reduce the resting vascular tone for laser catheter sizing and to prevent coronary vasospasm.

Catheter sizing should then be performed and should be based on the normal portion of the vessel with reference to the guide catheter after intracoronary nitroglycerin. To minimize the risk of perforation, the size of the laser catheter is selected so as to leave at least a 30% residual stenosis after a single pass. All de novo lesions exhibiting calcium or with a minimum lumen diameter of less than 1.0 mm should be prelased with the 1.3-mm laser catheter.

The lesion is then crossed with a 0.016- or 0.018-in coronary guidewire using standard angioplasty techniques under fluoroscopic guidance. It has not been necessary to protect major side branches with a second guidewire. As in balloon angioplasty, placement of the wire tip in the distal portion of the target artery is useful. This is particularly essential in ELCA where the solid mandrel portion of the wire must be across the lesion to allow for coaxial tracking of the catheter over the stiff body of the wire. For chronic total occlusions the use of a 0.018-in Terumo wire has improved crossability. Once a channel has been created with the Terumo wire, the lesion can be recrossed with a conventional 0.018-inch ACS wire for passage of the laser fiber.

Laser energy emitted from the catheter tip is calibrated at 45 to 60 mJ/mm^2 prior to insertion. Calibration is performed with a dry laser catheter to ensure accurate energy density calibration. Generally the energies for the 1.6-, 2.0-, 2.2-, and 2.4-mm laser fibers are in the range of 45 to 55 mJ/mm^2, and the tip energy for the 1.3-mm fiber is in the range of 50 to 60 mJ/mm^2. Recent results have suggested that restenosis rates may be lower at higher catheter-tip energies, perhaps due to increased mechanical trauma at lower energy densities (25).

After calibration, the central lumen of the laser fiber is flushed with saline and the laser catheter is advanced over the guidewire until its tip is 3 to 5 mm proximal to the lesion. The primary operator stands closest to the patient's groin and manipulates the laser catheter, the guiding catheter, and the laser foot pedal. The assistant operator controls the guidewire and the X-ray foot pedals. The primary operator holds the laser fiber 2 to 3 mm from the Y-adaptor, limiting the forward motion during each burst of pulses to this distance. Under fluoroscopic control the laser catheter is advanced at 1 mm/sec or less as laser pulses are delivered at 20 Hz. Rates of catheter advancement faster than 1 mm/sec may cause insufficient ablation, with additional mechanical trauma and resultant intimal dissection. Application of laser energy should occur for bursts of no longer than 2 sec with 3 to 5 sec between bursts to prevent vascular trauma secondary to buildup of gaseous ablation products in the subintimal tissue planes.

If the system fails to cross the stenosis and there is adequate guide catheter support, retraction of the guidewire while the laser catheter is being advanced may prove helpful. If the system continues to fail to cross the stenosis, the energy should be recalibrated and, if the reading is accurate, the energy may be increased by 5 mJ/mm^2. After passage through the lesion, the catheter is withdrawn well within the guide catheter, and angiographic contrast is injected. Because the complication rate appears to increase with multiple passes, no more than one pass should be undertaken with each size laser catheter. Care should be taken to withdraw the laser catheter several centimeters into the guide catheter before making test injections. This will prevent a high velocity jet of contrast material from injuring the arterial wall and potentially causing dissection. If the result appears satisfactory, the laser catheter is totally withdrawn from the guiding catheter and cineangiography is performed. When the posttreatment stenosis is visually estimated to be satisfactory, the guidewire is removed and completion angiograms are performed. If the residual stenosis is judged not to be sufficiently improved, a larger diameter laser fiber is attempted, or adjunctive balloon angioplasty is performed prior to completion angiography. Adjunctive balloon angioplasty is performed if the postlaser stenosis is more than 30%.

Following laser angioplasty, patients are transferred to a monitored unit for 24 hr. Postprocedure care, including anticoagulation and aspirin, is the same as for balloon angioplasty.

Two physicians are required to perform laser angioplasty. Because of the use of exchange-length guidewires, catheter exchanges are more complex than with PTCA and, in general, the performance of ELCA is technically more difficult than PTCA. Because the ELCA patient frequently has a more complicated and demanding anatomy than the routine PTCA patient, it is frequently useful to have another experienced operator with whom to discuss intraprocedural decisions. Additional input from a skilled operator can be very helpful in these difficult cases, and in the event of an emergency.

CLINICAL RESULTS

Preliminary data suggest that ELCA is most useful in complex lesions not well suited for balloon angioplasty. In the initial Cedars-Sinai Medical Center experience, 65% of patients treated with ELCA had lesions that were identified as not ideal for PTCA. These included lesions whose length was 10 mm or more with diffuse or tubular morphology, total occlusions or lesions in an ostial location. The overall acute laser success rate in this group of patients was 86%, with subgroup analysis revealing acute success in 72% of chronic total occlusions and 91% of partially occluded lesions. With adjunctive balloon angioplasty applied when indicated, the procedural success rate rose to 94% (defined as final diameter stenosis ≤50%). Notably, there were no acute side-branch occlusions in the 17 patients in this group who had one or more major branches originating within the lesion being treated. When grouped by ACC/AHA lesion type, laser and procedural success rates, respectively, were: type A lesions 83% and 97%; type B lesions 88% and 96%; type C lesions 85% and 88%. Major ischemic complications occurred in 3% of type A lesions, 2% of type B lesions and 0% of type C lesions. Success and complication rates for type B and type C lesions treated with laser angioplasty did not differ significantly from rates with type A lesions and exceeded ACC/AHA standards for expected outcomes (20). Based on these outcomes, it was suggested that excimer laser angioplasty may be a useful therapy in complex (type B and type C) lesions. Type B and type C morphologies which are unfavorable for balloon angioplasty may benefit from ELCA.

A recent multicenter investigation of 958 patients (1,151 lesions), using the 308 nm XeCl excimer laser system, showed an overall acute laser success rate (>20% reduction in residual stenosis or lumen size approximating catheter size) of 85%, and a procedural success rate (<50% residual stenosis) of 94%. Of the 1,151 lesions, 10% were in vein grafts, 10% were total occlusions, and 22% were greater than 20 mm in length (25). Results indicated that ELCA is safe and effective for coronary stenosis, with early results similar to those obtained for balloon angioplasty. Restenosis was identified as a persistent problem.

Data on ELCA of saphenous vein grafts suggest that procedural success rates of 96% can be achieved. In this group of 108 patients (127 saphenous vein graft lesions), 80% of the saphenous vein grafts were greater than 2 years old and were therefore considered high risk, with a decreased rate of success. No deaths or emergency coronary artery bypass operations were reported, 8 of 45 patients with 6 month follow-up required further intervention (21).

Recent results from the ELCA investigators suggests that the use of ELCA for aortoostial stenosis is a safe procedure with a high initial angiographic and clinical success rate. In 114 (114 lesions patients) the ELCA and procedural success rates were 90% and 96%, respectively. The aortoostial lesions approached consisted of 65 at the right coronary artery ostium, 12 at the left main ostium, and 37 at ostia in saphenous vein grafts. Percent stenosis improved from 84 ± 13 at baseline, to 43 ± 18 after ELCA, and 29 ± 17 after PTCA. At 1-month follow-up, 93% were clinically improved. Clinical or angiographic restenosis was present in 47% of 49 patients with 6-month follow-up. A repeat intervention was performed in 16 of these 49 patients with restenosis (22).

Complications of ELCA, with the exception of a perforation rate of 1.1% appear to be similar to those of balloon angioplasty. The most recently published complications rates of the Excimer Laser Coronary Angioplasty Registry are (patients may appear in more than one category): dissection 12.5%, acute occlusion 5.4%, spasm 2%, thrombus 1.9%, embolism 0.8%, aneurysm 0.5%, coronary artery bypass graft (CABG) 3.5%, myocardial infarction (MI) 1.4%, death 0.3% (26).

Because perforation is a complication that is exceedingly rare in balloon angioplasty, further discussion is indicated. The following are presently identified as risk factors for perforation:

1. Eccentric lesions on a bend.
2. Use of oversized laser catheters.
3. Multiple passes.
4. Lasing at true bifurcation sites.
5. In areas of previous dissections.

Approximately two-thirds of the perforations have had no hemodynamic compromise. The remaining one-third that have been hemodynamically unstable and have required immediate surgery have been in the setting of perforation of a native vessel in patients with an intact pericardium. Management of this complication will be discussed later in the chapter.

Although the preliminary follow-up data suggest that the restenosis rate is similar to that seen with balloon angioplasty, there exists recent intriguing work to suggest that higher tip energies, as well as a lower postlaser residual stenosis, may lead to a lower restenosis rate. Six-month angiographic and clinical follow-up on 446 patients has suggested a strong inverse relationship between catheter-tip energies and restenosis (25). This may be due to more precise cutting at higher energies with less mechanical disruption of the vessel wall. Quantitative coronary angiography has been performed on another group of 47 patients that underwent excimer laser angioplasty. Linear regression analysis demonstrated a significant correlation between the postlaser residual stenosis and the follow-up stenosis. A postlaser residual stenosis of less than 30% significantly improved the long-term angiographic outcome. A post–balloon angioplasty result of similar magnitude was not correlated with an improved long-term angiographic outcome (27). These data from a small group of patients suggest that the long-term outcome is related to the amount of plaque ablated by the laser catheter.

TROUBLESHOOTING

As noted above, there are significant differences between the performance of balloon angioplasty and ELCA. Among these are the management of acute occlusion, dissection, and perforation.

Should abrupt occlusion or severe dissection occur after passage of a laser catheter, exchange of the laser catheter for a balloon angioplasty catheter is indicated. Advancing a laser catheter across a dissection or recent occlusion may significantly worsen the pathology. The use of exchange-length wires or extension wires facilitates the placement of the balloon angioplasty catheter at the site of the occlusion or dissection. Management of

the acute occlusion or dissection then requires techniques similar to those used in balloon angioplasty. Prolonged inflations, perhaps with the use of perfusion catheters may be necessary. These techniques most often result in successful completion of the case with satisfactory results.

The technique for the management of hemodynamically significant perforations is as follows: After confirmation of contrast extravasation into the pericardium, the laser fiber is removed from the guidewire, leaving the wire in place across the lesion. Then an angioplasty balloon or autoperfusion balloon is placed across the area of the perforation and inflated to tamponade the bleeding. If the patient is hemodynamically stable, a pulmonary artery balloon flotation catheter is placed and echocardiography is performed. Should signs of pericardial tamponade be noted, pericardiocentesis is performed and the patient is taken to the operating room for repair of the perforation and bypass surgery. In the setting of severe hemodynamic instability, blind pericardiocentesis may need to be performed after the confirmation of tamponade hemodynamics by the flotation catheter.

CASE EXAMPLES

Ostial Stenosis: B.B., 78-year-old woman.

History:	1987	Gradual onset of exertional angina. Angiogram—Mild intimal irregularities of right and left coronary arteries. Medical therapy.
	March, 1991	Increasing angina, Tl 201 with reversible inferior defect. Angiogram with 80% ostial RCA stenosis, 3 mm in length.
Medications:		Cardizem, nitroglycerin, aspirin, Tenormin.

ELCA Procedure 3/29/91:

CASS segment	Guide catheter	Guide-wire	Laser catheter (mm)	Energy density (mJ/mm²)	Pulses	Balloon catheter	Number of inflations
1	9F JR3.5S	0.018' in ACS Hi Torque XTRA	1.3	60	230	—	—
1	9F JR3.5S	Torque XTRA	2.0	50	220	—	—

Discussion:

Aortoostial lesions have proven to be difficult to treat with PTCA. As discussed, aortoostial lesions may be more favorably treated with ELCA (6,22). In this case, previous diagnostic angiography had revealed an 80% ostial stenosis that was 3 mm in length. Because the use of a 2.0-mm laser fiber was anticipated, a 9F guide catheter was chosen. Care was taken to select a guiding catheter shape that would direct the laser fiber coaxial with the vessel lumen (Fig. 2A). A catheter with side holes was selected because damping was anticipated. In this case

the JR3.5 sat at the ostium, prevented from entering the vessel by the lesion. After the stenosis was crossed with a guidewire, a single pass with the guide catheter disengaged from the ostium was performed with the 1.3-mm laser fiber set at a relatively high energy level to minimize mechanical trauma. The smaller laser fiber was chosen to debulk the lesion for the 2.0-mm laser fiber. Then two passes of the 2.0-mm laser fiber were performed, after which no residual stenosis could be demonstrated by angiography (Fig. 2B). In aortoostial lesions up to three passes may be performed with the guide catheter angulated to change the catheter trajectory. Caution must be used to avoid perforation.

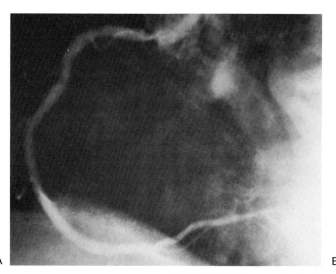 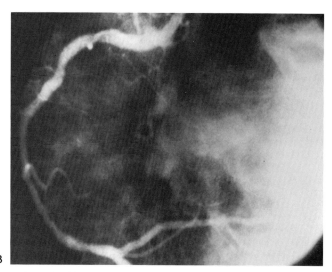

FIG. 2. Ostial stenosis. **A:** Preprocedure. **B:** After ELCA/PTCA.

Total Occlusion: R. D., 61-year-old man.

History:	April, 1991	Remote history of CABG with recent onset of unstable angina.
Past History:	1977	CABG
Medications:		ASA, calcium channel blocker.

ELCA Procedure 4/19/91:

CASS segment	Guide catheter	Guide-wire	Laser catheter (mm)	Energy density (mJ/mm²)	Pulses	Balloon catheter	Number of inflations
23	9F AL2	0.016 USCI Standard J with Tracker	—	—	—	—	—
23	9F AL2	0.018 Terumo Straight with Tracker	—	—	—	—	—
23	9F AL2	0.016 USCI Standard J with Tracker	1.3	55	900	—	—
23	9F AL2	J with Tracker	2.0	55	500	—	—
23	9F AL2	J with Tracker	—	—	—	3.5 MVP	1

Discussion:

Long total occlusions or recanalized lesions have lower acute success rates than subtotal occlusions due to difficulty crossing the occlusion with the guidewire. Excimer laser coronary angioplasty, an over-the-wire system, shares this limitation. Because long occlusions frequently involve major side branches, the low incidence of major side-branch occlusion may make ELCA superior to balloon angioplasty in this setting (22). Debulking

of the lesion may yield lower restenosis rates or restenosis in a focal area. In this case a 17-mm occlusion was present in the mid to distal portion of the circumflex coronary artery (Fig. 3A). No major side branches were involved. Because of the acute angle of origin of the circumflex coronary artery and the anticipated need for excellent guide catheter backup a 9F AL2 was selected. To obtain maximal support during attempts at crossing the lesion, a Tracker infusion catheter was used. Attempts at crossing the lesion with a 0.016-in standard J wire (USCI) were not successful. The wire would cross

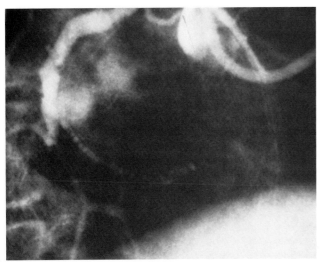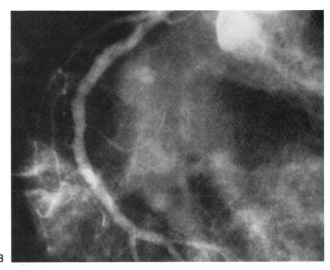

FIG. 3. Total occlusion. **A:** Preprocedure. **B:** After ELCA.

the initial portion of the lesion but, even with maximal support, no further progress could be made. Leaving the tracker in place down the circumflex, the USCI wire was replaced by a 0.018-in Terumo wire. Gentle continuous pressure on this wire created a channel into the distal lumen. The Terumo wire was then replaced by a 0.018-

in laser wire (ACS). This wire passed through the channel that was created by the Terumo wire with little manipulation. Single passes with 1.3- and 2.0-mm laser fibers resulted in a 2.0-mm lumen. A single inflation with a 3.0 mm balloon resulted in a 15% residual stenosis (Fig. 3B).

Diffuse Lesion: L. D., 71-year-old man.

History:	1983	Onset of angina, good response to medical therapy.
	1991	Increasing angina, Canadian Class III.
	March, 1991	Tl 201—infero-lateral ischemia Cath—Mild left disease, severe diffuse disease of the right coronary artery.
Medications:		Isordil, Inderal, Cardizem, aspirin

ELCA Procedure 6/3/91:

CASS segment	Guide catheter	Guide-wire	Laser catheter (mm)	Energy density (mJ/mm^2)	Pulses	Balloon catheter	Number of inflations
1	8F JR4	0.018″ ACS Hi Torque XTRA	1.3	50	540	—	—
1	8F JR4	XTRA	—	—	—	2.5 18K	3

Discussion:

This case illustrates the use of ELCA in a long, severe lesion. This 30-mm lesion is further complicated by occurring on a bend (Fig. 4A). Distal discrete disease is also present. Because this was not a tight radius bend, the risks of perforation using a 1.3-mm laser catheter were considered acceptable. After the wire was placed in the

distal portion of the right coronary artery, a single pass of the 1.3-mm fiber was performed. Mild dissection of the proximal and distal portions of the lesion were noted and it was elected to use a 2.5-mm balloon to perform PTCA on the distal lesions, as well as improve the post ELCA result. After PTCA there is a residual 10% stenosis and a mild distal dissection (Fig. 4B). Filling of the distal vessels is markedly improved.

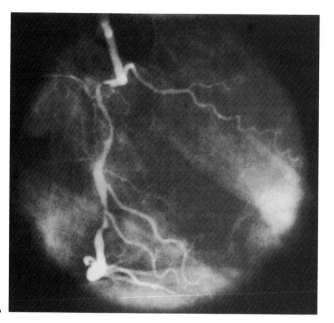
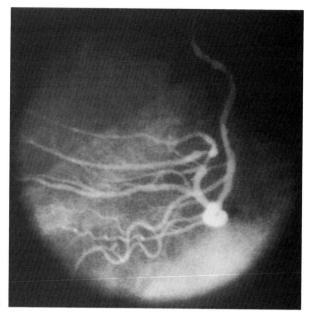

FIG. 4. Diffuse Lesion. **A:** Preprocedure. **B:** After ELCA/PTCA.

Saphenous Vein Graft: G. J., 64-year-old man.

History:	March 1991	Recent onset of Canadian Cardiovascular Class III angina.
Past History:	1983	CABG
Medications:		ASA, calcium channel blocker.

ELCA Procedure 3/25/91:

CASS segment	Guide catheter	Guide-wire	Laser catheter (mm)	Energy density (mJ/mm²)	Pulses	Balloon catheter	Number of inflations
	9F MP	0.018″ ACS Hi Torque	1.3	55	340	—	—
Graft to 1		XTRA					
Graft to 1	9F MP	XTRA	2.0	50	375	—	—

Discussion:

This case illustrates the use of ELCA in a saphenous vein graft. Angiography revealed a subtotal ostial lesion followed by a subtotal proximal shaft lesion that was 7 mm in length (Fig. 5A). After the lesion was crossed with the guidewire, ELCA was performed with 1.3- and 2.0-mm laser fibers. The post-ELCA result was excellent with a residual stenosis of 10% (Fig. 5B). Because the residual stenosis was less than 30% this was left as a stand alone laser.

Perforation: V. W., 59-year-old woman.

History:	January, 1991	Recent diagnosis of breast CA, developed unstable angina while undergoing radiation therapy. Thought nonoperative due to breast CA and recent radiation therapy.
Medications:		ASA, calcium channel blocker

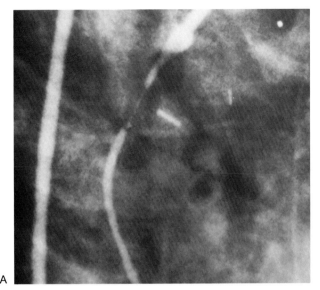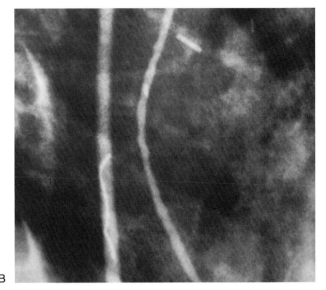

FIG. 5. Saphenous vein graft. **A:** Preprocedure. **B:** After ELCA.

ELCA Procedure 1/28/91:

CASS segment	Guide catheter	Guide-wire	Laser catheter (mm)	Energy density (mJ/mm²)	Pulses	Balloon catheter	Number of inflations
12	8fr SL 4	0.018″ ACS Hi Torque XTRA	1.3	55	160	—	—
12	8fr SL 4	XTRA	1.3	50	160	—	—
12	8fr SL 4	XTRA	—	—	—	2.5 mm Stack	2

Discussion:

Diagnostic angiography revealed a 90% lesion in the proximal portion of the left anterior descending coronary artery that was 3 mm in length (Fig. 6A). Because of the patients medical condition, she was thought not to be an operative candidate. After the lesion was crossed with the guidewire, ELCA was performed with a 1.3-mm laser fiber. The result was inadequate after the first pass, so a second pass with the same size laser fiber was elected. Dye extravasation was noted after the second passage of the laser catheter (Fig. 6B). While maintaining the wire position, the laser fiber was replaced by a 2.5-mm Stack Perfusion Catheter (ACS) and two dilations were performed. After PTCA the stenosis was 20%, without contrast extravasation (Fig. 6C). Because the patient was hemodynamically stable, she was observed clinically and with hemodynamic monitoring. At 6-month follow-up she has a normal exercise/thallium study. Angiography is pending.

CONCLUSIONS

Excimer laser coronary angioplasty is an evolving technique that is currently undergoing clinical study to define its utility in relationship to existing and emerging technologies available to the interventional cardiologist.

The performance of ELCA requires the presence of two physicians. The frequent exchanges necessitating the use of exchange-length or extended wires are more cumbersome than routine balloon angioplasty. Careful attention to the tip energy settings, catheter sizing, and rate of laser fiber advancement (<1 mm/sec) are mandatory to obtain optimal results and minimize complications.

Current data suggest that ELCA may be applied with risks similar to those of balloon angioplasty. Acute results may be superior when ELCA is applied to selected lesions that are considered to be unfavorable for balloon angioplasty. Ostial lesions, long segments or diffuse disease, saphenous vein grafts, and total occlusions are potential applications. Restenosis appears also to be similar

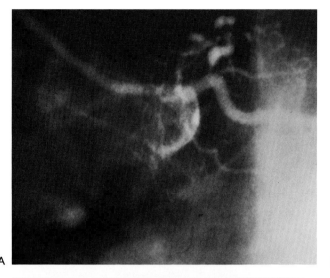

A

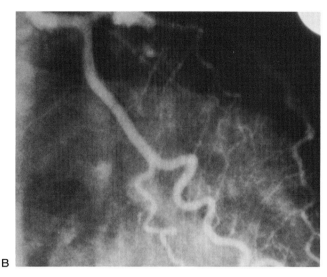

B

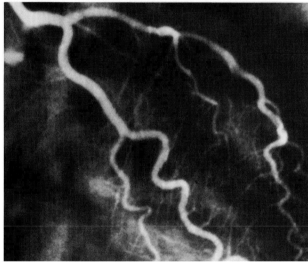

C

FIG. 6. Perforation. **A:** Preprocedure. **B:** After ELCA. **C:** After PTCA.

to that of balloon angioplasty with two recent exceptions: (i) The use of higher tip energies may be associated with a smoother residual lumen and less mechanical trauma to the vessel and may result in less injury induced smooth muscle cell proliferation. (ii) The use of larger laser fibers which minimizes postlaser stenosis (<30%) appears to result in a better long-term angiographic result. It is hypothesized that this results from a more effective debulking of the lesion by the larger catheter. Continued multicenter trials, including randomized studies, and improvement in the laser delivery systems will ultimately determine the role of excimer laser coronary angioplasty in the treatment of coronary artery disease.

REFERENCES

1. Hurst JW. The first coronary angioplasty as described by Andreas Gruentzig. *Am J Cardiol* 1986;57:185–186.

2. Gruentzig AR, Senning A, Seigenthaler WE. Nonoperative dilatation of coronary-artery stenosis: percutaneous transluminal coronary angioplasty. *N Engl J Med* 1979;301:61–68.
3. Holmes DR, Holubkov R, Vlietstra RE, et al. Comparisons of complications during percutaneous transluminal coronary angioplasty from 1977 to 1981 and from 1985 to 1986: the National Heart, Lung and Blood Institute Percutaneous Transluminal Coronary Angioplasty Registry. *Am J Cardiol* 1988;12:1149–1155.
4. Safian RD, McCabe CH, Sipperly ME, McKay RG, Baim DS. Initial success and long term follow-up of percutaneous transluminal coronary angioplasty in chronic total occlusions versus conventional stenosis. *Am J Cardiol* 1988;61:23G–28G.
5. Ellis SG, Shaw RE, Gershony G, Thomas R, Roubin GS, Douglas JS, Topol EJ, Sterzer SH, Myler RK, King SB. Risk factors, time course and treatment effect for restenosis after successful percutaneous transluminal coronary angioplasty of chronic total occlusion. *Am J Cardiol* 1989;63:897–901.
6. Topol EJ, Ellis SG, Fishman J, Lemgruber P, Myler RK, Sterzer SH, O'Neill WW, Douglas JS, Roubin GS, King SB. Multicenter study of percutaneous transluminal coronary angioplasty for right coronary ostial stenosis. *J Am Coll Cardiol* 1987;9:1214–1218.
7. Vandormael MG, Delignul U, Kern MJ, Harper M, Presant S, Gibson P, Galan K, Chaitman BR. Multilesion coronary angioplasty: clinical and angiographic follow-up. *J Am Coll Cardiol* 1987;10:246–252.

8. Sinclair IN, McCabe CH, Sipperly ME, Baim DS. Predictors, therapeutic options and long-term outcome of abrupt reclosure. *Am J Cardiol* 1988;61:61G–66G.

9. Kent KM, Bentivoglio LG, Block PC, et al. Long-term efficacy of percutaneous transluminal coronary angioplasty (PTCA): report from the National Heart Lung, and Blood Institute PTCA Registry. *Am J Cardiol* 1984;53:27C–31C.

10. Nobuyoshi M, Kimura T, Nosaka H, Mioka S, Ueno K, Yokoi H, Hamasaki N, Horiuchi H, Ohishi H. Restenosis after successful percutaneous transluminal coronary angioplasty: serial angiographic follow-up of 229 patients. *J Am Coll Cardiol* 1988;12:616–623.

11. Grundfest WS, Litvack IF, Goldenberg T, Sherman T, Morgerstern L, Carroll R, Fishbein M, Forrester J, Margitan J, McDermid S. Pulsed ultraviolet lasers and the potential for safe laser angioplasty. *Am J Surg* 1985;150:220–226.

12. Grundfest WS, Litvack F, Forrester JS, Goldenberg T, Swan HJC, Morgerstern L, Fishbein M, McDermid IS, Rider DM, Pacala TJ. Laser ablation of human atherosclerotic plaque without adjacent tissue injury. *J Am Coll Cardiol* 1985;5:929–933.

13. Levine S, Mahta S, Krauthamer D, Margolis JR. Excimer laser coronary angioplasty of calcified lesions. *J Am Coll Cardiol* 1991;17:206 (abst).

14. Litvack F, Grundfest WS, Goldenberg T, Laudenslager J, Forrester JS. In: Topol EJ, ed. *Textbook of interventional cardiology.* Philadelphia: WB Saunders; 1990:682–699.

15. Litvack F, Grundfest W, Eigler N, Tsoi D, Goldenberg T, Laudenslager J, Forrester J. Percutaneous excimer laser coronary angioplasty (Letter). *Lancet* 1989;2:102–103.

16. Litvack F, Grundfest WS, Segalowitz J, Papioanniou T, Goldenberg T, Laudenslager J, Hestrin L, Forrester JS, Eigler NA, Cook SL. Interventional cardiovascular therapy by laser and thermal angioplasty. *Circulation* 1990;81[Suppl IV]:IV-109–IV-116.

17. Litvack F, Grundfest WS, Goldenberg T, Laudenslager J, Forrester JS. Percutaneous excimer laser angioplasty of aortocoronary saphenous vein grafts. *J Am Coll Cardiol* 1989;14:803–808.

18. Karsh KR, Haase KK, Voelker W, Baumbach A, Mauser M, Sepel L. Percutaneous coronary excimer laser angioplasty in patients with stable and unstable angina pectoris. *Circulation* 1990;81:1849–1859.

19. Litvack F, Eigler NL, Margolis JR, et al. Percutaneous excimer laser coronary angioplasty. *Am J Cardiol* 1990;66:1027–1032.

20. Cook SL, Eigler NL, Shefer A, Goldenberg T, Forrester JS, Litvack F. Percutaneous excimer laser coronary angioplasty of lesions not ideal for balloon angioplasty. *Circulation* 1991;84:632–643.

21. Unteraker W, Roubin G, Margolis J, et al. Excimer laser coronary angioplasty of saphenous vein grafts. *J Am Coll Cardiol* 1991;17:23A (abst).

22. Eigler NL, Douglas JS, Margolis JR, Hestrin L, Litvack FI, and the ELCA Investigators. Excimer laser coronary angioplasty of aortoostial stenosis: results of the ELCA Registry. *Circulation* 1991;84(II):251 (abstract).

23. Ryan TI, Faxon DP, Gunnar RM, Kennedy JW, King SB, Loop FC, Peterson KL, Reeves TJ, Williams DO, Winters WL Jr. Guidelines for percutaneous transluminal coronary angioplasty: a report of the American College of Cardiology/American Heart Association Task Force on Assessment of Diagnostic and Therapeutic Cardiovascular Procedures (Subcommittee on Percutaneous Transluminal Coronary Angioplasty). *J Am Coll Cardiol* 1988;12:529–545.

24. Ellis SG, Roubin GS, King SB, Douglas JS, Weintraub WS, Thomas RG, Cox WR. Angiographic and clinical predictors of acute closure after native vessel coronary angioplasty. *Circulation* 1988;77:372–379.

25. Margolis JR, Krauthamer D, Litvack F, Rothbaum DA, Unteraker WJ, Breshnahan JF, Kent KM, Cummins FE, and the ELCA Registry Investigators. Six month follow-up of excimer laser coronary angioplasty registry patients. *J Am Coll Cardiol* 1991;17:218A (abstract).

26. Bresnahan JF, Litvack F, Margolis J, Rothbaum D, Kent K, Untereker W, Cummins F, and the ELCA Investigators. Excimer laser coronary angioplasty: initial results of a multicenter investigation in 958 patients. *J Am Coll Cardiol* 1991;17:30A (abstract).

27. Torre SR, Sanborn TA, Sharma S, Isreal D, Marmur J, Cohen M, Ambrose JA. Percutaneous coronary excimer laser angioplasty: quantitative angiographic analysis demonstrates a correlation between post-laser residual stenosis and six month follow-up stenosis. *J Am Coll Cardiol* 1991;17:22A (abstract).

CHAPTER 17

Intracoronary Ultrasound

Andrew P. Chodos and John E. Brush, Jr.

Intravascular ultrasound is a new imaging technique which utilizes an internal ultrasound catheter to visualize the vessel wall and related vascular structures. The initial impetus to develop this technology came in the early 1960s from the limited image quality provided by the then newly available transthoracic echocardiographic equipment (1). Within a decade of those first efforts, the feasibility of two-dimensional intravascular cross-sectional imaging was demonstrated, but improved transthoracic ultrasound imaging capabilities diminished the apparent need for these alternative devices. The recent advent of novel intravascular therapeutic devices has markedly renewed the interest in intravascular imaging. Because of the complexity of these devices, information regarding the integrity of the intimal surfaces, the presence or absence of thrombus, dissection, or ulceration, and the relative eccentricity of lesions is becoming increasingly important to adequately assess treatment efficacy and to guide clinical decision-making.

LIMITATIONS OF ANGIOGRAPHY

Coronary angiography has traditionally been the gold standard for assessing the severity of coronary artery disease, but it has several recognized limitations (Table 1). While an angiogram provides an outline of the vessel lumen, it only provides inferential information about the condition of the vessel wall. Vessel tortuously and overlap can limit the interpretation of a coronary angiogram. An angiogram, being a longitudinal lumenal silhouette, can obscure important cross-sectional lesion characteristics, and a severely stenotic eccentric lesion in one view can sometimes appear angiographically insignificant in other views. Autopsy studies have demonstrated discrepancies between pathologic and angiographically determined measurements (2,3). These factors can lead to considerable interobserver variability in the interpretation of coronary angiograms (4). Percent stenosis, measured angiographically, continues to guide most clinical decisions regarding coronary artery disease, but this measurement does not always predict the physiologic significance of a lesion (5,6). Intracoronary ultrasound imaging may circumvent many of these limitations of angiography.

Several devices for intravascular intervention have been recently developed and their use is increasing. Atherectomy, rotational ablation, and laser technologies all carry a small but measurable risk of vessel perforation, which is decreased with proper positioning of the device within the vessel. Deployment of intravascular stents also requires accurate knowledge of three-dimensional lumenal characteristics for correct placement and follow-up. Intracoronary ultrasound can provide real-time monitoring and catheter guidance during these interventions, thus increasing procedure efficacy and safety. Furthermore, it is frequently difficult for the angioplasty operator to discern from an angiogram whether there is dissection, thrombus formation, or both, following coronary angioplasty. Additional information provided by intravascular ultrasound may aid the angioplasty operator in determining the pathology of the coronary artery when the angiogram is ambiguous.

Finally, there has been recent interest in the relationship between lesion morphology and the clinical expression of coronary artery disease. Ambrose et al. have shown angiographically that ulcerated lesions are associated with more unstable symptoms (7). It is likely that further refinements in these observations, through the use of intravascular ultrasound imaging, will provide prognostic information. Moreover, there is evidence that atheroma composition and volume influences the outcome following coronary angioplasty (8). There are angiographic predictors of increased risk of dissection or

AP Chodos and JE Brush, Jr.: Evans Memorial Department of Clinical Research, and the Department of Medicine, Section of Cardiology, Boston University Medical Center, Boston, Massachusetts

TABLE 1. *Limitations of angiography*

Inability to accurately detect thrombus
Imaging eccentric lesions
Interobserver variability
No information on vessel wall characteristics
Problems with vessel overlap
Image attenuation due to chest wall and lung

restenosis, but these angiographic predictors are imprecise (9). Intravascular ultrasound appears to have the capability to define atheroma topography, volume, and composition. It will be important to develop new predictors of vessel dissection or restenosis based on more detailed morphologic information provided by intravascular ultrasound.

Thus, intravascular ultrasound imaging may circumvent many of the limitations of angiography and this new technology has the potential to add to our current understanding of coronary artery disease. In this chapter, we will review the currently available intravascular ultrasound technology, and discuss current use and potential applications.

INTRAVASCULAR ULTRASOUND DEVICES

All current intravascular ultrasound systems utilize a miniaturized piezoelectric element or elements located on the distal tip of an intravascular catheter. The piezoelectric material is either made of a crystal, usually lead zirconate titanate (PZT), or a polymeric material such as polyvinylidene difluoride. These piezoelectric elements, when excited with electrical current produce an ultrasound wave at a frequency which varies depending upon the type of material, the thickness of the material and the backing behind the material. Intravascular ultrasound devices commonly produce ultrasound with a central

frequency of 20 to 30 mHz. The frequency ranges of these devices have been chosen to optimize tissue resolution as well as tissue penetration; higher frequencies result in improved resolution, while lower frequencies result in improved tissue penetration. Current systems provide resolution to a tissue depth of approximately 3 to 4 mm.

There are currently two methods to direct the ultrasound beam outward from the catheter to produce the 360-degree circumferential image of the vessel wall. One approach uses a mechanically rotating transducer or acoustic mirror to direct the ultrasound signal roughly perpendicular to the longitudinal axis of the catheter. In this type of device, the transducer, the mirror, or both are mechanically rotated by a flexible drive shaft at 700 to 1,800 rpm. The second approach uses an array of multiple ultrasound elements (phased array) which are circumferentially mounted on the distal tip of the imaging catheter. In both types of systems, images are usually collected at 10 frames per second (10,11).

There are three mechanically rotating intravascular ultrasound systems (Fig. 1) which are currently commercially available. The device developed by Boston Scientific and Diasonics has a rotating transducer made of PZT which rotates within an catheter measuring 4.8 French (F). The external shell of the catheter can produce reflected echos on the rotating transducer, called the reverberation artifact, and to minimize this artifact, the transducer is tilted forward at a 10-degree angle. The near zone around the rotating transducer has a crystal artifact, known as the ring-down artifact, which makes the near zone unavailable for ultrasound interrogation. A second mechanical device developed by Cardiovascular Imaging Systems uses a stationary 30-MHz PZT transducer at the catheter tip and a more proximal acoustic mirror which rotates at 1,500 rpm. The catheter, which is 5F, is advanced over a guidewire, which

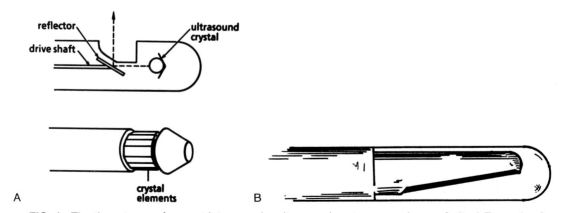

FIG. 1. The three types of current intravascular ultrasound systems are shown. **A:** (*top*) Example of a rotating imaging system where the ultrasound crystal is located at the tip of the catheter and the image is obtained by rotating a reflector 360 degrees; (*bottom*) Device composed of 64 stationary crystal elements that are electronically switched in order to create a 360-degree image. **B:** Device in which the transducer rotates within an external shell of the catheter.

produces an artifact in one sector of the ultrasound image. A third mechanical device, developed by Intertherapy, uses a 25-MHz PZT crystal and acoustic mirror which rotate together in a canoe configuration. The assembly rotates at 1,800 rpm within a catheter sheath. The purported advantage of having both the transducer and mirror rotate together is that the distance between the transducer and mirror, and the angle of the ultrasound beam and the mirror, remain constant as the catheter flexes and torques within the artery. The ring-down artifact is reduced in both of the mechanical devices that use an acoustic mirror, because the ultrasound beam travels a short distance from the transducer to the mirror and the crystal artifact is therefore contained within the catheter. The mechanical devices are all driven by a motor and flexible drive-shaft assembly. When the catheter is advanced and is flexed, there can be increased friction of the drive shaft causing nonuniformity in the rotating speed of the transducer or mirror, resulting in the so-called catch-and-slip artifact. Furthermore, the mechanical devices have a reverberation artifact from reflections from the outer catheter or from the catheter sheath which surrounds the rotating transducer/mirror. The mechanical devices have the advantage of being relatively simple in design and the images are considered to be of high quality.

The electronic device, developed by Endosonics Corporation has 64 piezoelectric elements made of polyvinylidene difluoride with a center frequency of 20 MHz. At the catheter tip, there are four integrated circuits to control the firing and receiving of the ultrasonic signals, which are transmitted down the catheter by four wires. The design, also called a dynamic aperture array, fires one or two of the ultrasound elements at a time, and the echo signals are electronically reconstructed and focused in computer memory. The design differs from a phased-array system, which is commonly used in external ultrasound imaging. A phased-array system fires multiple elements simultaneously to focus the transmitted ultrasound wave on a point at a specified distance from the transducer, rather than focusing the received signals in the computer's memory. The multiple element device is 5.5F and uses an over-the-wire design. A limitation of this device is the ring-down artifact which limits the ultrasound imaging adjacent to the catheter. It is possible to mask the ring-down artifact to improve the image appearance, but with the current device, imaging of vessels smaller than 2.2 mm is not possible. A newer 3.5F device is in the developmental stages and should improve imaging of smaller vessels. A device which combines the ultrasound array with a balloon on a single catheter has been developed and is currently undergoing clinical trials. The specifications of the currently available intracoronary ultrasound systems are seen in Table 2.

At present, it is unclear whether the mechanically rotating design or the array design is superior. The array design has the advantage of not requiring any rotational hardware. This generally allows for a more flexible catheter and space for a central lumen which can accommodate a 0.014-in movable guidewire. Both of these characteristics improve its use in distal and tortuous vessels. Depth of penetration and lateral resolution are theoretically superior in the mechanically rotated systems. In the mechanical systems, the full aperture with a single, larger element is always facing the tissue to be imaged, thus maximizing signal power. By comparison, the electronic system has a smaller aperture (and therefore a reduced signal power) with only a single, smaller element serving as the signal transducer. Additionally, the lack of ring-down artifact translates into superior imaging adjacent to the catheter in some of the mechanical systems.

IMAGE INTERPRETATION

Validation of Measurements *In Vitro*

The accuracy of ultrasound-derived lumenal measurements was studied by Hodgson et al., using the dynamic aperture array device (12). When compared with drilled

TABLE 2. *Specifications of current intravascular ultrasound systems*

Type of system (Company)	Catheter size	Delivery	Frequency (MHz)
Mechanical (Cardiovascular Imaging System)	Peripheral 5F (OD 1.7 mm)	Over-the-wire or fixed tip	30
	8F (OD 2.7 mm)	Fixed tip	20
	Coronary 4.3F (OD 1.42 mm)	Over-the-wire	30
Mechanical (Intertherapy)	4.9 (sheath FOD 1.6 mm)	Images through sheath	20
	3F imaging device (OD 1 mm)		
Phased array (Endosonics)	5.5F (OD 1.8 mm)	Over-the-wire	20
	3.5F (OD 1.1 mm)	Over-the-wire	20
Mechanical (Diasonics)	4.8F (OD 1.6 mm)	Rounded tip	20
	3.4F prototype (OD 1.1 mm)	Monorail	20
Mechanical (Dumed)	4.9F (OD 1.7 mm)	Rounded tip	30

OD, outer diameter.
Modified from Coy, (11), with permission.

holes in polyethylene phantoms ranging from 3.0 to 7.6 mm in diameter, the accuracy of the lumen measurements was found to be excellent (r = 0.99). *In vitro* studies of explanted animal arteries and human arteries have demonstrated a good correlation between measurements from ultrasound images and histologic preparations (r = 0.83 to 0.98) when comparing lumenal cross-sectional diameter and area, wall thickness, and relative percent narrowing (13–17). Tobis et al. compared the cross-sectional diameter measured using a mechanically rotating device to the area measured from histologic sections, and found a very good correlation (r = 0.88) (18,19). Potkin et al. also compared ultrasound measurements with those from histological sections of human coronary arteries and found a close correlation in the measurements of cross-sectional lumenal area (r = 0.85) and linear wall thickness (r = 0.92) (20). Both interobserver and intraobserver variability are reported to be acceptable (12,16,20).

Validation of Measurements *In Vivo*

Studies in man and animals demonstrate good correlation between intracoronary ultrasound and angiographically derived internal dimension measurements (r = 0.80 to r = 0.98), (21,22). Some investigators, however, have reported discrepancies between ultrasound-derived internal dimensions and those obtained by quantitative angiography. This has been particularly noted when imaging eccentric lesions (Fig. 2), and lesions following mechanical interventions (23). Nissen et al. compared vessel measurements determined by ultrasound and angiography in an animal angioplasty model and found better correlations before PTCA as compared to measurements obtained following dilation (r = 0.92 and r = 0.86, respectively), (21). In a follow-up study in man these investigators again noted close correlations when imaging normal (r = 0.92) or concentrically narrowed lesions (r = 0.93), but substantially less agreement when comparing images from eccentric lesions (r = 0.63), (22). Whether this reflects the known limitations of angiographic assessment of eccentric lesions or true errors by intravascular ultrasound is not yet known. There are also numerous other reports suggesting that intravascular ultrasound is actually more sensitive than angiography at detecting early or subclinical coronary artery disease (24,25).

Detection of the Intimal Leading Edge

The intima appears as an echo-bright signal, usually well demarcated from the darker (hypoechoic) central lumen and adjacent media. Identification of both the hypoechoic media and the echobright intima serve as important landmarks permitting definition of plaque

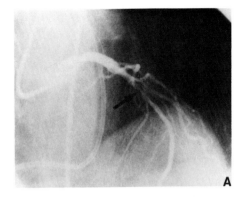

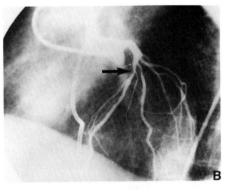

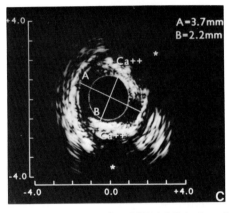

FIG. 2. **A, B:** Angiograms of a 60% LAD lesion viewed in orthogonal right anterior oblique (RAO) and left anterior oblique (LAO) projections. **C:** ICUS image of the same lesion. Note the large difference in luminal diameters demonstrated in the ICUS image. This lesion eccentricity was not apparent in the angiographic image.

boundaries and, therefore, quantitative analysis of plaque characteristics. Failure to clearly identify the intimal leading edge is an important cause of inadequate ultrasound image collection. This point is emphasized by a recent study in which images adequate to assess wall dimensions were obtained in less than 50% of segments imaged (26). The origin of this inner echo-bright signal was studied by Webb et al., who reported that when the internal elastic lamina is dissolved with elastase this bright leading edge is lost (27). Whether this echo-bright signal originates from the internal elastic lamina or represents acoustic reflections from the smooth intimal

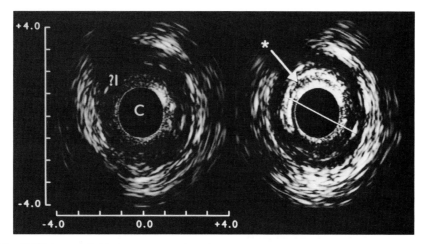

FIG. 3. The ICUS image (*left*) shows a poorly delineated intimal boundary. Intracoronary radiographic contrast (*right*) opacifies the lumen (arrow, *) and facilitates the identification of the lumen/intimal interface. This has potential to enhance internal vessel measurements.

boundary is currently unresolved. Our laboratory is currently investigating various methods, such as intracoronary radiographic contrast injections, to enhance the visualization of this lumen-intimal interface (Fig. 3).

Factors Affecting Image Quality

With most devices the catheter will appear as a circle within a dark lumen and the surrounding vessel wall. Image interpretation is intuitively obvious, since the cross-sectional ultrasound display is similar to the cross-sectional image from histologic sectioning. Several features affecting the quality and the reproducibility of image collection have been noted, however (Table 3). It is important to position the catheter coaxially in the center of the vessel. Failure to appropriately orient the catheter results in emitted echo signals that are not perpendicular to the vessels wall. This results in an artifactually elliptical image with blurring of distal and lateral wall surfaces, thus leading to erroneous measurements of internal dimensions (17). Eccentric catheter position will cause blooming of the vessel wall closest to the transducer and artificially increase near wall thickness measurements. Behind heavily calcified plaques, there is significant echo shadowing, which precludes ultrasound imaging of such sectors. Improper gain settings can result in an artificially thicker appearance of a vascular structure, if the gain is too high, or a thinner appearance,

TABLE 3. *Factors and artifacts affecting image quality*

Noncoaxial catheter position
Eccentric catheter position
Dropout and calcium blinding
Gain artifact
Videotape image degradation

if it is set too low and the intimal boundary is not appreciated. Because of the size of the currently available catheters, there can be some distortion of the shape of tight stenoses or smaller vessels. Catheter stiffness, which varies with different designs, may also limit imaging in vessels with marked tortuousity. Improvements in catheter design and technology will be necessary to overcome some of these limitations and to increase the clinical utility of these devices.

TISSUE CHARACTERIZATION

Three-Layered Appearance

A reproducible three-layered appearance is consistently seen when imaging muscular arteries (Fig. 4), and a more homogeneous appearance is seen in elastic arteries (14,15,20). Both muscular and elastic arteries have three distinct histologic layers defined by the intima, media, and adventitia. The major difference between these two types of arteries is in the composition of the media. The media in muscular arteries (i.e., coronary arteries) contains primarily smooth muscle cells, collagen, and ground substance. The media of elastic arteries also contains smooth muscle cells, but is also rich in densely packed elastin fibers (10). Several studies suggest that the three-layered ultrasound image of muscular arteries corresponds to the distinct anatomic layers seen histologically. In both muscular and elastic vessels the intima and adventitia appear as echo-bright reflections. In muscular arteries, the media is often echo-lucent so that there is visual separation of the inner intima from the outer adventitia (20). This three-layered appearance theoretically results from sharp acoustic impedance differences between the three tissue interfaces. Conversely, the

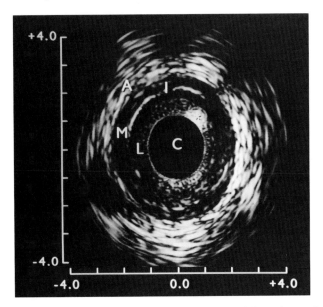

FIG. 4. This ICUS image illustrates the normal three-layered appearance of a muscular coronary artery. The catheter (C) is surrounded by the dark lumen (L). The echo-bright intima (I) and adventitia (A), are separated by the hypoechoic media (M). At one o'clock (*) is a bubble artifact.

regular array of elastin fibers located in the media of elastic arteries results in an echo-bright signal that is not easily distinguished from signals reflected from the adjacent histologic layers (14). Data from an *in vitro* study that shows loss of the three-layered appearance after disruption of the media by PTCA would support this interpretation regarding the significance of the three-layered appearance (18).

Other investigators submit that the three-layered appearance is not due to the three histological vessel layers. In fact, one study demonstrated that the same three-layered ultrasound image can be reproduced by imaging a fluid-filled plastic syringe (28). This suggests that reflections from a smooth surface such as the intima might cause this appearance. Furthermore, most *in vitro* intravascular ultrasound images are of undistended vessels which can dramatically influence mural spatial relationships causing an increase in the sonolucent zone due to elastic recoil. Fitzgerald et al. report that the three-layered appearance was infrequently seen when imaging normal vessels of young patients, and more frequently seen in older patients manifesting intimal thickening greater than 150 microns (29). Some of this controversy may result from a failure of these studies to consistently distinguish what type of vessel (muscular or elastic) is being imaged (10). Our clinical experience confirms that the three-layered appearance is frequently, but not universally, appreciated when imaging coronary vessels in patients with ischemic heart disease. Atherosclerotic disease within the media, and the previously described limitations of this imaging technology, probably account for the reported discrepancies.

Tissue Analysis

Three general tissue types have been identified by intravascular ultrasound imaging: calcium deposits appear as bright echo signals with distal shadowing (Fig. 5); fibrous plaques cause dense, homogeneously bright signals without distal shadowing; and lipid-filled lesions are hypoechoic (14,20). Fibrous plaque appears bright because of the high acoustic reflectivity of the high collagen content in the tissue (30), but it has less reflectivity than calcium and, therefore, no distal shadowing. In one study of 32 human arteries *in vitro*, there was a 96% agreement between the tissue type identified by ultrasound and that identified histologically (20). The identification of calcium by this technique appears to be quite accurate and potentially more sensitive than standard angiography. A study by Tobis et al. reported that following angioplasty 70% of the lesions had calcium when examined by intravascular ultrasound (usually located in the outer parameter of the atheroma adjacent to the media), whereas angiography suggested calcium in only 5% of the same lesions (19).

The important role of thrombosis in the clinical presentation of coronary artery disease has been well documented. However, the angiographic identification of thrombus is often ambiguous and imprecise. The ability to visualize and characterize thrombus by intravascular ultrasound would undoubtedly yield important information about the pathophysiology of the acute coronary insufficiency syndromes. Intravascular ultrasound can detect the development of thrombus formation in an animal model of low-flow vessel injury (31). Distinguishing thrombus from a soft plaque is, however, difficult due to

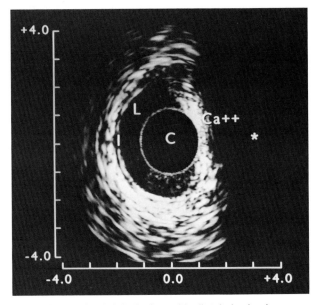

FIG. 5. This echo-bright lesion with distal shadowing represents a calcified lesion. Note the signal dropout (signified by *) which occurs with this type of lesion.

the similarly hypoechoic signals. Work by Fitzgerald et al. (32) using back-scatter analysis techniques shows some potential successes in identifying unique signals from thrombotic material. Using quantitative ultrasound techniques, Chandraratna et al. found that tissue attenuation coefficients were able to differentiate between fatty lesions and thrombus (33). Pandian et al. demonstrated 100% sensitivity in detecting freshly placed thrombus in an *in vitro* study using explanted dog arteries (34). In that study, measurement of the thrombus size by ultrasound correlated well with the histologic measurement. Whether it will be possible to accurately identify thrombus in diseased coronary arteries in patients, with sufficient sensitivity and specificity, remains to be established.

Problems in the Extrapolation of *In Vitro* Results

There are several inherent limitations when extrapolating results from *in vitro* and histologic studies to data obtained from *in vivo* image collections. First, there is the subjective nature of the terminology used to define an ultrasound image. This clearly predisposes to interobserver variability in the interpretation of intravascular sonograms and tends to complicate validation efforts. As with angiographic experiments, the processing and fixation of arterial segments during preparation for *in vitro* analysis may affect both specimen geometry and dimensions, and thus confound comparative studies (35). The absence of a distending pressure in most *in vitro* studies could also affect vessel spatial relationships and the acoustic properties of the tissue, both of which could potentially alter image appearance. Temperature, imaging medium (blood vs. saline), motion artifact in pulsatile vessels, and difficulties in achieving coaxial transducer position during *in vivo* studies, each have potential to alter images and, therefore, hinder correlation efforts. While temperature is thought to have limited impact on images, the effects of these other parameters are less clear (36).

OTHER APPLICATIONS

The ability to obtain cross-sectional images of coronary lesions for real-time assessment of coronary morphologies makes intravascular ultrasound potentially useful during invasive procedures. The ability to image flaps and dissections with intravascular ultrasound is presently being investigated. Two potential problems have been noted in this regard. First, echo dropout can create the false impression of a dissection. Second, the ultrasound device itself can expand the lumen, pushing the dissection flap aside and making visualization of the dissection plane impossible. Nevertheless, studies have demonstrated potential for imaging dissections flaps.

The ability of intravascular ultrasound to provide information following atherectomy, laser, stenting, or ablation procedures is also currently being studied. Attempts to use intracoronary ultrasound to assess the mechanism of atherectomy and to image postatherectomy intimal surfaces have been reported. Of note, as with angioplasty studies, is the correlation between angiography and intravascular ultrasound–derived lumenal measurements *in vivo* and after atherectomy sometimes show moderate discrepancies. The major problems in the application of intracoronary ultrasound during atherectomy are the difficulties in orienting the cutter to the intracoronary ultrasound image and the inability to precisely redirect the positioning of the atherectomy device.

Intravascular ultrasound has been used for early and late imaging of stented lesions. Stents characteristically appear highly refractile, casting small acoustic shadows above the compressed atheroma. Stent recoil has been demonstrated using intravascular ultrasound (37). Information on regional intimal hyperplasia in the proximal portion of the stented segment, which may be related to increased blood turbulence, has been reported (38). Stents placed in saphenous vein grafts have been successfully imaged as well. As anticipated, the three-layered appearance typically seen in muscular arteries has not been demonstrated when imaging saphenous vein grafts by intravascular ultrasound (39). It is of note that intravascular ultrasound has successfully imaged in situ saphenous vein grafts, as well as identifying the anastomotic site and documenting both the proximal lesion in the native vessel and its distal patency (40,41). Such intraoperative real-time assessment might potentially allow modification of the procedure at the time of the initial operation, thus improving outcomes and potentially diminishing the need for reoperation.

FUTURE DIRECTIONS

There are currently ongoing studies and clinical investigations attempting to define the clinical utility of the this new intravascular ultrasound technology. There are several areas where improvement in catheter design will undoubtedly enhance the use of this technique in clinical cardiology. The smallest catheters are currently approximately 3F in diameter, a factor which clearly limits the size of the vessels that this technology can image. Further improvements in miniaturization, mechanical hardware, and electronic circuitry will undoubtedly lead to smaller catheters which will make possible the imaging of smaller arterial segments. Additionally, forward-looking devices which would obviate the need to enter a lesion are currently being investigated (42). Improvements in imaging processing and display should facilitate future interpretations of these images. For example, simultaneous side-by-side display of cineangiography and intravascular ultrasound images on the same monitor should soon be available. Display of electrocardiographic and hemodynamic data obtained from catheters combining ultrasound and Doppler flow capabilities will facilitate studies of pressure-volume and elastic recoil relationships (43). On-line three-dimensional reconstruction is now feasible and should increase our ability to integrate the large quantity of information provided from multiple intracoronary ultrasound (ICUS) cross-sectional images (44). We can also expect more catheters that combine ultrasound imaging with a therapeutic device, such as a balloon, atherectomy device, or laser delivery system (45). Several combination balloon ultrasound imaging catheters are currently available and are undergoing clinical investigation. Image quality will also likely improve in the future due to advances in ultrasound catheter and computer technology. With these improvements, one would expect intravascular ultrasound to find increasing use in clinical and investigational cardiology.

REFERENCES

1. Pandian H. Intravascular and intracardiac ultrasound imaging: an old concept, now on the road to reality. *Circulation* 1989;80:1091–1094.
2. Grondin C, Dyrda I, Pasternac A, Campeau L, Bourrassa M, Lesperance J. Discrepancies between cineangiographic and postmortem findings in patients with coronary artery disease and recent myocardial revascularization. *Circulation* 1974;49:703–708.
3. Arnett E, Isner J, Redwood D, et al. Coronary artery narrowing in coronary heart disease: comparison of cineangiographic and necropsy findings. *Ann Intern Med* 1979;91:350–356.
4. DeRouen T, Murray J, Owen W. Variability in the analysis of coronary arteriograms. *Circulation* 1976;55:324–328.
5. Marcus M, Skorton D, Johnson M, Collins S, Harrison D, Kerber R. Visual estimates of percent diameter coronary stenosis: "A battered gold standard." *J Am Coll Cardiol* 1988;11:882–885.
6. White C, Wright C, Doty D, et al. Does visual interpretation of the coronary arteriogram predict the physiologic importance of a coronary stenosis? *N Engl J Med* 1984;310:819–824.
7. Ambrose J, Winters S, Stern A, et al. Angiographic morphology and the pathogenesis of unstable angina. *J Am Coll Cardiol* 1985;5:609–616.
8. Lee RT, Grodzinsky AJ, Frank EH, et al. Structure-dependent dynamic mechanical behavior of fibrous caps from human atherosclerotic plaques. *Circulation* 1991;83:1764–1770.
9. Ellis S, Roubin G, King S, Douglas J, Cox W. Importance of stenosis morphology in the estimation of restenosis risk after elective percutaneous transluminal coronary angioplasty. *Am J Cardiol* 1989;63:30–34.
10. Nissen S, Gurley J, DeMaria A. Assessment of vascular disease by intravascular ultrasound. *Cardiology* 1990;77:398–410.
11. Coy K, Maurer G, Siegel R. Intravascular ultrasound imaging: a current perspective. *J Am Coll Cardiol* 1991;18:1811–1823.
12. Hodgson JM, Graham S, Savakus A, et al. Clinical percutaneous imaging of coronary anatomy using an over-the-wire ultrasound catheter system. *Int J Card Imaging* 1989;4:187–193.
13. Pandian N, Kreis A, O'Donnell T. Intravascular ultrasound estimation of arterial stenosis. *J Am Soc Echocardiogr* 1989;2:390–397.
14. Gussenhoven E, Essed C, Lancee C, et al. Arterial wall characteristics determined by intravascular ultrasound imaging: an *in vitro* study. *J Am Coll Cardiol* 1989;14:947–952.
15. Mallery J, Tobis J, Griffith J, et al. Assessment of normal and atherosclerotic arterial wall thickness with an intravascular ultrasound imaging catheter. *Am Heart J* 1990;119:1392–1400.
16. Moriuchi M, Tobis J, Mahon D, et al. The reproducibility of intravascular ultrasound imaging *in vitro*. *J Am Soc Echocardiogr* 1990;3:444–450.
17. Nishimura RA, Edwards WD, Warnes CA, et al. Intravascular ultrasound imaging: *in vitro* validation and pathologic correlation. *J Am Coll Cardiol* 1990;16:145–154.
18. Tobis J, Mallery J, Gessert J, et al. Intravascular ultrasound cross-sectional arterial imaging before and after balloon angioplasty *in vitro*. *Circulation* 1989;80:873–882.
19. Tobis J, Mallery J, Mahon D, et al. Intravascular ultrasound imaging of human coronary arteries *in vivo*: analysis of tissue characterizations with comparison to *in vitro* histological specimens. *Circulation* 1991;83:913–926.
20. Potkin B, Bartorelli A, Gessert J, et al. Coronary artery imaging with intravascular high-frequency ultrasound. *Circulation* 1990;81:1575–1585.
21. Nissen S, Grines C, Gurley J, et al. Application of a new phased-array ultrasound imaging catheter in the assessment of vascular dimensions: *in vivo* comparison to cineangiography. *Circulation* 1990;81:660–666.
22. Nissen S, Gurley J, Grines C, et al. Intravascular ultrasound assessment of lumen size and wall morphology in normal subjects and patients with coronary artery disease. *Circulation* 1991;84:1087–1099.
23. Davidson C, Shelkh K, Kisslo K, et al. Intravascular ultrasound evaluation of coronary and peripheral interventional technologies. *J Am Coll Cardiol* 1991;17:93A.
24. Tobis J, Mahon D, Lehmann K, et al. The sensitivity of ultrasound imaging compared with angiography for diagnosing coronary atherosclerosis. *Circulation* 1990;82[Suppl III]:439.
25. Nissen S, Gurley J, Grines C, et al. Coronary atherosclerosis is frequently present at angiographically normal sites: evidence from intravascular ultrasound in man. *Circulation* 1990;82[Suppl III]:459.
26. Sheikh K, Davidson C, Kisslo K, et al. Limitations and utility of *in vivo*, catheter based ultrasound imaging for assessing peripheral arterial wall and lesion morphology. *Circulation* 1990;82[Suppl III]:442.
27. Webb JG, Yock PG, Slepian MJ, et al. Intravascular ultrasound: significance of the three-layered appearance of normal muscular arteries. *J Am Coll Cardiol* 1990;15:17A.
28. Junbo G, Erbel R, Seidel I, et al. Controversial conclusion of the wall structure in intravascular ultrasound imaging. *J Am Coll Cardiol* 1991;17:112A.
29. Fitzgerald P, St. Goar F, Kao A, et al. Intravascular ultrasound imaging of coronary arteries: Is three layers the norm? *J Am Coll Cardiol* 1991;17:217A.
30. Mimbs JW, O'Donnel M, Bauwens D, et al. The dependence of ultrasonic attenuation and backscatter on collagen content in dog and rabbit hearts. *Circ Res* 1980;47:49–56.
31. Ferguson J, Ober J, Edelman S, et al. Documentation of experimentally-induced thrombus formation using intravascular ultrasound. *J Am Coll Cardiol* 1991;17:217A.
32. Fitzgerald P, Connolly A, Watkins R, et al. Distinction between soft plaque and thrombus by intravascular ultrasound tissue characterization. *J Am Coll Cardiol* 1991;17:111A.
33. Chandraratna P, Choudhary S, Jones J, et al. Differentiation between fatty plaque and thrombus by quantitative ultrasonic methods. *Circulation* 1991;84:II–702.
34. Pandian N, Kreis A, Brockway B. Detection of intraarterial thrombus by intravascular high frequency two-dimensional ultrasound imaging *in vitro* and *in vivo* studies. *Am J Cardiol* 1990;65:1280–1283.
35. Siegel RJ, Swan K, Edwards G, et al. Limitations of postmortem assessment of human coronary artery size and luminal narrowing: differential effects of tissue fixation and processing on vessels with different degrees of atherosclerosis. *J Am Coll Cardiol* 1985;5:342–346.
36. Yock P, Linker D, Angelsen B. Two-dimensional intravascular ultrasound: technical development and initial clinical experience. *J Am Soc Echocardiogr* 1989;2:296–304.

37. Keren G, Bartorelli A, Hansch E, et al. Intracoronary ultrasound is an improved technique to assess acute and chronic changes after stent placement. *J Am Coll Cardiol* 1991;17:217A.

38. Zeiher A, Hohnloser S, Fritz R, et al. Intravascular ultrasound assessment of intimal hyperplasia after coronary stent implantation in humans: implications for mechanisms of in-stent restenosis. *Circulation* 1991;84[Suppl II]:721.

39. Karen G, Picahrd A, Satler L, et al. Intravascular ultrasound of saphenous vein grafts after PTCA and investigational angioplasty procedures. *J Am Coll Cardiol* 1991;17:126A.

40. Weintraub A, Schwartz S, Pandian N, et al. Intraoperative intravascular ultrasound imaging of coronary arteries, bypass grafts and anastomotic sites in humans—feasibility, methods, safety, and diagnostic ability. *J Am Coll Cardiol* 1991;17:218A.

41. Yeon E, Lima J, Hargrove W, et al. Size and shape of the anastomotic junction as seen with intravascular ultrasound during coronary bypass surgery. *Circulation* 1991;84[Suppl II]:702.

42. Evans J, Ng K, Vonesh M, et al. Arterial imaging utilizing a new forward viewing intravascular ultrasound catheter: initial studies. *J Am Coll Cardiol* 1992;19:140A.

43. Kaufman J, Resenfield K, Pieczek A, et al. Combined intravascular ultrasound and intravascular Doppler wire provide complementary anatomic and physiologic imaging during percutaneous revascularization. *J Am Coll Cardiol* 1992;19:293A.

44. Rosenfield K, Kaufman J, Pieczek A, et al. On-line three-dimensional reconstruction from 2D IVUS: utility for guiding interventional procedures. *J Am Coll Cardiol* 1992;19:224A.

45. Fitzgerald P, Sudir K, Gupta M, et al. Combined atherectomy/ultrasound imaging device reduces subintimal tissue injury. *J Am Coll Cardiol* 1992;19:223A.

CHAPTER 18

Percutaneous Support Techniques

Seth D. Bilazarian and Alice K. Jacobs

In this chapter we review the clinical data on a variety of mechanical support modalities used in conjunction with percutaneous transluminal coronary angioplasty (PTCA). The technology in support systems has evolved rapidly, in parallel with the evolution of PTCA. Some of these techniques have been advocated for use in a standby-ready mode or prophylactically in high-risk patients undergoing PTCA. Other techniques have been used in patients only after hemodynamic compromise or abrupt closure of the coronary artery. Each modality will be discussed from a practical viewpoint, with a review of the technical equipment required, the technique for insertion, and a summary of the available clinical data on safety and efficacy. Finally, a comparison of the techniques will be made to assist the practicing interventionalist in clinical decisions about their use.

IDENTIFICATION OF PATIENTS AT RISK FOR AN ADVERSE OUTCOME

Since the advent of PTCA in 1977, its application has expanded greatly to encompass patients with more advanced disease. Frequently, these patients are elderly and have significant comorbid diseases relevant to the procedures (i.e., peripheral vascular disease), severe left ventricular dysfunction, multivessel coronary artery disease and/or a single patent coronary artery or a target vessel for PTCA which serves a large portion of the myocardium (1). Often these patients are deemed inoperable for surgical revascularization, making PTCA the only therapeutic option (2–4). In this subset of patients, the risks of morbidity associated with PTCA are high but, more importantly, hemodynamic collapse with balloon inflation or abrupt closure may result in death.

With the availability of support devices, PTCA of pa-

tients at high risk for an adverse outcome may be accomplished with a greater margin of safety (5,6). Identifying the patient at high risk for hemodynamic compromise is difficult; several investigators have identified preprocedural clinical (7–9) and angiographic (10,11) characteristics associated with an increased risk of acute complications during PTCA. Clinical features which may place patients at higher risk of in-hospital death after PTCA include poor left ventricular function, absence of prior coronary bypass surgery, New York Heart Association Class IV angina, advanced age, and female gender. Angiographic factors associated with the risk of abrupt vessel closure include lesion length, lesion angulation, thrombus, bifurcation lesions, post-PTCA percent stenosis, branch point lesions, multilesion disease, and multivessel disease (12).

Left ventricular function prior to PTCA was not a predictor of mortality in the Emory-San Francisco Heart Institute study (13), although a report from the Mid-America Heart Institute found left ventricular ejection fraction of less than 30% to be an independent predictor of death (14). However, a later report of nearly 9,000 patients demonstrated similar angiographic success when comparing groups whose left ventricular ejection fraction was greater or less than 40%, and found no difference in the incidence of death, myocardial infarction, or emergency coronary artery bypass grafting (15). Kohli et al. reported a similar experience (16). Kahn et al. evaluated a single center experience in 9,175 patients and found that when adjusted for age and anginal symptoms, women were not at higher risk than men (17), refuting the earlier NHLBI PTCA Registry experience (18).

Despite several retrospective reports of factors associated with an adverse outcome during PTCA, there have been few prospective studies. Bergelson and colleagues prospectively validated a statistical model as an accurate and reproducible way to improve prediction of hemodynamic compromise (19). In this study population of 157 consecutive patients, angiographic character-

SD Bilazarian and AK Jacobs: Section of Cardiology, Boston University Medical Center, Boston, Massachusetts

istics including myocardium at risk, multivessel disease, diffuse disease of the segment, and pre-PTCA stenosis were independent predictors of hemodynamic compromise. These angiographic characteristics were assigned a weighted value, based on the strength of their relationship to hemodynamic compromise, to create a new scoring system for identifying patients at high risk (Table 1). Prospective evaluation of this risk score in another patient sample revealed that this scoring system more accurately predicted hemodynamic compromise than either severely reduced ejection fraction, or greater than 50% myocardium at risk, alone. The extent of myocardium at risk can be graded in a so-called jeopardy score, which can reliably predict the risk of in-hospital death after abrupt closure (20).

Since the use of each support device is associated with potential complications, it will be critical for practicing interventionalists to develop accurate and reliable methods to stratify patients undergoing PTCA, based on risk of abrupt closure, hemodynamic compromise, and death. With a more accurate prediction of outcome, support modalities can be used in selected patients who may benefit, and avoided in lower risk patients in whom the risk of morbid adverse consequences from the support technique is not justified.

REGIONAL MYOCARDIAL SUPPORT TECHNIQUES

Antegrade Perfusion

The simplest and most elegant form of myocardial protection during coronary occlusion at the time of PTCA is use of the commercially available autoperfusion, passive hemoperfusion, or perfusion balloon catheters. The possibility of preserving coronary flow during balloon inflations by use of a double-lumen catheter was first explored by Gruentzig and coworkers in 1977 (21). Since then, catheter-based antegrade perfusion techniques have achieved widespread use in patients undergoing PTCA. Based on both experimental (22–24) and clinical (25,26) efficacy in maintaining antegrade perfusion and reducing myocardial ischemia, these antegrade perfusion modalities have gained popularity due to their simplicity and ease of use (27).

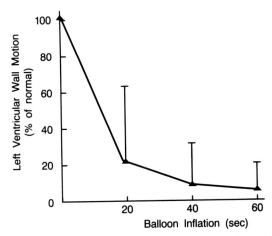

FIG. 1. Effect of balloon occlusion on regional left ventricular function. From Wohlgelernter et al. (29), with permission.

Physiology

In most patients, balloon occlusion time is limited by chest pain, electrical instability, or hemodynamic compromise (fall in systolic blood pressure or a rise in the pulmonary diastolic or wedge pressure). The myocardial oxygen consumption of the area distal to the balloon inflation depends on the size and viability of the territory, presence of collaterals, and pre-PTCA stenosis. Within 20 sec of balloon inflation, there is evidence of ischemic regional left ventricular dysfunction (Fig. 1). Regional akinesis and dyskinesis is present 60 sec after inflation (28). With balloon deflation there is prompt recovery of function within 60 sec, following periods of occlusion of less than 2 min (29). In the passive perfusion systems, the aortic pressure serves as the driving force, and a lumen with side holes before and after the balloon serves as a conduit for distal hemoperfusion (Fig. 2). Perfusion is dependent on catheter characteristics (length, lumen diameter, guidewire presence) and blood viscosity. The influence of these characteristics on flow rate is shown in Table 2. With any given catheter, flow is improved with guidewire removal, by limiting inflation pressure to prevent impingement of the central lumen, and by correcting hypotension (flow is linearly related to pressure). If residual ischemia is present, either from side-branch occlusion or inadequate flow rate to the distal myocardial bed, autoperfusion will not be adequate and inflation time must be limited.

Passive Hemoperfusion

Technique

The catheters are delivered as an over-the-wire or monorail system in the routine fashion. The balloon is inflated and the wire is withdrawn to a position proximal to the most proximal radiopaque marker (which marks

TABLE 1. Multivariate analysis of predictors of hemodynamic compromise

Angiographic characteristic	Unit	Odds ratio	p value
Myocardium at risk	10%	1.7	0.03
Multivessel disease	no, yes	4.3	0.03
Diffuse disease	no, yes	4.1	0.05
Pre-PTCA stenosis	10%	0.6	0.05

From Bergelson et al. (19), with permission.

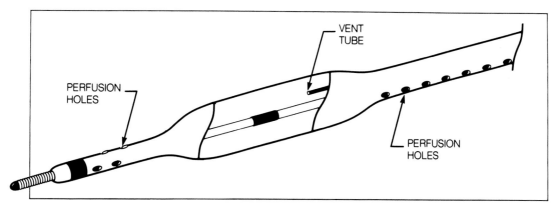

FIG. 2. Perfusion balloon catheter.

the most proximal side holes). The wire lumen should be gently flushed with heparinized saline every few minutes to prevent central lumen thrombus. Perfusion lumen patency and side-branch occlusion can be assessed with contrast media injection (Fig. 3). Proximal injection, however, is not a reliable indicator of distal flow, since hand injections can generate a higher pressure than normal aortic diastolic pressure.

After balloon deflation, the wire is carefully placed distally, with care to avoid the wire tip from exiting either proximal or distal side holes. If the wire becomes entrapped and cannot be withdrawn, gently advancing the balloon catheter may free the tip and allow wire placement distally. The catheter is then withdrawn over the wire, into the guide, in standard fashion.

Indication

The use of these catheters has increased as a larger proportion of patients undergoing PTCA are considered high risk, and because of an overall trend toward longer balloon inflations. The autoperfusion catheters have been advocated as first-line catheters for routine use because of the theoretical benefits of both prolonged and slow balloon inflation. These benefits include improved plaque remolding and dessication, reduction in elastic recoil, and compression of nutrient flow to the vasa vasorum thereby decreasing intimal hyperplasia. Improved patient comfort with less chest pain is a practical and real

benefit of the catheters. In addition, these catheters may be used as bail-out catheters when abrupt closure and/or coronary dissection complicate PTCA. The catheters usually permit prolonged balloon inflations which serve to tack up intimal flaps and dissections. In patients with persistent coronary occlusion, these catheters serve as an effective bridge to surgery when left inflated, since they reduce myocardial ischemia in preparation for emergency surgical revascularization. Factors which increase the necessity of maintaining antegrade flow during balloon inflation or abrupt vessel closure are listed in Table 3.

The disadvantages associated with routine use of the perfusion balloon catheters are related to the large shaft and balloon-crossing profiles which limit the ability to cross tortuous, small, diffusely diseased vessels, or to reach distal lesions. The relatively large profile results in suboptimal cineangiography and may result in more traumatic dilatation because of the Dotter effect. The stiff tip at the site of the distal side holes may traumatize sites distal to the lesion, and flow may be compromised in the presence of tandem lesions or side branches (Fig. 4).

Efficacy

During routine use there is no evidence that prolonged balloon inflation with antegrade perfusion balloons improves initial success or reduces late restenosis (30). In

TABLE 2. *Flow rates in auto-perfusion catheters (cc/min)[a]*

	Catheter type						
	Stack 40 S wire (in)				Stack perfusion wire (in)		
Balloon length	0	0.010	0.014	0.018	0	0.010	0.014	0.018
20	40	25	20	15	60	45	40	30
25					55	40	35	26
30					55	41	31	25
40					44.5	29.5	25.3	17

[a] Bench test data in steady flow model at 80 mmHg (Advanced Cardiovascular Systems, Santa Clara, CA).

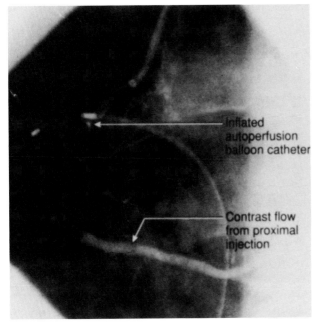

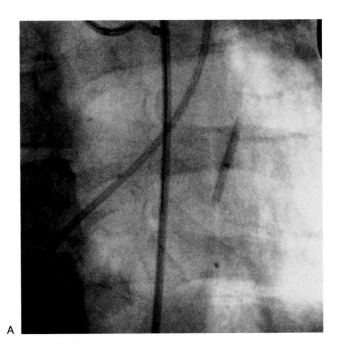

A

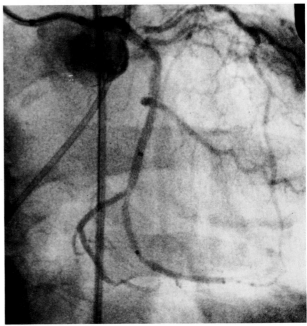

B

FIG. 3. Perfusion balloon catheter placed in the proximal right coronary artery (shown in the left anterior oblique projection) in a patient with a large dissection after PTCA. Proximal contrast injection demonstrates perfusion through the catheter into the distal artery. From Lincoff et al. (6), with permission.

FIG. 4. A: Inflation of a perfusion balloon catheter in the left circumflex artery (shown in the right anterior oblique projection with caudal angulation). **B:** Follow-up angiography reveals an obtuse marginal branch which was occluded during balloon inflation.

patients intolerant of balloon inflation because of angina or hemodynamic instability, these catheters provide improved safety and comfort. Clinical studies have documented that the perfusion balloon catheter can be tolerated for approximately 15 to 30 min with little electrocardiographic change, angina, or elevation in enzyme levels (31).

In patients in whom abrupt closure occurs during PTCA, there are several, nonrandomized reports of improved outcome using the perfusion balloon catheter. Sundram et al. reported that 31 patients with abrupt closure in whom 61% had a bail-out catheter successfully placed showed significant reduction in myocardial infarction, when compared with controls (9% vs. 75%) (32). Smith et al. reported on 28 patients at Duke University with abrupt closure; 57% of these patients had successful PTCA with the perfusion balloon catheter, and

the remainder in whom the perfusion balloon catheter could not be placed had emergency coronary artery bypass graft (CABG) surgery (33). Leitschuh et al. have reported similar results in 26 consecutive patients in whom abrupt closure occurred before the perfusion balloon catheter was available (34). The need for emergency CABG was 23%, compared to 5% in the consecutive series of patients with abrupt closure after the perfusion

TABLE 3. Angiographic predictors of the likelihood antegrade flow will be needed

Unlikely need
 Total, chronic occlusions
 Subtotal occlusion with collateral
 Myocardium served is old, completed or advanced infarct
Possible need
 Critical lesion associated with rest angina
Probable need
 Moderately severe lesion without collateral and serving
  viable myocardium

balloon catheter was in routine use. The added benefit of reducing myocardial ischemia in preparation for emergency surgical revascularization has been shown (35–37).

Active Hemoperfusion

Since the perfusion balloon catheter is limited by intrinsic perfusion pressure, methods to actively pump blood or perfusate to the distal myocardium have been developed. These pumping methods involve hand injection (38) and piston pump systems (39,40). The injectate may be either renal vein blood, or arterial blood obtained from the side arm of an oversized arterial sheath.

Physiology

In comparison with perfusion balloon catheters, active systems use catheters which have smaller and more flexible shafts and balloons, and have the ability to adapt distal flow as needed in the individual patient. Flow rates of up to 80 ml/min can be achieved (40).

Technique

The most promising of these devices is the piston pump system developed by Leocor Inc. (Corflo). This system consists of a thin-walled coaxial double lumen catheter with a crossing profile (0.032-in to 0.035-in), similar to that of most balloon catheters. The device is placed over a wire and renal vein blood is pumped through the wire lumen at pressures of up to 220 psi and at flows of up to 80 ml/min (or 25–30 ml/min with the guidewire in place). The physiologic anteroperfusion system is another device which delivers diastolic electrocardiographic-synchronized (flow-pressure controlled) autologous blood through a standard PTCA catheter (39).

Indication

The indications for these devices are the same as for the perfusion balloon catheter, but the active systems can be effective when the perfusion balloon catheter fails, or when it is likely to fail in the setting of hypotension, increased blood viscosity, or small and tortuous vessels.

Efficacy

DiSciascio et al. tested the efficacy of the Corflo system in 110 patients selected because of their inability to tolerate 3 min of balloon inflation (40). In this patient group, inflation time increased from 1.3 to 7.1 min, and ST-segment and chest pain score were decreased. Persistent ischemia occurred in only 2 patients in whom side branches arose near the treated lesion. There was insignificant systemic hemolysis and 2 patients undergoing right coronary artery PTCA had atrioventricular block, which resolved when hemoperfusion was discontinued (40). Promising preliminary results using the physiologic anteroperfusion system have been reported by Farcot et al. in 40 patients (39).

Oxygenated Perflurocarbons (Fluosol)

Physiology

Fluosol (Alpha Therapeutic, Los Angeles, CA) is a stable mixture of two perflurochemicals emulsified in water. When oxygenated and injected through the lumen of a PTCA catheter, fluosol provides an extensive capacity for dissolving oxygen, and transporting and delivering it to the myocardium. The potential advantages of fluosol over blood include its low viscosity, the absence of hemolysis at high flow rates, and the absence of thrombosis in small lumen catheters at low flow rates. Animal studies indicate that fluosol may limit reperfusion injury by suppression of neutrophils (41).

Technique

The commercially available product is provided as three solutions which must be thawed, mixed, oxygenated, and used within 8 hr.

Indication

Fluosol has been commercially approved as a distal coronary perfusate during angioplasty. The 30 to 60 min required to prepare this compound and oxygenate it may limit its clinical usefulness, but a new, more rapid preparation method has recently been introduced.

Efficacy

Several studies have demonstrated limitation of ischemic sequelae during PTCA with distal fluosol infusion. In comparison with control balloon inflations, fluosol perfusion reduces regional systolic wall motion abnormalities (Fig. 5), diastolic dysfunction, and ST-segment elevation (20,42,43). In animal studies, blood is a superior distal perfusate (44). A comparison between fluosol and hemoperfusion has not been made in a clinical trial.

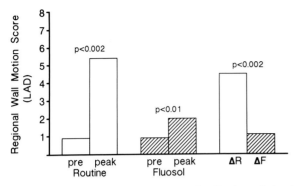

FIG. 5. Regional wall motion in the distribution of the left anterior descending artery prior to and at peak coronary balloon inflation, with and without distal Fluosol perfusion. LAD, left anterior descending artery; R, Routine; F, Fluosol. From Cowley et al. (42), with permission.

Retrograde Perfusion

Coronary Sinus Techniques

Technologic interventions to treat patients with coronary artery disease have evolved rapidly over the last decade and have been primarily focused on improving antegrade delivery of oxygen and nutrients to the myocardium. Meanwhile, techniques for delivery of blood in a retrograde manner via the undiseased cardiac venous system have evolved in parallel. There are several advantages to utilizing the coronary sinus:

1. The venous system is rarely diseased.
2. Skilled operators can cannulate the coronary sinus quickly and in over 85% of patients.
3. The procedure is performed in veins rather than arteries so that consequences of bleeding or serious arterial injury are reduced.
4. Coronary sinus pressure monitoring provides a continuous recording of left ventricular end diastolic pressure (45).
5. There is the potential to access ischemic microvasculature in a retrograde fashion when antegrade access is lost.

Based upon theoretical benefits, data from animal models, and preliminary clinical trials supporting the utility of coronary sinus retroperfusion for temporary support of acutely ischemic myocardium, the technique is under review by the Food and Drug Administration.

Coronary Sinus Anatomy and Physiology

Most cardiac venous blood drains into the right atrium via the coronary sinus, which is located inferior

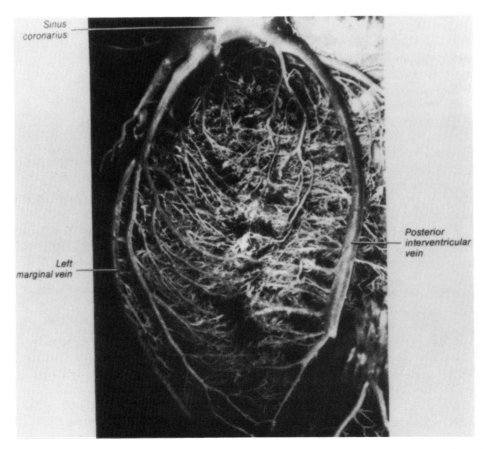

FIG. 6. Technovit cast demonstrating the intricate microvasculature and the dense anastomotic network of the cardiac veins. From Tschabitscher et al. (46), with permission.

to the fossa ovalis and posterior to the tricuspid valve. The posterior interventricular vein and small cardiac vein, which drain the inferior wall and right ventricle, respectively, enter near the coronary sinus ostium. The coronary sinus varies from 4 to 14 mm in diameter, but averages approximately 9 to 10 mm. The coronary sinus continues along the posterior atrio-ventricular groove for 2 to 3 cm and on the posterolateral margin bifurcates into the great cardiac vein and the left marginal vein. The great cardiac vein continues in the AV groove, initially with few branches, and is called the silent area. This silent area is an optimal position for coronary sinus catheter stability. The great cardiac vein continues to the anterior septum where it becomes the anterior interventricular vein.

The heart is served by a microcirculation with extensive veno- and arteriovenous anastomoses (Fig. 6), which allow retrograde delivery of oxygenated blood or pharmaceutical agents to reach the myocardium (46). These anastamoses may also permit more effective washout of toxic metabolites after release of coronary sinus occlusion. However, up to 30% of the venous return bypasses the coronary sinus and drains directly into the atria or ventricles via Thebesian veins (47). In fact, coronary blood flow decreases only 35% with total occlusion of the coronary sinus (48), therefore, these channels may be recruited to allow drainage of blood if coronary sinus pressure is elevated. This extensive Thebesian network, however, may prevent retrograde perfusion of ischemic myocardium by shunting retrograde flow from the capillary bed to direct drainage in the atrium and ventricle.

Normal coronary sinus pressure is similar to right atrial pressure, with discrete a, c, and v waves. With occlusion of the coronary sinus, the pressure waveform becomes more complex. Within 2 to 5 cycles, there is a rise in systolic pressure that reaches a plateau. This plateau of systolic pressure usually is 40 to 50 mmHg, and bears no consistent relationship to peak left ventricular systolic pressure. The plateau phase appears to represent complete filling of the venous capacitance circulation. In man, the diastolic waveform during coronary sinus occlusion resembles that of the left ventricle over a wide range of pressures, and at end-diastole is identical to left ventricular end-diastolic pressure (45).

Retrograde Perfusion Modalities

Retroinfusion

Retroinfusion of pharmacologic agents is the easiest and most widely used technique. Implementation requires only coronary sinus catheterization and a pump to deliver agents to the myocardium. The pumping is continuous and not synchronized to the cardiac cycle; it is often combined with coronary sinus occlusion to prevent reflux into the right atrium. With complete occlusion of venous outflow, high coronary sinus pressures

have been reported with subsequent myocardial edema and hemorrhage.

Animal and human experimental data suggest that retrograde delivery via the coronary sinus of streptokinase (49), diltiazem (50), lidocaine (51), procainamide (52), metoprolol (53), and recombinant tissue–type plasminogen activator (54) is as effective or more effective than intravenous administration. The greatest advantage of retroinfusion is its potential to achieve high myocardial tissue levels of drugs without accompanying high systemic levels, thereby reducing the risks of extracardiac side effects. The major clinical use of retroinfusion has been retrograde delivery of cardioplegia during cardiac surgery (55).

Pressure-controlled intermittent coronary sinus occlusion

Intermittent coronary sinus occlusion is based on the unique anatomic features of the myocardial venous system, particularly its extensive venovenous anastamoses. By filling the venous capacitance system, coronary sinus occlusion has the potential to redistribute nutrients from nonischemic to ischemic areas. Similarly, with deflation of the coronary sinus balloon, toxic metabolites are removed from areas of ischemic injury by a washout phenomenon (56).

Pressure monitoring during pressure-controlled intermittent coronary sinus occlusion is important for both efficacy and safety. It is necessary to elevate coronary sinus pressure sufficiently to fill the venous system and ensure retrograde delivery to the jeopardized myocardium. After the coronary sinus pressure reaches a plateau, deflation of the balloon allows a return to baseline. This facilitates washout and prevents development of the myocardial edema and hemorrhage seen with higher pressures, and in nonintermittent occlusion such as with retroinfusion.

The experimental data supporting the efficacy of pressure-controlled coronary sinus occlusion in reducing infarct size are extensive (57,58). However, their utility has not been established during brief ischemia (59). Pressure-controlled intermittent coronary sinus occlusion has been used during coronary surgery and has resulted in better preservation of myocardial function during reperfusion (60).

Synchronized retroperfusion

During synchronized retroperfusion arterial blood is pumped during diastole, and normal venous drainage occurs during systole. In this way, the myocardial edema and hemorrhage seen with earlier studies of retroinfusion and coronary sinus occlusion can be avoided. Balloon inflation occurs during each diastole, and arterial blood is pumped toward the jeopardized myocardium without reflux into the right atrium. Efficacy in reducing myocardial ischemia is based upon direct delivery of oxygenated blood to the myocardium, but enhanced myocardial washout may also occur (61).

A comparison of the retrograde perfusion techniques is shown in Table 4.

Synchronized Coronary Sinus Retroperfusion

Technique. Coronary sinus catheterization. Coronary sinus catheterization requires fluoroscopic guidance and pressure monitoring. The coronary sinus ostium is on the right side of the atrial septum, cephalad and posterior to the tricuspid valve. Cannulation is most successful from the right internal jugular vein. Once the catheter tip is positioned along the lateral wall of the mid right atrium, it is rotated counterclockwise (tip turned anteriorly) and advanced into the right ventricle. It is

then slowly withdrawn and rotated so the tip is posterior and above the tricuspid valve at the entrance of the coronary sinus. Gentle advancement will engage the coronary sinus ostium (or return the catheter into the right ventricle requiring additional counter-clockwise rotation during the next attempt). Once in the coronary sinus (right atrial pressure waveform maintained), the catheter is advanced along the AV groove into the great cardiac vein. Contrast media can be used to visualize the anatomy and variable tributaries. The great cardiac vein is demarcated by a small indentation produced by the venous valve of Vieussens. If the catheter does not move easily into the great cardiac vein, a standard soft tip guidewire through the endhole of the catheter may permit entry and facilitate advancement of the catheter. Cannulation of the great cardiac vein is successful in about 85% of attempts, within 5 min. It would be advantageous (especially during PTCA) if coronary sinus cannulation could be reliably achieved via the femoral vein.

TABLE 4. *Retrograde perfusion modalities*

Modality	Method	Advantages	Disadvantages
All		1. CS catheterization is simple to accomplish. 2. Avoids coronary artery manipulation and potential trauma. 3. No evidence of important vascular damage in published clinical reports.	1. Potential risk of damage to venous system. 2. During PTCA, additional time and equipment needed for CS catheterization.
Synchronized retroperfusion	Blood from femoral artery pumped into CS catheter synchronized to diastole and CS balloon occlusion	1. Normal venous drainage. 2. Delivery of pharmacologic agents to ischemic myocardium.	1. Arterial access required. 2. Potential for hemolysis with gated pumping. 3. Not effective in acute ischemia.
Retroinfusion	Transvenous cannulation of CS and delivery of pharmacologic agents using catheter with distal occlusive balloon	1. No arterial access. 2. Uniform delivery of cardioplegia (useful in severe CAD, left main disease and aortic valve disease).	1. Possible inadequate RV protection. 2. Myocardial edema and hemorrhage when CS occluded. 3. During cardiac surgery, longer time to diastolic arrest and RA incision required.
Pressure-controlled intermittent coronary sinus occlusion	Intermittent occlusion of CS without synchronization; occlusion maintained until CS pressure reaches a plateaus and then obstruction is released	1. No arterial access. 2. Simple system. 3. Facilitates washout of ischemic myocardium. 4. Continuous monitoring of LVEDP.	1. Not effective in acute ischemia.

CAD, coronary artery disease; CS, coronary sinus; LVEDP, left ventricular end-diastolic pressure; PTCA, percutaneous transluminal coronary angioplasty; RA, right atrium.

Retroperfusion system. The retroperfusion system consists of four basic components (Fig. 7): (i) a synchronized pneumatic pump for blood, triggered on the R wave of the electrocardiogram; (ii) an electropneumatic balloon inflation mechanism; (iii) the arterial cannula; and (iv) the coronary sinus catheter (62). The arterial cannula (placed in the femoral artery) connects to the pumping console; flow rate is selected and arterial blood is delivered to the distal port of the coronary sinus catheter while the balloon occludes the coronary sinus.

The pumping console has three basic functions: (i) maintenance of selected volumetric flow rates with a single pump stroke during diastole; (ii) electropneumatic balloon inflation with a fixed volume of gas in synchronization with each pump stroke; and (iii) pressure monitoring from the distal coronary sinus catheter. Flow rate is determined while coronary sinus pressure is closely monitored. Arterial flow is initiated at 50 ml/min and increased to 250 ml/min unless coronary sinus systolic pressure exceeds 60 mmHg. Balloon inflation and deflation can occur every cardiac cycle (synchronized retroperfusion) or the balloon can be left inflated for several cycles until a desired infusion pressure is reached before deflating (synchronized retroperfusion with pressure-controlled intermittent coronary sinus occlusion).

The retroperfusion catheter is a triple-lumen, 8.5 French (F) radiopaque catheter with a soft tip (Fig. 8). The balloon is located 10 mm from the distal end and, at full inflation, the balloon is oval-shaped with a 10 mm

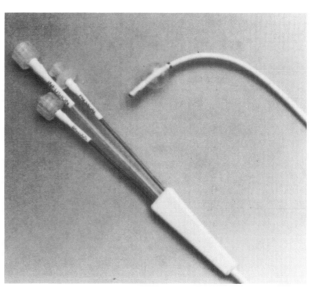

FIG. 8. Triple lumen, 8.5 French balloon-tipped retroperfusion catheter. From Kar et al. (62), with permission.

diameter. A radiopaque band proximal to the balloon aids fluoroscopic catheter placement.

The arterial catheter is a single lumen 7F or 8F catheter, equipped with a distal end and side holes to prevent intimal damage and to provide adequate arterial supply.

Indications. Preliminary clinical data support the use of synchronized retroperfusion on a prophylactic or standby basis in patients undergoing left anterior descending coronary artery angioplasty who are deemed to be at high risk for complications. In these patients, hemodynamic compromise is often seen and may be prevented or reversed with retroperfusion techniques. Based on experimental data, synchronized retroperfusion has potential use in the treatment of acute myocardial infarction in patients in whom thrombolytic therapy is contraindicated. In addition, retroperfusion may play a role in the treatment of refractory unstable angina. In each setting, it should be emphasized that retrograde perfusion would provide temporary support of ischemic myocardium while definitive revascularization is being established.

Contraindications. There are no a priori absolute contraindications to coronary sinus catheterization. In patients in whom right internal jugular venous access cannot be established, access from the subclavian or brachial vein can be attempted.

Efficacy. There are many published reports of the benefit of synchronized retroperfusion in salvaging ischemic myocardium during experimental myocardial infarction. In a canine model, synchronized retroperfusion that started 30 min after left anterior descending coronary artery occlusion reduced infarct size at 6 hr from 56% to 19% of myocardium at risk (63). Similarly, left ventricular ejection fraction during occlusion was pre-

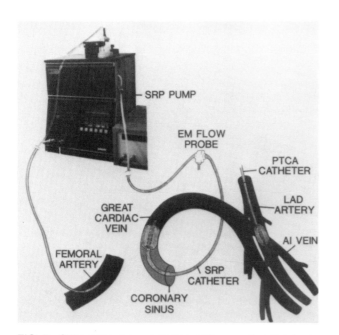

FIG. 7. Schematic representation of the synchronized retroperfusion system. SRP, synchronized retroperfusion; EM, electromagnetic; PTCA, percutaneous transluminal coronary angioplasty; LAD, left anterior descending artery; AI, anterior interventricular. From Kar et al. (62), with permission.

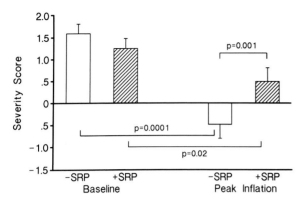

FIG. 9. Regional left ventricular function (based on echocardiographic severity score) during left anterior descending artery balloon inflation, with and without synchronized retroperfusion. SRP, synchronized retroperfusion.

served (64). Retrograde delivery of flow tracers and enhanced glucose metabolism in the risk region have been documented by positron emission tomography during synchronized retroperfusion (65).

The clinical use of synchronized retroperfusion was first reported in 1986 in five patients with refractory unstable angina. During synchronized retroperfusion, the frequency of anginal episodes was decreased, and no adverse effects were noted over the 12- to 50-hr duration of the study (66,67). Berland et al. reported a series of 14 patients undergoing left anterior descending PTCA and found significant reductions in angina and electro-cardiographic changes during synchronized retroperfusion (68). Echocardiography showed less severe reduction in left ventricular function when synchronized retroperfusion was used with balloon inflations. However, Beatt et al. were unable to demonstrate efficacy using similar criteria in three patients, but concern about the adequacy of the retroperfusion flow rates achieved was raised (69).

The preliminary results of a multicenter trial of synchronized retroperfusion have been reported (70). In 102 patients undergoing 485 coronary balloon inflations, angina occurred in 47% of the inflations with synchronized retroperfusion treated and 59% of the control inflations. In comparison with untreated coronary balloon inflations, there was less ST elevation (2.2 mm vs. 2.8 mm) and less decrease in left ventricular ejection fraction during coronary occlusion (Fig. 9). There were no significant complications, except at arterial and venous access sites; in 4 patients coronary sinus staining occurred without clinical consequences. A single center experience has also been reported (71).

Complications. Myocardial edema and hemorrhage may occur if there is an obstruction to coronary sinus drainage, excessive retrograde flow rates, or increased coronary venous pressure. Direct trauma to the coronary sinus from the catheter has also been reported without serious adverse sequelae. Damage to the formed ele-

ments of the blood has not been observed. In reported clinical studies of synchronized retroperfusion, there has not been a report of venous damage from the catheter, myocardial edema or hemorrhage, or hemolysis. As with any interventional technique, hematoma formation and vascular injury at catheter insertion sites is a potential, but manageable risk. Atrial fibrillation during catheter insertion has also been reported.

Conclusion. Retrograde perfusion techniques are promising therapies for treatment of prolonged ischemia or infarction. The clinical settings in which these techniques have the most potential are during PTCA complicated by abrupt vessel closure and during acute myocardial infarction in patients in whom thrombolytic therapy is contraindicated.

SYSTEMIC HEMODYNAMIC SUPPORT TECHNIQUES

Intraaortic Balloon Pump

After the perfusion balloon catheter, the most widely used support modality is intraaortic balloon counterpulsation (IABP). Its main attraction is its ease of implementation and reliable ability to relieve myocardial ischemia through a combination of increased coronary perfusion pressure and reduced myocardial oxygen demand through afterload reduction (Fig. 10) (72). The intraaortic balloon pump does not provide regional myocardial protection during PTCA balloon inflation or after abrupt closure, although theoretically it may be of some benefit due to improved collateral flow from increased coronary perfusion pressure (Fig. 11) (73). The intraaortic balloon pump can be used either prophylactically, in high-risk patients, or in a standby mode. To improve implementation times, patients at high risk

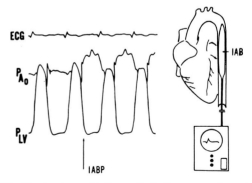

FIG. 10. Mechanism of intraaortic balloon counterpulsation. The intraaortic balloon is positioned in the thoracic aorta and inflated in diastole by monitoring to the electrocardiogram or arterial pressure waveform. Aortic pressure is augmented during diastole. Left ventricular systolic pressure decreases during pumping. ECG, electrocardiogram; P_{Ao}, aortic pressure; P_{LV}, left ventricular pressure; IAB, intraaortic balloon. From Weber et al. (72), with permission.

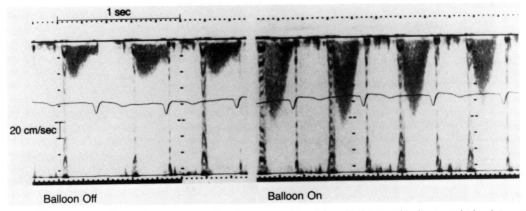

FIG. 11. Transesophageal measurements of coronary blood flow in the proximal artery during intraaortic balloon pumping; note the blood flow augmentation. From Kern (73), with permission.

may undergo femoral artery cannulation in the contralateral groin prior to PTCA with a small caliber sheath (5F). While deployed, the intraaortic balloon pump is deflated when PTCA catheters are introduced or withdrawn through the descending thoracic aorta; otherwise, the balloon actively pumps during the PTCA procedure.

Efficacy

Several small series without concurrent control groups have reported beneficial effects of the intraaortic balloon pump during high-risk PTCA. Kahn et al. studied 28 high-risk patients who had prophylactic placement of an intraaortic balloon (74). In these patients (mean left ventricular ejection fraction of 28%; 93% with three-vessel disease, 39% with a single patent vessel or left main disease), the intraaortic balloon resulted in hemodynamic stability, a 95% procedural success, and no myocardial infarction or death up to 72 hr after PTCA. Three patients (11%) required surgery for repair of vascular complications. Alcan et al. reported 14 patients who had an intraaortic balloon pump during PTCA (75). In 9 patients the intraaortic balloon was placed before PTCA (in 2 for shock; in 7 for unstable angina); all of them had a successful PTCA; one patient died in the hospital and 1 required coronary artery bypass surgery. In 5 patients, in the series by Alcan et al., the intra-aortic balloon was placed after PTCA (in 3 for late abrupt closure; in 2 after unsuccessful PTCA) as a bridge to emergency surgery. All patients survived. Voudris et al. reported on 27 patients who had a prophylactic intraaortic balloon placed for a left ventricular ejection fraction of less than 40%, or for multivessel PTCA (76). All patients had successful PTCA without myocardial infarction, surgery, or death. Anwar et al. reported the two-center experience of elective intraaortic balloon insertion in 97 patients undergoing PTCA who had a left ventricular ejection fraction of less than 35% (77). The PTCA success rate was 86%, and 7% of patients suffered a major cardiac event. Kreidish et al. reported 21 patients who had an intraaortic balloon inserted electively prior to PTCA (78% with a left ventricular ejection fraction <30%); the procedural success rate was 90% (78). The only complication related to the intraaortic balloon was a local hematoma in 2 patients.

Based on these series, the intraaortic balloon pump is a safe and effective modality to stabilize high-risk patients undergoing PTCA. Early procedural success rates are encouraging and complication rates related to intraaortic balloon use are low. Since none of the studies were randomized, it is unclear which patients actually required support, since the definitions of high risk varied, and the single parameter risk stratification used is limited. In the series which report long-term outcomes (76,77), the prognosis is less favorable, with high rates of cardiac and noncardiac deaths which are likely related to the underlying poor prognosis in these patients.

Future directions in counterpulsation now under investigation include percutaneous placement of an intraascending aortic balloon for improved circulatory support (78) and pulmonary artery balloon counterpulsation for the management of right heart failure (79). Neither of these newer devices have been evaluated for support during high-risk PTCA.

Percutaneous Bypass

One recent technological advance which allows PTCA to be performed on unstable and higher risk patients is percutaneous cardiopulmonary bypass support. This procedure, performed prophylactically in some centers, has allowed the angiographer to proceed on certain patients who formerly were not candidates for PTCA. Early feasibility studies concluded that cardiopulmonary bypass could support high-risk PTCA with a high likelihood of initial success, and with an acceptable, though not insignificant, incidence of morbidity (80,81). A detailed treatise on the operation and function of cardiopulmonary bypass support is available (82).

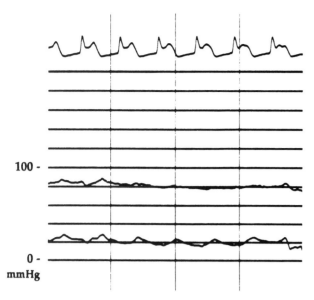

FIG. 12. Absence of pulsatile aortic pressure during successful PTCA of the right coronary artery in a patient on cardiopulmonary bypass support. Note the persistence of ST-segment elevation which denotes ongoing regional myocardial ischemia. From Mooney et al. (83), with permission.

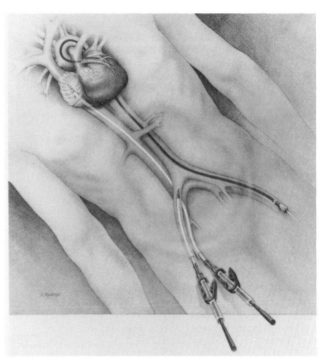

FIG. 13. Appropriate position of the arterial and venous cannulae during cardiopulmonary bypass support. Note the placement of the tip of the venous cannula just above the junction of the inferior vena cava and the right atrium. From Shawl (82), with permission.

Physiology

The cardiopulmonary bypass support system aspirates blood from the right atrium–inferior vena cava junction and returns oxygenated blood, under pressure, to the femoral artery. In this way, preload is reduced and total circulatory support is provided, regardless of the intrinsic cardiac rhythm or output. Despite the systemic perfusion support, there is no perfusion of the jeopardized myocardium during balloon inflation or coronary occlusion (Fig. 12) (83). Segmental wall motion abnormalities have been demonstrated during balloon inflation with cardiopulmonary bypass support, although fewer patients experience chest pain or ST-segment changes (84,85). The primary benefit of this modality is derived from a reduction in preload and cardiac work.

Technique

After aortoiliac angiography to exclude significant tortuosity or atherosclerosis, thin-walled, large-bore (20F) catheters are placed, after serial, progressive local site dilation (Fig. 13). The patient is fully anticoagulated with 300 U/kg of intravenous heparin. Venous blood is aspirated from the right atrium via a centrifugal, nonocclusive pump (Fig. 14); passed in series through a membrane oxygenator and a heat exchanger; and then returned to the ipsilateral femoral artery. As bypass is initiated, intravenous fluid administration is frequently

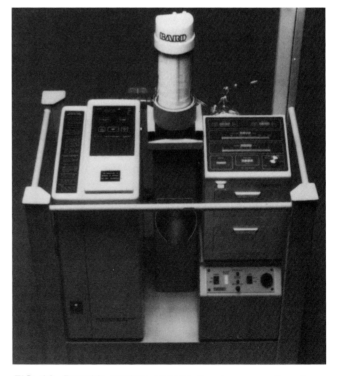

FIG. 14. Portable cardiopulmonary bypass support system. From Shawl (82), with permission.

required to compensate for the fall in preload pressure; subsequently intravenous fluid is used to compensate for the fall in systemic pressure. Percutaneous transluminal coronary angioplasty is then performed from the contralateral femoral site. After bypass is discontinued, the cannulas are removed percutaneously (or under direct surgical repair) and hemostasis is achieved with an external groin clamp for several hours.

Indication

The cardiopulmonary bypass support system has been advocated for prophylactic or standby support in patients who are at high risk because of severe left ventricular dysfunction, when the target vessel for PTCA is the only patent coronary artery, or in unprotected left main PTCA. The most frequent morbid event associated with cardiopulmonary bypass support is vascular trauma at entry sites; it occurs in 39% of patients (86). Some authors have reported equal efficacy with less morbidity using a protocol of standby-supported PTCA instead of prophylactic cardiopulmonary bypass, in patients classified as high risk (87). Tommaso et al. retrospectively compared the outcomes of 27 patients considered high risk for PTCA (88). These patients had (i) stenosis of 75% or more and left ventricular ejection fraction less than 25%, or (ii) more than 50% of the viable myocardium in jeopardy, and were treated with either supported, prophylactic cardiopulmonary bypass or standby-ready support (88). Using this definition of high risk, there was no difference in morbidity and mortality between groups. The authors concluded that these definitions of high-risk PTCA were too liberal and suggested that PTCA supported by cardiopulmonary bypass be reserved for patients who (i) have periprocedure hemodynamic instability or who have sustained prior hemodynamic collapse during an invasive procedure, (ii) are undergoing PTCA of the only patent vessel, (iii) have unprotected left main PTCA, or (iv) have a left ventricular ejection fraction of 15% or less. This is the only published report which tests the adequacy of prophylactic standby support, and conclusions based on it are limited due to a small patient population and a retrospective and nonrandomized comparison. The preliminary report of the Cardiopulmonary Support Registry, however, substantiates the efficacy of standby support in a report of 455 patients. Overall mortalities in these groups were the same (6%) despite similar risk characteristics (87).

Shawl et al. have reported successful initiation of the cardiopulmonary bypass support system in patients with cardiogenic shock (89), and in patients who sustained cardiac arrest while in the catheterization laboratory (90). Of these, cardiopulmonary bypass support was initiated in a mean of 21 min, with an 75% survival in those patients in whom revascularization was attempted (n = 5).

Efficacy

In the initial report of the Cardiopulmonary Bypass Support National Registry, 95% of attempted vessels were successfully dilated and there was an overall in-hospital mortality rate of 6%. The rates of vascular trauma were high (39%), and 43% of patients required transfusions due to blood loss (84). In the most recent preliminary report from this registry, the mortality rate remains constant (86). In these series it has been concluded that patients undergoing PTCA of an unprotected left main do not benefit from cardiopulmonary bypass support. In this subset, this technique makes PTCA technically feasible, but does not reduce the catastrophic risk of out-of-lab abrupt closure.

Hemopump

The Nimbus Hemopump (Fig. 15) is a new innovation in circulatory assist devices for critically ill patients. This device is a temporary left ventricular assist device which uses an axial flow pump to draw blood out of the left ventricle and expel it into the aorta. The pump is an Archimedes screw pump which rotates at 25,000 rpm to provide a flow rate of up to 3.5 l/min.

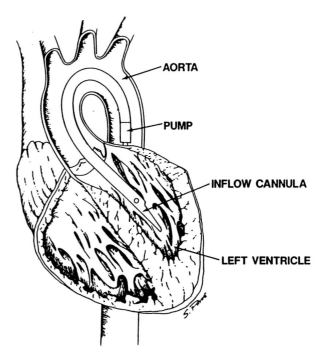

FIG. 15. Schematic representation of the position of the Hemopump across the aortic valve. From Wampler et al. (92), with permission.

Physiology

The Hemopump catheter is placed into the ventricle and results in significant left ventricular decompression by unloading the left ventricular cavity and discharging blood into the descending aorta in a nonpulsatile manner. In this way, up 3.5 l/min of nonpulsatile perfusion to the systemic circulation is provided. Compared to intraaortic balloon counterpulsation, there is significantly better reduction in the myocardial oxygen consumption (50% vs. 17%) and better systemic support compared to the modest 15% improvement in cardiac output seen with intraaortic balloon pumping. The maximal flow rates provided with this device are lower than those obtained with cardiopulmonary bypass support. Efficacy of the Hemopump is based on adequate left ventricular filling.

Technique

The device requires a surgical cutdown and placement of a 12-mm vascular graft (sidewinder) for insertion in the femoral artery. The 21F cannula is passed retrograde up the aorta and into the left ventricle through the aortic valve. Once inserted, the monitoring console is easily managed by catheterization laboratory personnel; it does not require supervision of specialized perfusion teams.

Indication

This device is investigational, but, compared with cardiopulmonary bypass support, several potential advantages exist for its use in supported PTCA. These advantages include minimal anticoagulation requirements, no additional requirement for in-lab personnel, safe use for support for up to 7 days, and direct left ventricular decompression. Trials in small numbers of patients in cardiogenic shock (91–93) and supported PTCA (84,85) have been reported. Peripheral vascular disease and aortic valve disease are contraindications to its use.

Efficacy

Loisance et al. reported the use of the Hemopump in supported PTCA in eight patients (94). The Hemopump was successfully placed in five. In the supported patients, there was an improvement in hemodynamic parameters during the procedure, despite arrhythmia and left ventricular dysfunction during balloon inflation. Long-term outcome was excellent (94). Lincoff et al. reported that two patients underwent PTCA during cardiogenic shock. The Hemopump permitted hemodynamic stabil-

ity and successful PTCA, but both patients died while in hospital (95).

Partial Left Heart Bypass

In an effort to provide systemic support with a simpler system, methods to provide oxygenated blood to the systemic circulation under pressure have been devised. Preliminary reports using partial left heart bypass in PTCA have been reported (96,97).

Physiology

The physiology of this modality is similar to the cardiopulmonary bypass support system. Preload, cardiac work, and oxygen consumption are all reduced.

Technique

Using a transseptal approach a 14F to 20F catheter is placed in the left atrium. Oxygenated blood is pumped to a femoral artery cannula which provides support similar to the cardiopulmonary bypass support system, without the requirement for a membrane oxygenator.

Indication

The device is investigational, but its attraction, in comparison with cardiopulmonary bypass support, is that a membrane oxygenator is not required and that lower doses of heparin may be used.

Efficacy

In preliminary reports in four (96) and five (97) high-risk patients, hemodynamic support has been provided during PTCA. Issues about the overall success of this modality, success in transseptal cannulation, and potential long-term incidence of atrial septal defect have not been addressed.

APPROACH TO THE HIGH-RISK PATIENT

Selection of patients who are at high, but acceptable, risk for PTCA requires careful prelaboratory preparation and a careful strategy anticipating periprocedural hemodynamic collapse (Table 5). Discussion with cardiac surgery consultants concerning the patient's suitability for emergency surgery revascularization should be undertaken. In addition, consideration by the surgeons should

TABLE 5. *Approach to the high risk patient before PTCA*

1. Discussion risks with patient and/or family.
2. Consideration "higher-level" cardiac surgery standby.
3. PTCA limited to most experienced operators.
4. Placement of small-caliber sheaths in contralateral femoral artery.
5. Careful predilation strategy.
6. Adequate hemodynamic monitoring with pacing PA catheter.
7. Anticipation of potential need for out-of-lab support system.

be given to a higher level of readiness, with immediately available portable support modalities.

Once consensus is reached among the clinical cardiologist, the interventionalist, and the cardiac surgeon, the risks of death, morbidity, and the need for emergency surgical revascularization should be discussed with the patient and family. Anticipation of the potential need for long-term and/or out-of-lab dependence on support systems should also be discussed.

Percutaneous transluminal coronary angioplasty for this subset of patients should be limited to the most experienced laboratories and operators. Consideration should be given to referring high-risk patients to specialized centers with expertise in support modalities. In these patients, careful clinical evaluation of the vascular access site should be made prior to PTCA, and should include measurement of the systolic pressure in each limb. When femoral arterial access is achieved, iliac and femoral screening angiography should be considered to assess the vascular adequacy for placement of large cannulas in the contralateral femoral site. In selected patients, placement of small caliber sheaths (5F) is indicated to improve the speed of deployment of these modalities.

The dilatation strategy should be well planned. Assessment of pre-PTCA medications, adequate hydration, lesion-specific equipment selection, and choice of distal wire placement can result in significantly safer salvage PTCA, or safe transfer to the operating room, should abrupt closure occur. Adequate hemodynamic monitoring with placement of a pacing pulmonary artery (PA) catheter permits monitoring of the PA diastolic pressure and controlled pacing for improved heart rate and cardiac output in unstable situations.

CHOOSING SUPPORT MODALITIES

The goal of all the support modalities is to provide oxygenated blood to ischemic myocardium and/or support to the systemic circulation (Table 6). Other than the secondary gains from improvement in left ventricular ejection fraction, the perfusion catheters and retroperfu-

sion do not provide the direct peripheral circulatory support provided by percutaneous bypass systems or the Hemopump, and do not improve the peripheral hemodynamic profile as does the intraaortic balloon pump.

When abrupt closure complicates PTCA, the antegrade perfusion catheter techniques have been effectively used for treatment of flow-limiting coronary dissections and as a bailout therapy to limit ischemia and infarction prior to emergent coronary artery bypass surgery. When antegrade access to the artery is lost, retroperfusion may be effective in limiting myocardial ischemia in the left anterior descending distribution pending surgical revascularization.

During PTCA, in a high-risk patient or a high-risk lesion which serves a large region of myocardium, the contralateral femoral artery may be accessed with a 5F sheath. In this way, rapid insertion of an intraaortic balloon pump can be accomplished. In some patients with proximal lesions and a large territory at risk, the operator may choose to perform the procedure with a perfusion balloon catheter. This option has become more popular with the newer generation, lower profile perfusion catheters, such as the ACS RX perfusion and ACS Stack 40S (Advanced Cardiovascular Systems, Santa Clara, CA) which can be delivered to more tortuous and distal sites.

In failed, standard PTCA, abrupt closure is managed first with the perfusion balloon catheter. However, during PTCA, an intraaortic balloon is placed if significant myocardial ischemia, hypotension, or arrhythmia develop and if these are not resolved with balloon deflation, fluid resuscitation (as guided by the pulmonary artery diastolic pressure), and low-dose sympathomimetic (e.g., dopamine, 5–10 mcg/kg per min) agents. The intraaortic balloon pump will permit longer balloon inflations and prepare the patient for a stable transition to emergency coronary artery bypass grafting. If regional antegrade or retrograde perfusion is maintained, this approach allows placement of optimal conduits (internal mammary artery) during coronary artery bypass surgery.

When a patient is brought to the lab in an unstable condition from severe ongoing ischemia, or from an evolving myocardial infarction and/or cardiogenic shock, an intraaortic balloon pump is placed prior to diagnostic angiography. Percutaneous transluminal coronary angioplasty of the culprit or infarct artery is then undertaken. Portable cardiopulmonary bypass may then be instituted if hemodynamic compromise persists, or if emergency coronary artery bypass grafting is anticipated. In these critically ill patients, a combination of support techniques appear theoretically attractive as a means of providing systemic hemodynamic support and perfusion of the ischemic myocardium, but these combination therapies have not been rigorously tested in clinical trials.

TABLE 6. *Support modalities—comparitive*

Support modality	Percutaneous insertion/removal	Size (F)	Ease of implementation	Success	Complication	
					Rate	Types
Ideal	Yes/yes	8	Yes	100%	Low	Minor
Perfusion catheter (PBC)	Yes/yes	4.5	Yes, simple blood perfusate; no added vascular access	Routine 95% Failed PTCA 57–82%	Low	Central lumen thrombus
Active hemoperfusion	Yes/yes	4.3	Yes simple blood perfusate from renal vein or femoral artery; no added vascular access	Routine 92%; pts intolerant to long PTCA inflation 98%	Low	Hemolysis; complete AV block
Fluosol	NA	NA	30–60-min preparation; no added vascular access	Modest	1–2%	Ventricular arrhythmia
Synchronized retroperfusion (SRP)	Yes/yes (venous and arterial)	8.5	Moderate; requires coronary sinus cathetization	85%	10%	Bleeding, hematoma, myocardial edema and hemorhage
Intraaortic balloon pump (IABP)	Yes/yes	8.5–10.5	Yes; in-lab; no added personnel	90%	9–43% (10%)	Limb ischemia, emboli, aorta damage, thrombocytopenia
Cardio-pulmonary bypass support (CPS)	Yes/yes	18	No; requires specialized personnel	80–95%	40%	Vascular site blood loss, hemolysis, thrombocytopenia
Hemopump	No/no	21	No; high placement failure rate	75%	60% 10% 10% 14%	Dysrhythmia Embolus Thrombocytopenia significant blood loss

NA, not applicable; SBP, systolic blood pressure; pts, patients; RBC, red blood cell; LAD, left anterior descending coronary artery; PTCA, percutaneous transluminal coronary angioplasty; PVD, peripheral vascular disease; bpm, beats per minute; CO, cardiac output; MVO_2, myocardial oxygen consumption; PTA, percutaneous transluminal angioplasty; LV, left ventricle; RCA, right coronary artery; CPS, cardiopulmonary bypass support.

advantages and disadvantages

Complication risk group	Contraindication	Beneficial effects	Indications	Limitation/requirement
None or well-defined	None or well-defined	Afterload preload coronary perf. regional support systemic support	Prophylactic in high-risk pts For pre-operative stability after failed PTCA	None
	Polycythemia, hypotension	Maintains perfusion and oxygenation to at-risk myocardium Patient comfort	Routine PTCA Prohylactic in high-risk pts (large area of myocardium at risk with inflation) For preoperative stability after failed PTCA Coronary dissection requiring long balloon inflation Drug delivery to jeopardized myocardium	Tortuous vessels, distal or tandem lesions. No perfusion to sidebranches with inflations Perfusion ineffective with hypotension (SBP <75 mmHg Requires wire removal from distal vessel High-pressure inflation limits flow Large profile may Dotter lesion and limits angiogram quality
RCA PTCA		Maintains perfusion and oxygenation to myocardium at risk Capable of adapting flow rate to prevent/resolve ischemia May be beneficial in no-reflow after recanalization of total occlusion Patient comfort	Routine PTCA Prohylactic in high-risk pts (large area of myocardium at risk with inflation) For preoperative stability after failed PTCA Coronary dissection requiring long balloon inflation Drug delivery to jeopardized myocardium	No perfusion to sidebranches with inflations May require wire removal from distal vessel
		High O_2 carrying capacity Neutrophil suppression (may limit reperfusion injury) Small particle size (10^{-4} of RBC) No hemolysis or thrombosis	High-risk PTCA PTCA with active high pressure and flow perfusion reperfusion of occluded vessels	30–60-min prep. time No clinical data demonstrating superiority to hemoperfusion No perfusion to sidebranches with inflations
		Coronary perfusion, regional support	Prohylactic in high-risk pts For pre-operative stability after failed PTCA; may facilitate cardioplegia delivery Permits drug delivery to jeopardized myocardium	CS catheter and added apparatus Only proven for LAD distribution Investigational
Diabetes, PVD (31% vascular complication), women Iliofemoral atheroslerosis, prolonged CPS use	Aortic regurgitation, PVD, s/p PVD surgery, Extreme ileofemoral disease	Afterload preload coronary perfusion, systemic support Systemic hemodynamic support, cardiac work oxygen demand MVO_2 by 50% 1–6 l/min output	Prophylactic in high-risk pts For preoperative stability after failed PTCA Prophylactic in extremely high risk Shock or arrest during PTCA	Stable rhythm HR < 120 bpm Only 15% CO increase Only 17% MVO_2 reduction Difficult to insert in iliofemoral disease (may require PTA preinsert) High-dose heparin required Skilled perfusionist Unable to wean some patients
Ventricular mural thrombus PVD	Severe aortic stenosis Severe aortic insuff. Mechanical prosthetic valve Severe right heart failure Severe PVD	Decompress LV Maintain systemic circulation CO up to 5 l/min collaterals less anticoag. req'd compared to CPS	Shock or arrest (doesn't req. elec. stability) Prolonged use possible (up to 7 days)	CO limited to 3.5 l/min Dependent on adequate LV filling Unable to wean some pts Investigational

REFERENCES

1. Holmes DR, Holubkov R, Vlietstra RE, Kelsey SF, Reeder GS, Dorros G, Williams DO, Cowley MJ, Faxon DP, Kent KM, Bentivoglio LG, Detre K. Comparison of complications during percutaneous transluminal coronary angioplasty from 1977 to 1981 and from 1985 to 1986: the National Heart, Lung, and Blood Institute Percutaneous Transluminal Coronary Angioplasty Registry. *J Am Coll Cardiol* 1988;12:1149–1155.
2. Taylor GJ, Rabinovich E, Mikell FL, Moses HW, Dove JT, Batchelder JE, Wellons HA, Schneider JA. Percutaneous transluminal coronary angioplasty as palliation for patients considered poor surgical candidates. *Am Heart J* 1986;111:840–844.
3. Colle JP, Delarche N. Clinical factors affecting the immediate outcome of PTCA in patients with unstable angina and poor candidates for surgery. *Cathet Cardiovasc Diagn* 1991;23:155–163.
4. Feldman RL, Carmichael M, Domingo M, Dresen W, Eligeti R, Fox R, Jesrani M, Kuykendall L, Maffei V, Martin S, Mittal V, Passalacqua D, Potu P, Rai S, Sackin D, Savage K, Singh M, Smith K, Stone I, Urban P, Vasudevan R, Walker D, Kaizer J, Standley M. Coronary angioplasty in patients who were considered poor bypass surgery candidates. *J Invas Cardiol* 1991;3:170–174.
5. Myler RK, Stertzer SH. Cardiopulmonary support: the risk and benefits of assisted coronary angioplasty. *J Am Coll Cardiol* 1990;15:30–31.
6. Lincoff AM, Pompa JJ, Eliis SG, Vogel RA, Topol EJ. Percutaneous support devices for high risk or complicated coronary angioplasty. *J Am Coll Cardiol* 1991;17:770–780.
7. Dorros G, Cowley MJ, Janke L, Kelsey SF, Mullin SM, Van Raden M. In-hospital mortality rate in the National Heart, Lung, and Blood Institute Percutaneous Transluminal Coronary Angioplasty Registry. *Am J Cardiol* 1984;53:17C–21C.
8. Dorros G, Cowley MJ, Simpson J, Bentivoglio LG, Block PC, Bourassa M, Detre K, Gosselin AJ, Gruentzig AR, Kelsey SF, Kent KM, Mock MB, Mullin SM, Myler RK, Passamani ER, Stertzer SH, Williams DO. Percutaneous transluminal coronary angioplasty: report of complications from the National Heart, Lung, and Blood Institute PTCA registry. *Circulation* 1983;67:723–730.
9. Brendlau CL, Roubin GS, Leimgruber PP, Douglas JS, King SB, Gruentzig AR. In-hospital morbidity and mortality in patients undergoing elective coronary angioplasty. *Circulation* 1985;72:1044–1052.
10. Ischinger T, Gruentzig AR, Meir B, Galan K. Coronary dissection and total coronary occlusion associated with percutaneous transluminal coronary angioplasty: significance of initial angiographic morphology of coronary stenosis. *Circulation* 1986;74:1371–1378.
11. Myler RK, Shaw RE, Stertzer SH, Hecht HS, Ryan C, Rosenblum J, Cumberland DC, Murphy MC, Hansell HN, Hidalgo B. Lesion morphology and coronary angioplasty: current experience and analysis. *J Am Coll Cardiol* 1992;19:1641–1652.
12. Ellis SG, Roubin GS, King SB III, Douglas JS Jr, Weintraub WS, Thomas RG, Cox WR. Angiographic and clinical predictors of acute closure after native vessel coronary angioplasty. *Circulation* 1988;77:372–379.
13. Ellis SG, Roubin GS, King SB III, Douglas JS Jr, Shaw RE, Stertzer SH, Myler RK. In-hospital cardiac mortality after acute closure after coronary angioplasty: analysis of risk factors from 8,207 procedures. *J Am Coll Cardiol* 1988;11:211–216.
14. Park DD, Laramee LA, Teirstein P, Lignon RW, Giorgi LV, Hartzler GO, McCallister BD. Major complications during PTCA: analysis of 5113 cases. *J Am Coll Cardiol* 1988;11:237(abstract).
15. Stevens T, Kahn JK, McCallister BD, Ligon RW, Spaude S, Rutherford BD, McConahay DR, Johnson WL, Giorgi LV, Shimshack TM, Hartzler GO. Safety and efficacy of percutaneous transluminal coronary angioplasty in patients with left ventricular dysfunction. *Am J Cardiol* 1991;68:313–319.
16. Kohli RS, Disciascio G, Cowely MJ, Nath M, Goudreau E, Vetrovec GW. Coronary angioplasty in patients with severe left ventricular dysfunction. *J Am Coll Cardiol* 1990;16:807–811.
17. Kahn JK, Rutherford BD, McConahay DR, Johnson WL, Giorgi LV, Shimshak TM, Ligon RW, Hartzler GO. Comparison of procedural results and risks of coronary angioplasty in men and women for conditions other than acute myocardial infarction. *Am J Cardiol* 1992;69:1241–1242.
18. Cowley MJ, Mullin SM, Kelsey SF, Kent KM, Gruentzig AR, Detre KM, Passamani ER. Sex differences in early and long-term results of coronary angioplasty in the NHLBI PTCA Registry. *Circulation* 1985;71:90–97.
19. Bergelson BA, Jacobs AK, Cupples LA, Ruocco NA, Kyller MG, Ryan TJ, Faxon DP. Prediction of risk for hemodynamic compromise during coronary angioplasty. *Am J Cardiol* 1992;70:1540–1545.
20. Ellis SG, Myler RF, King SB III, Douglas JS Jr, Topol EJ, Shaw RE, Stertzer SH, Roubin GS, Murphy MC. Causes and correlates of death after unsupported coronary angioplasty: implications for use of angioplasty and advanced support techniques in high-risk settings. *Am J Cardiol* 1991;68:1447–1451.
21. Anderson HV, Leimgruber PP, Roubin GS, Nelson DL, Gruentzig AR. Distal coronary artery perfusion during percutaneous transluminal coronary angioplasty. *Am Heart J* 1985;110:720–726.
22. Turi ZG, Campbell CA, Gottimukkala MV, Kloner RA. Preservation of distal coronary perfusion during prolonged balloon inflation with an autoperfusion angioplasty catheter. *Circulation* 1987;75:1273–1280.
23. Cambell CA, Rezkalla S, Kloner RA, Turi ZG. The autoperfusion balloon angioplasty catheter limits myocardial ischemia and necrosis during prolonged balloon inflation. *J Am Coll Cardiol* 1989;14:1045–1050.
24. Christensen CW, Lassar TA, Daley LC, Reider MA, Schmidt DH. Regional myocardial blood flow with a reperfusion catheter and an autoperfusion balloon catheter during total coronary occlusion. *Am Heart J* 1990;119:242–248.
25. Hinohara T, Simpson JB, Phillips HR, Behar VS, Peter RH, Kong Y, Carlson EB, Stack RS. Transluminal catheter reperfusion: a new technique to reestablish blood flow after coronary occlusion during percutaneous transluminal coronary angioplasty. *Am J Cardiol* 1986;57:685–686.
26. Quigley PJ, Hinohara T, Phillips HR, Peter RH, Behar VS, Kong Y, Simonton CA, Perez JA, Stack RS. Myocardial protection during coronary angioplasty with an autoperfusion balloon catheter in humans. *Circulation* 1988;78:1128–1134.
27. Bourassa MG. Is the leaking balloon angioplasty catheter a better catheter? *J Am Coll Cardiol* 1989;14:1051–1052.
28. Serruys PW, Wijns W, van den Brand M. Left ventricular performance, regional blood flow, wall motion and lactate metabolism during transluminal angioplasty. *Circulation* 1984;70:25–36.
29. Wohlgelernter D, Cleman M, Highman HA, Fetterman RC, Duncan JS, Zaret BL, Faffee CC. Regional myocardial dysfunction during coronary angioplasty: evaluation by two-dimensional echocardiography and 12-lead electrocardiography. *J Am Coll Cardiol* 1986;7:1245–1254.
30. Ohman EM, Marquis JF, Ricci DR, Brown RIG, Knudtson ML, Kereiakes DJ, Samaha JK, Margolis JR, Niederman AL, Dean LJ, Gurbel PA, Sketch MH, Wildermann NM, Lee KL, Califf RM. Effect of gradual prolonged inflation during angioplasty on inhospital and longterm outcome: results of multicenter randomized trial. *J Am Coll Cardiol* 1992;19:33A(abst).
31. Quigley PJ, Kereiakes DJ, Abbottsmith CW, Bauman RP, Tcheng JE, Muhlestein JB, Phillips HR, Stack RS. Prolonged autoperfusion angioplasty: immediate clinical outcome and angiographic follow-up. *J Am Coll Cardiol* 1989;13:155(abst).
32. Sundram P, Harvey JR, Johnson RG, Schwartz MJ, Baim DS. Benefit of the perfusion catheter for emergency coronary artery grafting after failed percutaneous transluminal coronary angioplasty. *Am J Cardiol* 1989;63:282–285.
33. Smith JE, Quigley PJ, Tcheng JE, Bauman RP, Thomas J, Stack RS. Can prolonged perfusion balloon inflations salvage vessel patency after failed angioplasty? *Circulation* 1989;80[Suppl II]:373(abstract).
34. Leitschuh ML, Mills RM, LaRosa D, Jacobs AK, Ruocco NA, Faxon DP. Outcome after major dissection during coronary angioplasty using the perfusion balloon catheter. *Am J Cardiol* 1991;67:1056–1060.
35. Ciampricotti R, Dekkers PJ, el Gamal MI, van der Krieken AM, Relik T II. Catheter reperfusion for failed emergency coronary angioplasty without subsequent bypass surgery. *J Cathet Cardivasc Diagn* 1989;18:159–164.

36. Kusachi S, Takata S, Iwasaki K, Nishiyama O, Kita T, Namba H, Hata T, Taniguchi G, Saito D, Haraoka S. Reperfusion through balloon catheter to minimize myocardial infarction during the interval between failed percutaneous transluminal coronary angioplasty and emergency coronary artery bypass grafting. *J Heart and Vessels* 1989;5:59–63.

37. Tomaki H, Simpson JB, Phillips HR, Stack RS. Transluminal intracoronary reperfusion catheter: a device to maintain coronary perfusion between failed coronary angioplasty and emergency coronary bypass surgery. *J Am Coll Cardiol* 1988;11:977–982.

38. Banka VS, Trivedi A, Patel R, Ghusson M, Voci G. Prevention of myocardiol ischemia during coronary angioplasty: a simple new method for distal antegrade arterial blood perfusion. *Am Heart J* 1989;118:830–836.

39. Farcot JC, Berland J, Derumeaux G, Merchant S, Koning R, Cribier A, Bourdarias JP, Letac B. Results of physiologic anteroperfusion system to support prolonged PTCA inflations in 40 patients. *J Am Coll Cardiol* 1992;19:34(abstract).

40. Di Sciascio G, Angelini P, Vandormael MG, Brinker JA, Cowley MJ, Dean LS, Douglas JS, (CHIPS) investigators. Reduction of ischemia with a new flow-adjustable hemoperfusion pump during coronary angioplasty. *J Am Coll Cardiol* 1992;19:657–662.

41. Bajaj AK, Cobb AM, Virman R, Gay JC, Light RT, Forman MB. Limitation of myocardial reperfusion injury by intravenous perfluorochemicals: role of neutrophil activation. *Circulation* 1989;79:645–656.

42. Cowley MJ, Snow FR, DiSciascio G, Kelly K, Guard C, Nixon JV. Perfluorochemical perfusion during coronary angioplasty in unstable and high-risk patients. *Circulation* 1990;81[Suppl IV]:IV-27–IV-34.

43. Jaffee CM, Wohlgelernter D. Prevention of ischemia during percutaneous transluminal coronary angioplasty by transcatheter infusion of oxygenated flusol DA 20%. *Circulation* 1986;74:555–562.

44. Christensen CW, Reeves WC, Lassar TA, Schmidt DH. Inadequate subendocardial oxygen delivery during perfluorocarbon perfusion in a canine model of ischemia. *Am Heart J* 1988;115:30–37.

45. Faxon DP, Jacobs AK, Kellett MA, McSweeney SM, Coats WD, Ryan TJ. Coronary sinus occlusion pressure and its relation to intracardiac pressure. *Am J Cardiol* 1985;56:457–460.

46. Tschabitscher M. Anatomy of the coronary vessels. In: Mohl W, Wolner E, Glogar D, eds. *The coronary sinus: proceedings of the 1st International Symposium on Myocardial Protection via the Coronary Sinus.* Darmstadt: Steinkopff Verlag;1984:8–10.

47. Wearn JT. The role of the Thebesian vessels in the circulation of the heart. *J Exp Med* 1928;47:293.

48. Jacobs AK, Faxon DP, Apstein CS, Coats WD, Gottsman SB, Ryan TJ. The hemodynamic consequences of coronary sinus occlusion. In: Mohl W, Wolner E, Glogar D, eds. *The coronary sinus: proceedings of the 1st International Symposium on Myocardial Protection via the Coronary Sinus.* Darmstadt: Steinkopff Verlag;1984:430–436.

49. Meerbaum S, Lang T, Provzhitkov M, Haendchen RV, Uchiyama T, Corday BJE. Retrograde lysis of coronary artery thrombus by coronary venous streptokinase administration. *J Am Coll Cardiol* 1983;51:1262–1267.

50. Tadokoro H, Miyazaki A, Satomura K, Kaul S, Fishbein MC, Corday E. Profound infarct size reduction with coronary venous retroinfusion of diltiazem in pigs. *J Am Coll Cardiol* 1988;11:65(abstract).

51. Simon P, Jacobs AK, Faxon DP, Minihan AC, Coats WD, Ryan TJ. Lidocaine delivery via the coronary sinus results in high concentrations in ischemic myocardium. *J Am Coll Cardiol* 1988;11:87(abstract).

52. Karagueuzian HS, Ohta M, Drury KJ, Fishbein MC, Meerbaum S, Corday E, Mandel WJ, Peter T. Coronary venous retroinfusion of procainamide: a new approach for the management of spontaneous and inducible sustained ventricular tachycardia during myocardial infarction. *J Am Coll Cardiol* 1986;7:551–563.

53. Ryden L, Tadokoro H, Sjoquist P, Regardh C, Kobayashi S, Corday E, Drury JK. Pharmacokinetic analysis of coronary venous retroinfusion: a comparison with anterograde coronary artery drug administration using metoprolol as a tracer. *J Am Coll Cardiol* 1991;18:603–612.

54. Miyazaki A, Tadokoro H, Drury JK, Ryden L, Haendchen RV, Corday E. Retrograde coronary venous administration of recombi-

nant tissue-type plasminogen activator: a unique and effective approach to coronary artery thrombolysis. *J Am Coll Cardiol* 1991;18:613–620.

55. Menasche P, Piwnica A. Cardioplegia by way of the coronary sinus for valvular and coronary surgery. *J Am Coll Cardiol* 1991;18:628–636.

56. Mohl W. The development and rationale of pressure-controlled intermittent coronary sinus occlusion—a new approach to protect ischemic myocardium. *Wien Klin Wochenschr* 1984;96:20–25.

57. Mohl W, Glogar D, Mayr H, Losert U, Sochor H, Pachinger O, Kaindl F, Wolner E. Reduction of infarct size induced by intermittent coronary sinus occlusion. *Am J Cardiol* 1984;53:923–928.

58. Jacobs AK. The effect of pressure-controlled intermittent coronary sinus occlusion during reperfusion. In: Mohl W, Faxon D, Wolner E, eds. *Clinics of CSI: proceedings of the 2nd International Symposium on Myocardial Protection via the Coronary Sinus.* Darmstadt: Steinkopff Verlag;1986:345–347.

59. Jacobs AK, Faxon DP, Coats WD, Vogel RM, Ryan TJ. Coronary sinus occlusion: effect on ischemic left ventricular dysfunction and reactive hyperemia. *Am Heart J* 1991;121:442–449.

60. Mohl W, Simon P, Neuman F, Schreiner W, Punzengruber C. Clinical evaluation of pressure-controlled intermittent coronary sinus occlusion: randomized trial during coronary artery surgery. *Ann Thorac Surg* 1988;46:192–201.

61. Chang BL, Drury KJ, Meerbaum S, Fishbein MC, Whiting JS, Corday E. Enhanced myocardial washout and retrograde blood delivery with synchronized retroperfusion during acute myocardial ischemia. *J Am Coll Cardiol* 1987;9:1091–1098.

62. Kar S, Jacobs AK, Faxon DP. Synchronized coronary venous retroperfusion during coronary angioplasty. In: Shawl FA, ed. *Supported complex and high risk coronary angioplasty.* Norwell, MA: Kluwer Academic Publishers; 1991:215–230.

63. Drury JK, Yamazaki S, Fishbein MC, Meerbaum S, Corday E. Synchronized diastolic coronary venous retroperfusion: results of a preclinical safety and efficacy study. *J Am Coll Cardiol* 1985;2:328–335.

64. Yamazaki S, Drury JK, Meerbaum S, Corday E. Synchronized coronary venous retroperfusion: prompt improvement of left ventricular function in experimental myocardial ischemia. *J Am Coll Cardiol* 1985;5:655–663.

65. O'Byrne GT, Nienaber CA, Miyazaki A, Araujo L, Fishbein MC, Corday E, Schelbert HR. Positron emission tomography demonstrates that coronary sinus retroperfusion can restore regional myocardial perfusion and preserve metabolism. *J Am Coll Cardiol* 1991;18:257–270.

66. Gore JM, Weiner BH, Benotti JR, Sloan KM, Okike ON, Ceunoud HF, Gaca JMJ, Alpert JS, Dalen JE. Preliminary experience with synchronized coronary sinus retroperfusion in humans. *Circulation* 1986;74:381–388.

67. Constantino C, Sampaolesi A, Serra CM, Pacheco G, Neuburger J, Conci E, Haendchen RV. Coronary venous retroperfusion support during high risk angioplasty in patients with unstable angina: preliminary experience. *J Am Coll Cardiol* 1991;18:283–292.

68. Berland J, Farcot JC, Barrier A, Dellac A, Gamra H, Letac B. Coronary venous synchronized retroperfusion during percutaneous transluminal angioplasty of left anterior descending coronary artery. *Circulation* 1990;81[Suppl IV]:IV-35–IV-42.

69. Beatt KJ, Serruys PW, Defeyter P, Van Den Bernad M, Verdouw PD, Hugenholtz PG. Haemodynamic observations during percutaneous transluminal coronary angioplasty in the presence of synchronized diastolic coronary sinus retroperfusion. *Br Heart J* 1988;59:159–167.

70. Kar S, for the Investigators of the Multicenter Coronary Venous Retroperfusion Clinical Trial Group. Coronary venous retroperfusion reduces ischemia during LAD angioplasty. *J Am Coll Cardiol* 1990;15:250(abst).

71. Kar S, Drury JK, Hajduczki I, Eigler N, Wakida Y, Litvack F, Buchbinder N, Marcus H, Nordlander R, Corday E. Synchronized coronary venous retroperfusion for support and salvage of ischemic myocardium during elective and failed angioplasty. *J Am Coll Cardiol* 1991;18:271–282.

72. Weber KT, Janicki JS. Intra-aortic balloon counterpulsation: a review of physiological principles, clinical results, and device safety. *Ann Thorac Surg* 1974;17:602–636.

73. Kern MT. Intra-aortic balloon pumping post-angioplasty: docu-

mentation of increased coronary blood flow. *Cardiac Assists* 1992;6:1–6.

74. Kahn JK, Rutherford BD, McConahay DR, Johnson WL, Giorgi LV, Hartzler GO. Supported "high risk" coronary angioplasty using intraaortic balloon pump counterpulsation. *J Am Coll Cardiol* 1990;15:1151–1155.

75. Alcan KE, Stertzer SH, Wallsh E, DePasquale NP, Bruno MS. The role of intra-aortic balloon counterpulsation in patients undergoing percutaneous transluminal coronary angioplasty. *Am Heart J* 1983;105:527–530.

76. Voudris V, Marco J, Morice MC, Fajadet J, Royer T. "High-risk" percutaneous transluminal coronary angioplasty with preventive intraaortic balloon counterpulsation. *Cathet Cardiovasc Diagn* 1990;19:160–164.

77. Anwar A, Mooney MR, Stertzer SH, Mooney JF, Shaw RE, Madison JD, VanTassel RA, Murphy MC, Myler RK. Intra-aortic balloon counterpulsation support for elective coronary angioplasty in the setting of poor left ventricular function: a two center experience. *J Invas Cardiol* 1990;2:175–180.

78. Kreidieh I, Davies DW, Lim R, Nathan AW, Dymond DS, Banim SO. High-risk coronary angioplasty with elective intra-aortic balloon pump support. *Int J Cardiol* 1992;35:147–152.

79. Skillington PD, Couper GS, Peigh PS, Fitzgerald D, Cohn LH. Pulmonary artery balloon counterpulsation for intra-operative right ventricular failure. *Ann Thorac Surg* 1991;51:658–660.

80. Vogel RA, Tommaso CL, Gundry SR. Initial experience with coronary angioplasty and aortic valvuloplasty using elective semipercutaneous cardiopulmonary support. *Am J Cardiol* 1988;62:811–813.

81. Shawl FA, Domanski MJ, Hernandez TJ, Punja S. Emergency percutaneous cardiopulmonary bypass support in cardiogenic shock from acute myocardial infarction. *Am J Cardiol* 1989;64:965–970.

82. Shawl FA. Percutaneous cardiopulmonary bypass support: technique, indications, and complications. In: Shawl FA, ed. *Supported complex and high risk coronary angioplasty.* Norwell, MA: Kluwer Academic Publishers; 1991:65–130.

83. Mooney MR, Mooney JF, Mathias DW, Sawicki E, Madison JD, Gobel FL, Goldenberg MD, Rogers JW, Brandenburg RO, Van Tassel RA. Clinical application of percutaneous cardiopulmonary bypass for high risk coronary angioplasty. *J Invas Cardiol* 1990;2:161–167.

84. Vogel RA. Initial report of the national registry of elective cardiopulmonary bypass supported coronary angioplasty. *J Am Coll Cardiol* 1990;15:23–29.

85. Pavlides GS, Stack RK, Dudlets PI, Hauser AM, O'Neil WW. Echocardiographic assessment of global and regional myocardial function during supported angioplasty. *Circulation* 1989;80[Suppl II]:271(abstract).

86. Vogel RA, Shawl FA. Report of the national registry of elective supported angioplasty: comparison of the 1988 and 1989 results. *Circulation* 1990;82[Suppl III]:653(abst).

87. Teirstein PS. Cardiopulmonary support. *Am J Cardiol* 1992;69:19F–21F.

88. Tommaso CL, Johnson RA, Stafford JL, Zoda AR, Vogel RA. Supported coronary angioplasty and standby supported coronary angioplasty for high-risk coronary artery disease. *Am J Cardiol* 1990;66:1255–1257.

89. Shawl FA, Domanski MJ, Wish M, Punja S, Hernandez TJ. Emergency percutaneous cardiopulmonary support in cardiogenic shock: long term follow-up. *Circulation* 1989;80[Suppl II]:258(abst).

90. Shawl FA, Domanski MJ, Wish M, Punja S, Hernandez TJ. Emergency percutaneous cardiopulmonary bypass in patients with cardiac arrest. *Circulation* 1989;80[Suppl II]:271(abst).

91. Frazier OH, Nalcatan T, Duncan JM, Parnis SM, Fuqua JM. Clinical experience with the Hemopump. *ASAIO Trans* 1989;35:604–606.

92. Wampler RK, Riehle RA. Clinical experience with the Hemopump left ventricular assist device. In: Shawl FA, ed. *Supported complex and high risk coronary angioplasty.* Norwell, MA: Kluwer Academic Publishers; 1991:231–249.

93. Smalling RW, Sweeney MJ, Cassidy DB, Barrett RL, Morris RE, Lammermeier DE, Key PG, Hayne MP, Frazier OH, Wampler K. Hemodynamics in cardiogenic shock after acute myocardial infarction with the Hemopump assist device. *Circulation* 1989;80[Suppl II]:624(abstract).

94. Loisance D, Duboise-Rande JL, Deleuze P, Okude J, Rosenval O, Geschwind H. Prophylactic intraventricular pumping in high risk coronary angioplasty. *Lancet* 1990;335:438–440.

95. Lincoff AM, Popma JJ, Bates ER, Deeb GM, Bolling SF, Meagher JS, Kelly AM, Wampler RK, Nicklas JM. Successful coronary angioplasty in two patients with cardiogenic shock using the Nimbus Hemopump support device. *Am Heart J* 1990;120:970–972.

96. Babic UU, Grujicic S, Djurisic Z, Vucinic M. Percutaneous left atrial aortic bypass with a roller pump. *Circulation* 1989;80[Suppl II]:II-272(abstract).

97. Glassman E, Chinitz L, Levite H, Slater J, Winer H. Partial left heart bypass support during high-risk angioplasty. *Circulation* 1989;80[Suppl II]:11-272(abstract).

CHAPTER 19

Percutaneous Transluminal Coronary Angioplasty and the Cardiac Surgeon

Richard J. Shemin

There has been exponential growth of percutaneous transluminal coronary angioplasty (PTCA) procedures treating coronary artery disease. These procedures have resulted in new challenges for cardiac surgeons. The momentum for PTCA expansion has been fueled by the efficiency of the procedure, its overwhelming acceptance as a procedure of choice for most patients with single-vessel coronary artery disease, and the perceived advantage of lower costs and greater convenience for the patient. However, many of these advantages are still controversial, especially when the procedure is utilized for the treatment of patients with multivessel disease and other subsets of patients.

Nevertheless, the increased utilization of PTCA has had a significant impact on the practice of coronary artery bypass surgery. Uniformly, cardiac surgical centers have documented a trend toward the referral of patients with more advanced coronary artery disease, reduced left ventricular function, and a marked increase in the number of patients who have had a prior (often multiple) PTCA procedure. This trend has dramatically shifted the baseline characteristics of the cardiac surgical population (1).

More importantly, the cardiac surgeon has had to learn to deal effectively with the acute complications of the PTCA procedure that often require emergency surgery. When restenosis occurs, the patient usually re-presents electively for either a repeat PTCA or coronary artery bypass graft operation. However, more challenging is the need to perform emergency coronary artery bypass surgery on patients with acute ischemia involving

a myocardial infarction (2–8). Patients with hemodynamic instability or frank cardiovascular collapse pose the ultimate challenge.

There exists a subset of patients who present for urgent coronary artery bypass grafting after failure of the PTCA procedure, or after PTCA complications, where the patient may not be a surgical candidate. Identification of these patients is extremely important so that expectations of the patient, family, and cardiologist are realistic. The overall impact upon the health care system for inappropriate CABG surgery is detrimental. We must accept the responsibility of making the hard but prudent choices.

SURGICAL BACKUP

Central to the issue of surgical coverage of acute complications that require emergency coronary artery bypass grafting is the logistical problem of providing surgical backup for the PTCA procedure. The definition of surgical backup has evolved over the past decade. However, the standards of surgical backup for PTCA are not well defined and vary greatly from institution to institution (9). It is likely that this situation will continue to evolve as the interplay of factors, such as risk of the individual PTCA patient for complications, health care costs, and volume of PTCA procedures performed by individual operators or institutions, changes over the next several years. It is difficult at this time to predict the ultimate outcome. However, the trend has been to move away from providing, for each individual PTCA patient, one-to-one backup with an open, waiting operating room and complete surgical team consisting of nurses, perfusionists, and surgeons. This situation may provide the ultimate safety for the patient but is economically unsatisfactory (10–12).

RJ Shemin: Department of Cardiothoracic Surgery, Boston University School of Medicine; Department of Cardiothoracic Surgery, The University Hospital, Boston University Medical Center; and Department of Thoracic Surgery, Boston City Hospital, Boston, Massachusetts

Ideally, patients with coronary artery disease who have been scheduled for an angioplasty procedure should have a formal surgical consult. Only in this way would the cardiac surgeon be able to totally prepare for a potential operation under urgent conditions. Without this formal preoperative evaluation, alternatives to the PTCA procedure will not be presented by the expert cardiac surgeon. Furthermore, with the consult, informed consent regarding the potential emergency procedure and its risk would be frankly discussed. More importantly, because of the ease of PTCA, the evaluation of comorbid conditions and other medical issues that might be critical if an urgent operation was necessary are not adequately investigated prior to the operation. These factors play a role in the different outcomes between elective CABG and emergency CABG after failed PTCA (12–17).

PATIENT SUBSETS

The current large volume of PTCA procedures, coupled with the current practice of same-day admission for PTCA, further complicates the ability to perform a proper surgical consult prior to the PTCA procedure. This is unfortunate because of the increasing level of risk of many PTCA patients, especially those with multivessel disease, prior procedures, advanced age, and multiple medical problems.

Percutaneous transluminal coronary angioplasty and CABG should be complimentary procedures for the treatment of coronary artery occlusive disease. However, for multivessel disease patients the procedures are competitive. Inadequate data and bias often drive the decision made between a PTCA versus a primary CABG procedure for a patient with multivessel disease and favorable anatomy for either procedure. The choice is increasingly being made independently by the cardiologist, without the input of the cardiac surgeon and this issue will need to be addressed increasingly in the future.

Current PTCA practice includes an increasing number of patients who have had prior PTCA or coronary artery bypass graft (CABG) surgery (18). The challenges of operating on a patient who has had a prior CAB procedure and develops an acute complication in the catheterization laboratory during PTCA, can be formidable. This example emphasizes the need for prior notification of the cardiac surgical team so that proper planning and evaluation can be performed. There will also be a group of patients in whom angioplasty is being performed as a heroic procedure. If complications occur, the overall risks of surgical intervention are prohibitive. When a patient is deemed not to be a surgical candidate under elective conditions they should clearly not be considered a candidate in an emergency situation. Therefore, it is necessary to identify these patients preoperatively (i.e., prior to PTCA) so that the expectations of the cardiologist and the patient are appropriate.

INCIDENCE OF EMERGENCY SURGERY

Approximately 2% to 8% of PTCA patients require surgical intervention for complications (19) (Table 1).

TABLE 1. *Results of emergency CABG after failed PTCA*

Author (ref.)	Year	Number of PTCAs	Emergency CABG	Q-Wave MI	Deaths
Akins (4)	1984	125	11 (8.8%)	1 (9.1%)	0
Crowley (34)	1984	3,079	202 (6.6%)	90 (45%)	13 (6.4%)
Jones (17)	1984	777	41 (5.3%)	9 (18%)	1 (2.4%)
Kabbani (35)	1984	600	27 (4.5%)	0	2 (7.7%)
Reul (36)	1984	518	70 (13.5%)	23 (32.8%)	4 (5.7%)
Bredleau (37)	1985	3,500	96 (2.7%)	47 (49%)	2 (2.1%)
Killen (6)	1985	3,000	115 (3.8%)	46 (40%)	13 (11.3%)
Pelletier (7)	1985	299	35 (11.7%)	10 (29%)	0
Shiu (38)	1985	240	14 (5.8%)	5 (36%)	1 (7.1%)
Golding (8)	1986	1,831	81 (4.4%)	35 (57%)	2 (2.5%)
Page (39)	1986	750	31 (4.1%)	13 (41%)	3 (10%)
Lazar (30)	1987	1,045	24 (2.3%)	15 (63%)	3 (12.5%)
Connor (16)	1988	996	146 (14.7%)	57 (39%)	4 (2.7%)
Parsonnet (13)	1988	958	67 (7.0%)	19 (28%)	8 (11.9%)
Greene (14)	1989	1,214	53 (4.4%)	27 (51%)	2 (3.8%)
Naunheim (15)	1989	2,418	103 (4.3%)	23 (22%)	11 (10.7%)
Talley (40)	1989	5,941	202 (3.4%)	54 (27%)	5 (2.5%)
Tebbe (41)	1989	950	34 (3.6%)	15 (44%)	3 (8.8%)
Buffet (33)	1990	2,576	100 (4%)	57 (57%)	19 (19%)
Doud (42)	1990	2,180	51 (2.4%)	13 (26%)	2 (3.9%)
Hochberg (43)	1990	1,625	53 (3.3%)	0	14 (26%)
Stark (23)	1990	859	42 (5.0%)	16 (44%)	5 (12%)
Total		35,481	1,598 (4.5%)	575 (36%)	117 (7.3%)

Results of surgical intervention after a PTCA failure have varied widely, with a range in operative mortality from 2% to 36% (13–17). It has been well documented that major determinants for operative mortality are the degree of left ventricular dysfunction, the patient's hemodynamic status when he reaches the operating room, and the extent of coronary artery disease. The amount of time the patient has been ischemic and the severity of ischemia often determine whether myocardial infarction will develop and the extent of myocardial salvage.

The earliest reports of surgical intervention after failed PTCA are vastly different from current reports due to changes in the angioplasty patient population and the more selective referral of only severely ischemic and hemodynamically unstable patients for emergency surgery. In early studies patients had preserved ventricular function, only single- or at most double-vessel disease, and the patients were younger and in better general medical condition. There was a low threshold for surgical intervention and the patients were usually hemodynamically stable. The operative mortality in these early series were not substantially greater than for elective patients (20).

MANAGEMENT OF EMERGENCY

In the Laboratory

Current practice in managing acute PTCA complications has changed due to new technologies. In general, there is an attempt to delay surgery or avoid emergency surgery under most circumstances. A variety of techniques has been developed to treat acute thrombosis and or dissection of the dilated vessel. These maneuvers are often successful. However, they also have the potential to delay prompt operative intervention and prolong ischemic time before surgical revascularization can be accomplished. Many patients have been stabilized and heparinized only to again experience abrupt closure and require emergency surgical intervention within hours of the original PTCA procedure. Recent surgical series for operative intervention after acute PTCA complications, therefore, and not surprisingly, document higher operative mortality (13–17).

The surgical team is promptly alerted when a procedural complication occurs (2% to 8% of cases). The standard approach to these complications includes the possible use of thrombolytic agents and/or redilatation of the occluded segment (21). Techniques using prolonged balloon inflations, laser welding, atherectomy, and intracoronary stents are under evaluation for the management of these PTCA complications (22–26). The reperfusion bail-out catheter is the most useful device for providing distal perfusion in an attempt to minimize myocardial ischemia (27).

The application of these techniques must be balanced evaluation with the patient's clinical status. The techniques are often time-consuming and their rational use requires more data on outcome to predict success. Only in this way will patients in whom surgery should be performed not be further delayed in the catheterization lab with futile attempts to mechanically manipulate the lesion.

In the Operating Room

A variety of other devices have been developed to help the surgical team respond to the variety of emergencies arising during PTCA. The intraaortic balloon pump has been found to be invaluable in stabilizing acute ischemia and hemodynamic compromise. A further technological improvement has been the perfection of percutaneous cannulas that can be inserted into the femoral artery and vein in the catheterization lab, or even at the bedside. The use of portable centrifugal pumps and oxygenators allows bypass to be instituted expeditiously in a variety of circumstances. Successful institution of this type of technology in the catheterization lab requires cooperation and close communication between the catheterization lab and surgical teams. The decision to institute bypass is made jointly by the cardiologist and surgeon, and according to established protocol. The cannulation should be available in the lab so that placement of the cannula can be performed by the cardiologist while the surgeon and perfusionist prepare the cardiopulmonary bypass circuit. Heparinization of the patient with 4 mg/kg of heparin to elevate the activated clotting time (ACT) to a minimum of 400 sec should be performed prior to cannula insertion. Cardiopulmonary bypass is ideal in a patient who has sustained a cardiac arrest in the catheterization lab; or when profound cardiogenic shock persists after placement of a bail-out catheter, intubation of the trachea and inotropic support, or an intraaortic balloon pump do not stabilize the patient's hemodynamics (28).

Some centers have investigated the use of elective cardiopulmonary bypass in the catheterization laboratory during angioplasty for high-risk patients termed supported angioplasty. Recent data from the registry on these patients suggest that this approach is costly and unnecessary in most patients. Most of the patients who are deemed high risk never develop a hemodynamic complication. Instead, we recommend having the pump on standby and only initiating the protocol when necessary. The use of percutaneous cardiopulmonary bypass combined with the intraaortic balloon pump will provide adequate oxygenation and systemic circulation. However, if myocardial ischemia continues to be present, further delays in proceeding to the operating room cannot be tolerated. If the heart has fibrillated and cannot be defibrillated, the possibility that distention of the left ventricle will be present is quite high and this situation markedly enhances ongoing injury. In this situation, continued external cardiac compression helps decompress the cardiac chambers until the chest can be opened and proper venting techniques instituted. Patient management on cardiopulmonary bypass is the responsibility of the perfusionist directed by the cardiac surgeon. They are the only specialists trained to use this technology.

The conduct of the operative procedure should be expeditious. Avoidance of time-consuming monitoring line placement should be individualized to the patient's status. In general, if the patient is hemodynamically stable and there is no evidence of ongoing ischemia, the operation can proceed in a routine manner. Optimal use of bypass conduits such as the internal mammary artery (IMA) should be routine. However, if there is any evidence of hemodynamic compromise and the ongoing electro-cardiogram (ECG) changes, the patient should be placed on cardiopulmonary bypass as soon as possible. It is possible, in selected cases, to harvest the IMA while on cardiopulmonary bypass. One of the most difficult situations arises when a patient has no venous conduit readily available, especially the patient with a prior coronary artery bypass operation. These patients need to be carefully selected for PTCA. In some cases if they arrest in the catheterization lab, operation should not be offered.

The bail-out catheter is not withdrawn until just prior to aortic crossclamping and the delivery of cardioplegia. Several options exist when considering the type of cardioplegia solution and its route of administration. In general both crystalloid cardioplegia and blood cardioplegia are available. There is some evidence to suggest that blood cardioplegia is superior but this remains controversial. There is also an emerging trend to perform coronary bypass surgery using warm cardioplegia. However, this has not been adequately tested in the setting of acute myocardial infarction with ongoing ischemia. We use hyperkalemic cold crystalloid or cold blood cardioplegia. The route of administration of cardioplegia can be either antegrade into the aortic root, retrograde via the coronary sinus, or a combination of both. This should be individualized.

In general, the delivery of cardioplegia to the muscle supplied by an acutely occluded vessel is most reliably accomplished with retrograde administration. Reoperation patients with diffuse disease or occluded grafts, or patients with a left main dissection would also theoretically benefit from the retrograde route of administration. The cardioplegia should be administered intermittently at least every 20 min during the crossclamp period and down the individual grafts. Other significant considerations include the use of warm induction cardioplegia in severely injured and ischemic ventricles. With this method, the aorta is crossclamped and warm substrate-enhanced cardioplegia containing glutamate or aspartate is administered to enhance and/or replenish myocardial high-energy phosphate stores. Another consideration for selective patients is modification of the reperfusate to modulate reperfusion injury.

RESULTS OF EMERGENCY SURGERY

In 1987 Satter reviewed 82 emergency and 113 elective coronary artery bypass procedures performed after unsuccessful PTCA (29). The operative mortality for emergency coronary artery bypass grafting was 10.9%, compared with an operative mortality of 1.2% in elective cases. Evidence of sustained ischemia after PTCA failure further increased operative mortality in some groups to 12.6%, and the perioperative myocardial infarction rate in this subgroup to 70%. For single-vessel coronary artery disease, patients with failed PTCA had an operative mortality of 3.5%, but the operative mortality markedly increased to 38% in patients with multivessel disease.

In 1987, our group at Boston University Medical Center published an experience with emergency coronary artery bypass grafting after failed PTCA; the report focused upon the periinfarction rate (33). The operative mortality for the emergency coronary artery bypass procedure was 11%. A 63% perioperative myocardial infarction rate was found. The significant determinants of perioperative myocardial infarction included attempted multivessel PTCA and evidence of ischemic ECG changes in the catheterization lab prior to transfer to the operating room. In a follow-up study in 1992, we reemphasized that placement of the reperfusing bail-out catheter did not decrease the incidence of myocardial infarctions following a failed PTCA that required CABG surgery (31). Experimental animal and clinical studies demonstrate myocardial salvage can be achieved when coronary reperfusion can be instituted within 4 hr (32). Therefore, we strongly favor expeditious surgical revascularization, instead of continued mechanical manipulation of the damaged artery that may increase the amount of ischemic damage or convert a hemodynamically stable situation into an unstable emergency patient. The infarct rate may not significantly decrease but the potential to salvage myocardium and potentially improve left ventricular (LV) function and prognosis may be significant.

Parsonette et al. published, in 1988, a comparative study of emergency coronary artery bypass grafting after failed PTCA with a computer-matched elective coronary artery bypass group (13). These patients were matched for all preoperative surgical risk factors. The failed PTCA emergency bypass group had an operative mortality of 12% compared to the elective coronary artery bypass group of 1.5%. Postoperative hemorrhage was present in 28% of the emergency group, versus 13% in the elective group. Perioperative myocardial infarction was present in 28% of the emergency group versus 9% in the elective group. The length of hospital stay was 15.3 days compared to 13.4 days in the elective group.

This study further emphasizes the erroneous but commonly held concept that a PTCA failure followed by coronary artery bypass surgery has a similar risk to elective surgery. The philosophy that an attempted PTCA is in the patient's interest because there is little to lose since emergency coronary artery bypass surgery can always be performed, is clearly inappropriate and, if it is so presented to the patient, is extremely misleading. No surgical series since the early reports of surgical revascularization in patients who have had failed percutaneous transluminal angioplasty in the early 1980s have been able to have a comparable operative mortality for these emergency PTCA failure patients requiring surgery and elective coronary artery bypass surgery patients. Clearly, the early series reflected low-risk patients with mostly single-vessel disease. Emergency cases in current series are vastly different than the patients requiring surgery in the earlier reports.

Long-term outcomes after emergency coronary artery bypass surgery for failed PTCA are being reported with increasing frequency. Clearly the long-term results of patients who do survive the perioperative period and hospital discharge is of great interest. In 1988, the Mayo Clinic group reported on the cumulative risks of angina recurrence and of a need for additional coronary artery bypass or PTCA, in patients that had an emergency operation for PTCA failure (16). These patients had a probability of angina recurrence of 21%, with a probability of requiring a repeat PTCA at 5 years of 2%, and a probability of requiring a coronary artery bypass operation of 6%. This was compared to a group of PTCA patients that were similar but had successful PTCA and did not require emergency coronary artery bypass grafting. In this group the probability of angina reoccurrence was 56%, the probability of requiring repeat PTCA was 21%, and 16% of patients crossed over to coronary artery bypass surgery during the 5-year follow-up. The probability of late myocardial infarction was 4% versus 9%, and the probability of late death was 6% versus 9%, when the emergency CABG for failed PTCA group was compared to the successful PTCA group. The highest late event rates occurred in the patients who had successful PTCA but incomplete revascularization. This subgroup is becoming more common with the increasing number of PTCA patients with multivessel disease. This subgroup remains the most controversial regarding treatment strategy.

Buffet et al., in 1991, reported late follow-up of 100 patients who underwent coronary artery bypass grafting for failed PTCA (33). In this current series, 83% of the patients had ischemic ECG changes in spite of the insertion of bail-out catheters upon entering the operating room. Twenty-three percent of the patients were in cardiogenic shock or had undergone cardiac massage until

cardiopulmonary bypass could be instituted. The in-hospital mortality was 19%. A Q-wave myocardial infarction evolved in 57% of patients. Actuarial survival at 7 years was 94%. One patient has required reoperative coronary artery bypass grafting and four required subsequent PTCA. Seventy-seven percent of all patients were angina free at 7 years. Seventy-three percent of the patients that were employed prior to their PTCA resumed work after the coronary operation.

The subgroup of patients who were operated upon in cardiogenic shock and were hospital survivors were followed up. It was found that 92% of these patients were symptom-free, and that no late deaths or repeat procedures had been required. There was an 8% late myocardial infarction rate. Eighty-five percent of the patients reported similar or improved quality of life status and 40% of the previously employed patients had returned to work.

These long-term results are encouraging. However, the challenge remains to appropriately select patients initially for either coronary artery bypass grafting or PTCA. The controversy over the appropriate procedure, especially in the subsets of patients that have multivessel coronary artery disease, varying degrees of left ventricular dysfunction, and acute ischemic syndromes require better data to guide treatment strategy. The current multicenter clinical trials have been slow to recruit patients and it will be several years before their data are available. In addition, the direct application of their data to current populations of patients may be difficult.

The surgical challenge to reduce the operative mortality requires further improvements in myocardial protection and control of reperfusion. Reductions in myocardial infarcts and improved myocardial salvage will result in reduced left ventricular damage, postoperative left ventricular dysfunction, and enhanced late prognosis.

Improved collaboration between the surgeon and cardiologist in patient selection is mandatory to appropriately assign risk and properly inform the patient. Instead of the usual what do we have to lose, approach and the understandable desire to delay surgery into the future, we need to focus less on short-term benefits and more on long-term outcomes. Survival is not the only important endpoint. All cardiovascular events need to considered. Long-term event-free survival is increasingly being studied. The preliminary data strongly favor coronary artery bypass surgery as an initial strategy instead of PTCA for multivessel diseased patients.

Once the complication in the catheterization lab occurs, the surgeon and cardiologist must cooperate as the operating room is readied to receive the emergency patient. The emergency portable cardiopulmonary bypass circuit must be prepared and, if percutaneous cardiopulmonary bypass is necessary in the cath lab, a rational approach to its application must be utilized. In addition, rational decisions should be made as to whether or not any further manipulation of the vessel is necessary or whether the patient should be sent immediately to the operating room. Ischemic time will affect myocardial salvage. Extra time taken in futile attempts at mechanical manipulation of the vessel may not only increase the ischemic time by delaying surgical revascularization but also may take a relatively stable patient to hemodynamic instability, a development which markedly escalates surgical risks.

Intraoperatively the surgeon must be experienced in acute revascularization and apply a variety of techniques to protect the myocardium and control reperfusion.

The surgical survivors have experienced excellent relief of angina and freedom from late cardiovascular events. Future knowledge regarding patient selection and risk stratification will hopefully reduce the number of high-risk patients currently having PTCA. These patients will be referred for surgical revascularization as an initial strategy for optimal long-term cardiovascular, event-free survival.

REFERENCES

1. Naunheim KS, Fiore AC, Wadley SS, et al. The changing profile of the patient undergoing caronary artery bypass surgery. *J Am Coll Cardiol* 1988;11:494–498.
2. Murphy DA, Carver JM, Jones EL, Curling PE, Guyton RA, King SB III, Gruentzig AR, Hatcher CR Jr. Surgical management of acute myocardial ischemia following percutaneous transluminal coronary angioplasty. Role of intra-aortic balloon pump. *J Thorac Cardiovasc Surg* 1984;87:332–339.
3. Jones EL, Craver JM, Gruentzig AR, et al. Percutaneous transluminal coronary angioplasty: role of the surgeon. *Ann Thorac Surg* 1982;34:493–503.
4. Akins CW, Block PC. Surgical intervention for failed percutaneous transluminal coronary angioplasty. *Am J Cardiol* 1984;53:108C–111C.
5. Brahos GJ, Baker NH, Ewy G, et al. Aortocoronary bypass following unsuccessful PTCA: experience in 100 consecutive patients. *Ann Thorac Surg* 1985;40:7–10.
6. Killen DA, Hamaker WR, Reed WA. Coronary artery bypass following percutaneous transluminal coronary angioplasty. *Ann Thorac Surg* 1985;40:133–138.
7. Pelletier LC, Pardini A, Renkin J, David PR, Hebert Y, Bourassa MG. Myocardial revascularization after failure of percutaneous transluminal coronary angioplasty. *J Thorac Cardiovasc Surg* 1985;90:265–271.
8. Golding LA, Loop FD, Hollman JL, et al. Early results of emergency surgery after coronary angioplasty. *Circulation* 1986;74 [Suppl 3]:26–29.
9. Cameron DE, Stinson DC, Greene PS, Gardner TJ. Surgical standby for percutaneous transluminal coronary angioplasty: a survey of patterns of practice. *Ann Thorac Surg* 1990;50:35–39.
10. Ullyot DJ. Surgical standby for coronary angioplasty. *Ann Thorac Surg* 1990;50:3–4.
11. Bonchek LI. Should surgical support within the same institution be required for percutaneous transluminal angioplasty. *Ann Thorac Surg* 1989;48:159–160.
12. Fred HL. Surgical standby arrangements for elective percutaneous transluminal coronary angioplasty. *South Med J* 1990;83:1459–1462.
13. Parsonnet V, Fisch D, Gielchinsky I, et al. Emergency operation after failed angioplasty. *J Thorac Cardiovasc Surg* 1988;96:198–203.
14. Greene MA, Gray LA, Slater AD, et al. Emergency aortocoronary bypass after failed angioplasty. *Ann Thorac Surg* 1991;51:194–199.
15. Nanuheim KS, Fiore AC, Fagan DC, McBride LR, Barner HB, Pennington DG, Willman VL, Kern MJ, Deligonul U, Vandormael MC, Kaiser GC. Emergency coronary artery bypass grafting for failed angioplasty: risk factors and outcome. *Ann Thorac Surg* 1989;47:816–823.
16. Connor AR, Vlietstra RE, Schaff HV, Ilstrup DM, Orszulak TA. Early and late results of coronary artery bypass after failed angioplasty. *J Thorac Surg* 1988;96:191–197.
17. Jones EL, Murphy DA, Carver JM. Comparison of coronary artery bypass surgery and percutaneous transluminal coronary angioplasty including surgery for failed angioplasty. *Am Heart J* 1984;107:830–835.
18. The BARI Investigators. BARI survey of revascularization practice. *Circulation* 1991;84[Suppl 4]:II-251.
19. Holmes DR, Holubkov R, Vlietstra RE, et al. Comparison of complications during percutaneous transluminal coronary angioplasty form 1977 to 1981 and from 1985 to 1986: the National Heart, Lung, and Blood Institute percutaneous transluminal coronary angioplasty registry. *J Am Col Cardiol* 1988;12:1149–1155.
20. Murphy DA, Craver JM, Jones EL, Gruentzig AR, King SB, Hatcher CR. Surgical revascularization following unsuccessful percutaneous transluminal coronary angioplasty. *J Thorac Cardiovasc Surg* 1982;84:342–348.
21. deFeyter RV, van den Brand M, Jaarman G, et al. Acute coronary artery occlusion during and after percutaneous transluminal coronary angioplasty: frequency, prediction, clinical course, management and follow-up. *Circulation* 1991;83:927–936.
22. Sinclair IN, McCabe CH, Sipperly ME, Baim DS. Predictors, therapeutic options and long-term outcome of abrupt reclosure. *Am J Cardiol* 1988;61:61G–66G.
23. Stark KS, Satler IF, Krucoff MW, et al. Myocardial salvage after failed coronary angioplasty. *J Am Coll Cardiol* 1990;15:78–82.
24. Sundram P, Harvey JR, Johnson RG, et al. Benefit of the perfusion catheter for emergency coronary artery grafting for failed percutaneous transluminal coronary angioplasty. *Am J Cardiol* 1989;63:282–285.
25. Topol EJ. Emerging strategies for failed percutaneous transluminal coronary angioplasty. *Am J Cardiol* 1989;63:249–250.
26. Sigwart U, Puel J, Mirkovitch V, Joffre F, Kappenberger L. Intravascular stents to prevent occlusion and restenosis after transluminal angioplasty. *N Engl J Med* 1987;316:701–706.
27. Hinohara T, Simpson JB, Phillips HR, Stack RS. Transluminal intracoronary reperfusion catheter: a device to maintain coronary reperfusion between failed coronary angioplasty and emergency coronary bypass surgery. *J Am Coll Cardiol* 1988;11:977–982.
28. Borkon MA, Killen DA, Piehler JM, Reed WA. Management of complications following failed angioplasty. In: Spence PA, Chitwood WR, eds. *Cardiac surgery: state of the art review.* Philadelphia: Hanley and Belfus; 1991;5:479–485.
29. Satter P, Krause E, Skupin M. Mortality trends in cases of elective and emergency aorto-coronary bypass after percutaneous transluminal coronary angioplasty. *Thorac Cardiovasc Surg* 1987;35:2–5.
30. Lazar HL, Haan CK. Determinants of myocardial infarction following emergency coronary artery bypass for failed percutaneous coronary angioplasty. *Ann Thorac Surg* 1987;44:646–650.
31. Lazar HL, Faxon DP, Paone G, Rajaii-Khorasani A, Jacobs A, Fallon MP, Shemin RJ. Changing profiles of failed angioplasty patients: impact on surgical results. *Ann Thorac Surg* 1992;53:269–273.
32. Reimer KA, Lowe JE, Rasmussen MM, Jennings RB. The wavefront phenomenon of ischemic cell death, I. Myocardial infarct size vs. duration of coronary occlusion in dogs. *Circulation* 1977;56:786.
33. Buffet P, Danchin N, Villemot JP, Amrien D, Ethevenot G, Julliere Y, Mathien P, Cherrier F. Early and long term outcome after emergency coronary artery bypass surgery after failed coronary angioplasty. *Circulation* 1991;84[Suppl 3]:254–259.
34. Crowley MJ, Dorros G, Kelsey SF, et al. Emergency coronary artery bypass surgery after coronary angioplasty: the National Heart Lung and Blood Institute's Percutaneous Transluminal Coronary Angioplasty experience. *Am J Cardiol* 1984;53:22C–26C.

35. Kabbani SS, Bashour TT, Jones R, et al. Surgical experience following percutaneous transluminal coronary angioplasty. *J Texas Heart Inst* 1984;2:112–116.

36. Reul GJ, Cooley DA, Hallman GL, et al. Coronary artery bypass for unsuccessful percutaneous transluminal coronary angioplasty. *J Thorac Cardiovasc Surg* 1984;88:685–694.

37. Bredleau CE, Roubin GS, Leimgruber PP, et al. In-hospital morbidity and mortality in patients undergoing elective coronary angioplasty. *Circulation* 1985;72:1044–1052.

38. Shiu MR, Silverton NP, Oakly D, Cumberland D. Acute coronary occlusion during percutaneous transluminal coronary angioplasty. *Br Heart J* 1985;54:129–133.

39. Page US, Okies JE, Colburn LQ, et al. Percutaneous transluminal coronary angioplasty. *J Thorac Cardiovasc Surg* 1986;96:198–203.

40. Talley JD, Jones EL, Weintraub WS, King SB. Coronary artery bypass surgery after failed elective percutaneous transluminal coronary angioplasty. *Circulation* 1989;79[Suppl I]I126–131.

41. Teebe U, Ruschewski W, Knake W, et al. Will emergency coronary bypass grafting after failed elective percutaneous transluminal coronary angioplasty prevent myocardial infarction? *Thorac Cardiovasc Surg* 1989;37:308–321.

42. Doud DN, Killian DM, Johnson SA, et al. Emergency myocardial revascularization after failed angioplasty. Abstract presented at the American College of Chest Physicians, 56th Annual Scientific Assembly.

43. Hochberg MS, gregory JJ, McCullough JN, et al. Outcome of emergency coronary artery bypass following failed angioplasty. *Circulation* 1990; [Suppl III]82:III-362.

Practical Angioplasty,
edited by David P. Faxon.
Raven Press, Ltd., New York © 1993.

CHAPTER **20**

Clinical Features of Restenosis Following Coronary Angioplasty

John E. Brush, Jr.

Restenosis, or early renarrowing after coronary angioplasty, has stimulated much research concerning wound healing and arterial response to injury. Beyond being an issue for important basic research, restenosis continues to be a significant clinical problem for the practicing cardiologist. Restenosis has resulted in increased angioplasty volume at many centers, necessitating major adjustments in hospital resources and manpower. In addition, the problem of restenosis has diminished, to a degree, the enthusiasm for angioplasty, vis-à-vis medical and surgical approaches. Nevertheless, restenosis is a treatable problem and despite this major drawback, angioplasty continues to be the preferred treatment strategy for many patients with coronary artery disease.

DEFINITION OF RESTENOSIS

Clinical restenosis can be defined as the recurrence in ischemic symptoms within approximately 6 months of a coronary angioplasty. Most of the clinical observational studies of restenosis have used clinical restenosis rather than angiographic restenosis as the major endpoint (1–6). Indeed, it can be argued that clinical restenosis is the most important issue in treating patients, since the recurrence or lack of recurrence of anginal symptoms has the most important implications for the care of the patients. However, for research purposes, clinical restenosis may be too insensitive to detect important differences in study groups, and angiographic restenosis is a more important endpoint for interventional studies of restenosis.

Typically, a patient will describe an angina-free pe-

riod, followed by a period in which the angina becomes progressively more severe. Symptoms usually progress gradually, allowing adequate warning and alerting the patient to seek medical attention. As discussed below, restenosis usually results from progressive neointimal proliferation that causes gradual narrowing of the artery. Unlike unstable angina, which is often due to a disrupted plaque or thrombus, restenosis rarely progresses to myocardial infarction.

When symptoms recur early following coronary angioplasty, without a symptom-free period, the symptoms are more likely due to subacute vessel closure as a result of coronary spasm, thrombosis, or an intimal flap, and not due to neointimal proliferation. When symptoms recur later than 6 months after coronary angioplasty, the symptoms become increasingly likely to be due to progression of a lesion at another site in the coronary vasculature (Fig. 1). In a cohort of 53 patients with 3-year angiographic and clinical follow-up following angioplasty, Rosing et al. found that none had restenosis at the angioplasty site (7). In another report of 133 patients followed for 6 years, Gruentzig et al. found that only 15% had clinical and angiographic evidence of restenosis (8). Conventional clinical wisdom bears out these findings: a patient with an initial successful angioplasty who does not develop restenosis in the initial 6 months has an excellent prognosis and is unlikely to need a repeat procedure for restenosis.

Angiographic restenosis usually causes recurrent symptoms (and, therefore, clinical restenosis), but angiographic restenosis can also occur in the absence of symptoms. The most common definition of angiographic restenosis is the definition used by the National Heart, Lung, and Blood Institute Registry: a loss of greater than or equal to 30% of the cross-sectional luminal diameter, or a loss of greater than or equal to 50% of the initial gain

JE Brush, Jr.: Evans Memorial Department of Clinical Research and Department of Medicine, Boston University Medical Center, Boston, Massachusetts

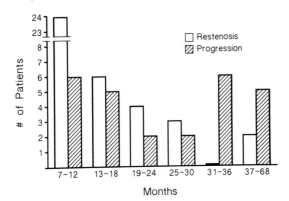

FIG. 1. The incidence of late restenosis after 6 months declines rapidly and by 1 year repeat procedures are done for restenosis as commonly as they are for progression of coronary disease. By 2 years the dilation of new lesions due to progression of disease is more common than restenosis.

in cross-sectional luminal diameter. In other words, if the residual stenosis following angioplasty is 30%, but the patient returns with a 60% stenosis, the patient would have restenosis. Alternatively, if an 80% stenosis is dilated to 40% and the patient returns with a 60% stenosis, the patient would have restenosis.

Another criterion for defining angiographic restenosis is a repeat angiogram which shows a greater than 50% narrowing. This method favors lesions with a poorer initial result as shown in Fig. 2. In the top example, a 70% stenosis is dilated to a 15% residual stenosis. There is a large deterioration in the vessel diameter, but because the initial result is so good, the residual stenosis is 45%, less than the 50% cutoff. In the bottom example, a 70% stenosis is dilated to a residual stenosis of 40%. There is a small deterioration in the vessel diameter, but because of the poor initial result, the residual stenosis is 55%, more than the 50% cutoff. Therefore, using 50% stenosis as a cutoff to define restenosis eliminates a great deal of useful information that is important for the interpretation of study results.

These angiographic definitions are based on an estimation of the percent stenosis of a narrowing as compared with the adjacent vessel. Serruys' group has pointed out that this may be an imprecise method for quantifying restenosis (9). There may be progression of disease in the adjacent vessel segments during the 2 to 6 months between angiograms. Also, the reference arterial segment is often also dilated, causing vessel trauma and endothelial denudation. Progression of disease or neointimal proliferation in the reference segment could result in a decrease in the percent stenosis and an underestimation of the angiographic restenosis rate. Furthermore, in patients with diffusely diseased arteries, it is often difficult to determine an appropriate length of vessel to use as a reference. Serruys et al. have recommended using an absolute measurement of the minimal luminal diameter as a measure of restenosis and have found that a decrease in luminal diameter of 0.72 mm measured by quantitative angiography represents a true deterioration in vessel diameter and should define angiographic restenosis (9). This definition was derived from the standard deviation of minimal lumen diameter measured by quantitative angiography. The error of repeated measurements was 0.36 mm; thus, 0.72 mm represent two standard deviations from the mean. It was also observed by this group and others that the minimal lumen diameter, when plotted for a large group of patients before, after, and at the 6-month follow-up angiogram, assumed a Gaussian distribution (9a). Likewise the change in minimal lumen diameter between the 6-month follow-up period and the period immediately after also followed a Gaussian distribution. A small number of patients demonstrated no significant change in minimal lumen diameter, but the majority showed at least some degree of renarrowing. In order to take into account the change in vessel disease, this group and others have used the term relative gain and relative loss, that is, the ratio between the change in minimal lumen diameter and the reference diameter (9b). While this method of defining restenosis may not reflect the incidence of clinical restenosis, it is the most

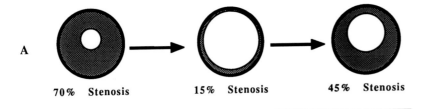

A

70% Stenosis   15% Stenosis   45% Stenosis

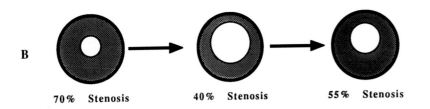

B

70% Stenosis   40% Stenosis   55% Stenosis

FIG. 2. A schematic drawing showing the difficulties in using a 50% stenosis rule to define restenosis. **A:** a 70% stenosis is dilated to 15%. There is a large amount of neointimal proliferation, but it results in only a 45% stenosis. **B:** a 70% stenosis is dilated to 40%. Less neointimal proliferation occurs as compared with example A, but the resultant stenosis is 55% and is defined as restenosis.

sensitive method of defining the process for restenosis trials and the testing of new pharmacological therapy (9c).

The timing of the repeat angiogram is also important in determining angiographic restenosis. Surreys et al. studied 400 angioplasty patients with repeat angiography at 1, 2, 3, and 4 months (10). The angiographic follow-up rate was 86%. The actual restenosis rates varied according to the definition used, but it appeared that the incidence of restenosis was progressive until the third month. At 4 months, there was slight further increase in the restenosis rate defined in terms of absolute lumen diameter. Nobuyoshi et al. also found that stenosis diameter decreased between 1 and 3 months, but reached a

TABLE 1. *Incidence of clinical restenosis*

Study	Incidence (%)	Reference
Gruentzig et al.	25	12
Bertrand et al.	27	13
Kent et al.	17	14
Kaltenbach et al.	17	15
Leimgruber et al.	30	16
Mabin et al.	22	17

plateau at 3 months and did not deteriorate significantly thereafter (11), (Fig. 3).

INCIDENCE OF RESTENOSIS

The incidence of clinical restenosis is reported to be 17% to 33% (Table 1) (12–17). The incidence of angiographic restenosis in various published series is approximately 30% to 34% (Table 2) (6,8,18,34). The discrepancy between the incidence of angiographic restenosis and clinical restenosis raises some interesting issues (Fig. 4). Does this mean that a large number of patients experience silent ischemia following angioplasty? Or do collateral vessels form and mature in some patients following angioplasty with the result that there is less myocardial ischemia when the angioplastied lesion becomes hemodynamically significant? In patients with previous myocardial infarction, is the myocardial region served by the angioplastied vessel too small to produce ischemia when angiographic restenosis occurs? Any one of these explanations could provide an answer in individual patients.

PATIENT CHARACTERISTICS LEADING TO RESTENOSIS

There are certain characteristics of patients that are predictive of higher clinical restenosis rates. These characteristics and the approximate relative risk of restenosis for each characteristic are listed in Table 3. These predictors of restenosis can be used by the clinician to estimate the probability of restenosis when deciding whether to proceed with an angioplasty for an individual patient. These clinical predictors are also important because they may provide some insight into the pathophysiology of restenosis in patients. Caution must be used when interpreting predictors of clinical restenosis, however, since detection bias may result in certain types of patients ap-

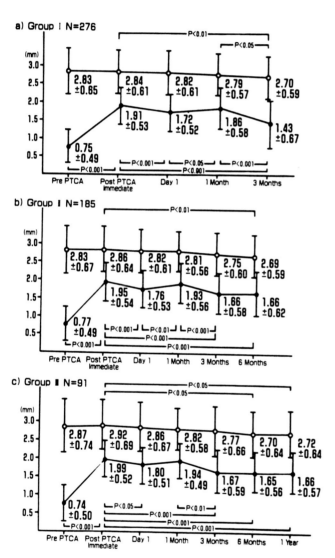

FIG. 3. The change in minimal lumen diameter (MLD) and reference diameters for three groups of patients serially studied over time. Group 1 patients were studied at 1 day, 1 month, and 3 months. Group 2 patients at 1 day, 3 months, and 6 months. Group 3 patients at 1 day, 1 month, 3 months, 6 months and 1 year. The change in MLD was greatest after 3 months following a successful angioplasty. From Nobuyoshi (11), with permission.

TABLE 2. *Incidence of angiographic restenosis*

Study	% Angio follow-up	Incidence (%)	Reference
Gruentzig et al.	93	31	8
Holmes et al.	84	34	18
Roubin et al.	83	30	6
Simonton et al.	89	30	34

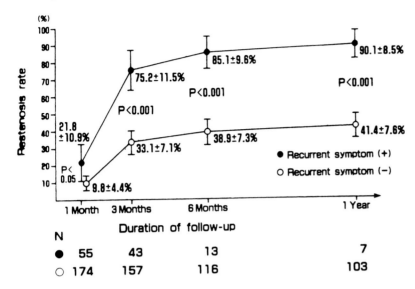

FIG. 4. The incidence of restenosis (defined as >50% stenosis at follow-up) is significantly higher in symptomatic patients than in asymptomatic patients. However, narrowing is evident even in patients without symptoms. From Nobuyoshi (11), with permission.

pearing to have higher restenosis rates. For example, angioplasty of the left anterior descending (LAD) artery usually involves a larger area of myocardium, which may cause more extensive myocardial ischemia. Therefore, a patient with an LAD angioplasty may be more likely to return and have restenosis detected. Such potential sources of bias should be considered before concluding that a certain factor is associated with a higher rate of restenosis.

Men have been shown to have a higher restenosis rate. Cowley reported data from the National Heart, Lung, and Blood Institute (NHLBI) Angioplasty Registry indicating that the clinical restenosis rate for men is 36%, as compared with a rate of 22% in women (20).

Patients who continue to smoke have a higher restenosis rate. Galan et al. reported an angiographic restenosis rate of 55% in patients who continued to smoke, as compared with a 38% rate in patients who stopped smoking at the time of angioplasty (21). Kaltenbach et al. reported a very low restenosis rate of 15% among patients who were required to stop smoking before undergoing angioplasty (22). It is likely that platelets have an important causative role in restenosis, and smoking has been shown to increase platelet adhesiveness (23).

Diabetic patients have a higher restenosis rate. Holmes et al. reported from the NHLBI Angioplasty Registry that the angiographic restenosis rate in diabetic pa-

tients is 47%, as compared with a rate of 32% in nondiabetic patients (24). Margolis et al. reported an extraordinarily high restenosis rate of 75% in patients with insulin-dependent diabetes, as compared with a rate of 22% in controls (25). Insulin is a known growth factor (26) and it may be that diabetic patients with hyperinsulinemia have a greater propensity to develop restenosis because of the proliferative effects of insulin.

Hypercholesterolemia may be a risk factor for restenosis, although studies that have evaluated this issue have revealed mixed results. Jacobs et al. studied 165 consecutively treated angioplasty patients and found that the cholesterol level was not different in patients who developed restenosis, as compared with patients without restenosis (27). These investigators subsequently studied the lipoprotein profiles of 250 patients who developed restenosis, compared with a randomly chosen sample of 350 patients who did not develop restenosis (28). In this analysis, the cholesterol was slightly but significantly higher in male patients who developed restenosis. Furthermore, high-density lipoprotein (HDL) cholesterol was significantly lower and apoprotein B and apoprotein A1 were significantly higher in male patients who developed restenosis. Among female patients, apoprotein A1 was significantly higher in patients developing restenosis. Harlan et al. recently reported the lipoprotein profile from a cohort of 2,100 patients undergoing first-time native coronary angioplasty, 86% of whom had angiographic followup (29). In this study, serum cholesterol levels were not predictive of restenosis. There was a linear decline in the restenosis rate with increasing HDL levels above 40 mg/dl. Thus, lipoproteins appear to have some effect on restenosis, although further studies will be necessary to clarify this issue.

It is interesting that several of the risk factors for atherosclerosis, namely, male gender, smoking, diabetes, and hypercholesterolemia, have been associated with higher restenosis rates. Although there are major differences between the pathologic appearance of restenosis

TABLE 3. *Patient characteristics affecting restenosis*

Characteristic	Relative risk	Reference
Male gender	1.6	20
Continued smoking	1.5	21,22
Diabetes mellitus	1.5–3.4	24,25
Hypercholesterolemia	variable	27–29
Chronic dialysis	high	30
Unstable angina	1.5	24,31–33
Acute infarction	0.6	34
Previous infarction	1.4	24
Variant angina	2.9	36–38

and atherosclerosis, both processes may represent an abnormal vessel healing response. In the case of restenosis, this healing response is secondary to an abrupt insult at the site of an atherosclerotic plaque. In the case of atherosclerosis, this healing response is perhaps due to chronic low-grade vessel injury in a previously normal vessel. It is quite possible that many of the same mechanisms, involving growth factors and cell-to-cell communications, are operative in both of these pathologic processes.

Kahn et al. recently reported that restenosis is particularly prevalent in chronic dialysis patients (30). Follow-up angiography in 12 chronic dialysis patients revealed restenosis in 26 of 32 (81%) of the angioplasty sites. These authors postulated that platelet hyperaggregability contributed to the extraordinarily high restenosis rates in these chronically ill patients.

Patients who undergo angioplasty for treatment of unstable angina have a higher restenosis rate. Data from the NHLBI registry indicated that patients with new onset angina have a restenosis rate of 44%, as compared with a restenosis rate of 29% in patients with chronic angina (24). Results from many other studies have revealed similar results (31–33). Again, platelets and thrombosis may contribute to the higher restenosis rate in these patients. Angiographic and angioscopic studies have demonstrated the presence of thrombus in patients with unstable symptoms. The higher incidence of restenosis in patients with unstable angina provides another clue that thrombus may contribute to the restenosis process. The restenosis rate following angioplasty for acute myocardial infarction, however, does not appear to be increased. In a study of 91 patients, Simonton et al. found that the in-hospital abrupt closure rate was significantly higher in patients with acute myocardial infarction undergoing angioplasty, but the long-term restenosis rate was actually lower (19%), as compared with patients undergoing elective angioplasty, who had a 33% restenosis rate (34). The reason for the lower restenosis rate in these acute myocardial infarction patients is unclear, but may be related to concomitant use of thrombolytic therapy, which may have produced an antiplatelet effect by causing systemic fibrinolysis.

Patients with no previous myocardial infarction have a slightly higher clinical restenosis rate. In the NHLBI registry, patients without previous infarction have a restenosis rate of 37%, as compared with a restenosis rate of 26% in patients with a history of previous infarction (24). It is possible that this apparent increase in restenosis in these patients reflects detection bias. Patients with prior infarction may have less viable myocardium served by the angioplastied vessel or may have more collateral vessels to the angioplastied vessel and, therefore, may be more prone to develop silent restenosis. It is not known whether the angiographic restenosis rate is higher in patients with no previous infarction.

Patients with variant angina have a higher restenosis rate. Corcos et al. reported a 58% restenosis rate in patients with variant angina (35). This finding has been confirmed in other studies (36–38) and may reflect an ineffective initial procedure rather than true restenosis. In such patients, angioplasty will not affect the tendency for vascular smooth muscle spasm and in fact may worsen the tendency for spasm because of the endothelial denudation caused by the angioplasty. Endothelial denudation exposes the underlying vascular smooth muscle to circulating platelets and vasoactive substances which can potentially precipitate or worsen coronary vasospasm. Alternatively, vasospasm may increase the tendency for true restenosis caused by neointimal proliferation. Bertrand et al. showed that patients who had arterial spasm provoked by ergonovine 6 months after angioplasty had a 43% to 58% restenosis rate, as compared with a 20% restenosis rate in patients who did not show coronary artery spasm before or after angioplasty (39). It is possible that recurrent vessel spasm in the setting of variant angina may cause repeated reductions in blood flow and that this may adversely affect vessel remodeling and result in restenosis.

VESSEL CHARACTERISTICS LEADING TO RESTENOSIS

There are certain anatomic characteristics of coronary vessels that are predictive of higher clinical restenosis rates. These characteristics and the relative risk of restenosis for each characteristic are listed in Table 4.

Angioplasty of the left anterior descending artery has been associated with a higher restenosis rate. Leimgruber et al. found that the clinical restenosis rate was 34% for LAD angioplasty, as compared with 18% for the circumflex artery and 27% for the right coronary artery (33). A potential limitation of the study by Leimgruber et al. and of other studies is a low rate of angiographic follow-up. The Leimgruber study had an angiographic follow-up rate of 57%. The NHLBI angioplasty registry had an 84% angiographic follow-up rate, and this study did not report that LAD angioplasty was associated with a higher restenosis rate (24). A higher clinical restenosis rate following LAD angioplasty could be explained by detection bias. Usually, the LAD supplies a large amount of myocardium, and stenosis here is more likely to cause symptomatic ischemia or a positive exercise test than in a smaller artery. Therefore, restenosis of the LAD is more

TABLE 4. *Vessel characteristics affecting restenosis*

Characteristic	Relative risk	Reference
LAD	1.3–1.9	33
Ostial LAD	1.7	40
Saphenous vein grafts	1.5–2.0	41–45
Ostial RCA	high	46
Long lesions	2.1–7.3	47–49
Lesions at bend points	1.4	50
Chronic total occlusions	2.0	51,52

likely to come to the attention of the patient and the clinician. Further studies with angiographic follow-up will be necessary to clarify whether the LAD is intrinsically more prone to restenosis.

The ostium of the LAD appears to be particularly prone to restenosis. Whitworth et al. studied 172 patients undergoing angioplasty of the LAD (40). Patients with ostial LAD angioplasty had a restenosis rate of 63%, as compared with a 38% restenosis rate in patients with nonostial LAD angioplasty.

Restenosis following angioplasty of saphenous vein grafts has been studied extensively. Patients with graft stenoses are particularly appealing angioplasty candidates, since reoperation carries a higher operative mortality and morbidity than an initial bypass operation and since medical therapy is often inadequate. Unfortunately, angioplasty of saphenous vein grafts carries a higher clinical restenosis rate, which ranges, in various studies, from 37% to 50% (41–45). Block et al. reported that proximal to mid saphenous vein grafts have a 56% restenosis rate, whereas mid to distal grafts have a 15% restenosis rate (41). Platko et al., however, found a 50% restenosis rate in proximal vein grafts, a 45% restenosis rate in the body of vein grafts and a 42% restenosis rate in distal vein grafts (42). Other studies have suggested that angioplasty of the distal saphenous vein at the site of the distal anastomosis has a restenosis rate that is similar to that of native coronary arteries. Cote et al. studied 26 patients angiographically, after saphenous vein angioplasty, and found that, in patients with patent vessels, the average balloon to graft ratio was 1.00, significantly larger than a ratio of 0.83 in patients with restenosis, a finding which suggested that larger balloon sizing may be important for reducing the restenosis rate (45). These investigators also found that the residual stenosis immediately following angioplasty in nonrestenosed grafts was 22%, as compared with a residual stenosis of 34% in restenosed grafts.

Ostial lesions of the right coronary artery, saphenous vein grafts and protected left main arteries appear to behave differently than native coronary arteries in several ways. In such lesions, the balloon is dilating the atherosclerotic plaque in the aortic root in a transverse fashion, rather than in a longitudinal fashion as in a straight segment of a native coronary artery. The mechanism of dilation may be different in such lesions and the primary success rate is lower. Topol et al. studied 42 patients undergoing right coronary ostial angioplasty at three centers and reported that the primary success rate in ostial right coronary artery lesions was 79%, and that 9.4% required emergency bypass surgery (46). Furthermore, these investigators found a 48% clinical restenosis rate for right coronary ostial lesions. Of 22 patients (52%) undergoing repeat angiography, angiographic restenosis occurred in 16 (73%, or 38% of the total study population). The authors speculated that the higher primary

failure rate and the higher restenosis rate in these patients may be due to technical factors, including a requirement for higher balloon inflation pressures, difficulty in adequately dilating lesions, and difficulty with guiding catheters.

Long lesions are associated with a higher restenosis rate. Hall and Gruentzig reported a 45% clinical restenosis rate in patients with lesions longer than 16 mm, as compared with a 21% to 28% restenosis rate for lesions less than 10 mm (47). Other studies have confirmed this finding (48,49), and Uebis et al. (49) found that lesions with a length of less than 2 mm had an angiographic restenosis rate of only 4.5%, as compared with a rate of 33% for longer lesions. Ellis et al., however, did not find lesion length to be a significant predictor of restenosis (50). Dilation along multiple balloon lengths causes a greater amount of endothelial denudation and exposes greater amounts of underlying tissue to circulating growth factors. This may increase the chances of restenosis.

There are data suggesting that bifurcation lesions and lesions at bend points have a higher restenosis rate (50). It is possible that these areas in the coronary vasculature have higher shear forces which affect vascular healing and result in higher restenosis rates.

Angioplasty of chronic total occlusions has been shown to have a higher restenosis rate. In a multicenter study of 484 patients, Ellis et al. reported an angiographic restenosis rate of 41% at 6 months and a 66% restenosis rate at 12 months (51). In these patients, who frequently have well-developed collateral vessels, silent restenosis leading to total reocclusion was common, although myocardial infarction was rare. Finci et al. reported restenosis in 45% of patients with angioplasty of chronic total occlusions (52).

PROCEDURAL FACTORS LEADING TO RESTENOSIS

There are certain procedural factors that are predictive of higher clinical restenosis rates. These factors and the relative risk of restenosis for each characteristic are listed in Table 5.

The most obvious and important procedural factor affecting restenosis rates is multivessel angioplasty. Initially, angioplasty was restricted to patients with single-vessel disease. More recently, multivessel angioplasty has been performed with increased frequency. Patients

TABLE 5. *Procedural factors affecting restenosis*

Factor	Relative risk	Reference
Multivessel disease	1.4	54–58
Residual lesion	1.4	33
Intimal dissection	0.8	69,70
High coronary wedge pressure	2.3	72

undergoing multivessel angioplasty have a higher restenosis rate than patients with single-vessel angioplasty. Interestingly, the restenosis rates in multivessel angioplasty are not multiples of the restenosis rates of individual vessels (53). In other words, a patient undergoing two-vessel angioplasty is not twice as likely to develop restenosis as a patient undergoing one-vessel angioplasty. This finding underscores the concept that multiple risk factors lead to restenosis, and that these factors lead to restenosis in a complex fashion. In a single patient with multivessel angioplasty, these factors may lead to restenosis in one vessel, while other vessels will not develop restenosis. Several studies have shown that the clinical restenosis rate following multivessel angioplasty is approximately 34% (54–58). Follow-up studies with more complete angiographic follow-up report a higher restenosis rate of approximately 50% (59–62). Of the patients who develop restenosis, over half develop single-vessel restenosis and less than half develop multivessel restenosis (58,63). Vandormael et al. (60) found that patient-related variables were not predictive of multivessel restenosis; however, Lambert et al. (59) found multivessel restenosis more common in patients with diabetes and recent onset angina, and Shaw et al. (64) found multivessel restenosis more common in patients with diabetes, hypercholesterolemia, smokers, and patients with recent onset angina.

Lambert et al. (65) and DiSciascio et al. (66) found that multilesion angioplasty (that is, dilatation of multiple lesions in the same vessel) had the same clinical restenosis rate as multivessel restenosis, approximately 30%.

There are several other procedural factors that influence restenosis rates. In general, the better the angioplasty result, the lower the clinical restenosis rate. In procedures where the resultant lesion is less than 30%, and the translesional pressure gradient is low, the restenosis rate tends to be lower (33). Whether this finding indicates that underdilated lesions are more prone to neointimal proliferation is open to question. It is possible that an underdilated vessel is simply more prone to produce a hemodynamically significant lesion and symptoms than a vessel that is more completely dilated. For example, a patient with a residual stenosis of 45% following angioplasty may have a hemodynamically significant lesion of 65% after a deterioration of only 20%. Another patient with a residual stenosis of 20% following angioplasty may have a hemodynamically insignificant lesion of 40% following a similar deterioration of 20%. Therefore, patients with a residual stenosis of 45% would have a higher clinical restenosis rate without having a larger amount of neointimal proliferation. As a practical point, the angioplasty operator should always strive for the best possible angiographic result by carefully measuring the vessel size and using the appropriately sized balloon. If this balloon results in inadequate dilation, the balloon size and inflation pressure can be progressively and grad-

ually increased to achieve a better angiographic result, while carefully avoiding vessel dissection.

Roubin et al. examined whether using purposefully oversized balloons would result in a lower restenosis rate (67). Unfortunately, larger balloon sizing resulted in a higher abrupt closure rate and the trial was prematurely halted. A higher incidence of dissection with larger balloon sizes was also seen by Nichols et al., but undersized balloons resulted in a larger residual stenosis and a higher restenosis rate (68).

Leimgruber et al. reported that intimal dissection seen after angioplasty was associated with a lower restenosis rate (69). In a study of 986 patients, clinical restenosis was seen in 24% of patients with intimal dissection, as compared with 30% of patients without intimal dissection. Matthews et al., however, reported that intimal dissection was not predictive of a lower restenosis rate in a study of 273 patients (70). It is possible that a small intimal dissection is a marker of more complete dilatation, and as noted above, patients with less residual stenosis are less likely to develop restenosis.

DiSciascio et al. found that the length of balloon inflation time did not influence restenosis rates in patients with total occlusions (71). Angioplasty with 1-min inflations had a similar restenosis rate to that for angioplasty with 5-min inflations.

Coronary wedge pressure, that is the balloon lumen pressure during balloon inflation, was evaluated as a predictor of restenosis. The coronary wedge pressure is thought to reflect the adequacy of collateral vessels. Urban et al. (72) found that patients with a coronary wedge pressure of greater or equal to 30 mmHg have a 52% restenosis rate, as compared with a 23% restenosis rate in patients with a coronary wedge pressure of less than 30. Thus, competitive flow through collateral channels may have a negative impact on vessel remodeling and result in higher restenosis rates.

EXERCISE STRESS TESTING TO DETECT ANGIOGRAPHIC RESTENOSIS

Several investigators have evaluated the use of exercise stress testing to detect angiographic restenosis. The accuracy of exercise stress testing in predicting restenosis is influenced by the timing of the stress test, the extent of coronary disease in other vessels, as well as other factors which influence exercise stress test results. Wijns et al. found the positive predictive value of ST depression or angina during stress testing to detect restenosis to be 50% and the negative predictive value to be 65% (73). Deligonul et al. evaluated 196 patients with exercise stress testing 1 month following angioplasty and found that the test was more likely to be positive in patients with multivessel disease or with incomplete revascularization, but was not predictive of restenosis (74). These investigators found that exercise stress testing at 1 month was indicative of future cardiac events, but they recommended performing stress testing at a later date to detect restenosis. Bengtson et al. performed 6-month exercise stress tests in 228 patients who did not have cardiac events or early repeat revascularization in the interval since the angioplasty (75). In this study with 92% angiographic follow-up, exercise-induced angina, recurrent angina, and a positive treadmill test were independent predictors of restenosis. Although the exercise stress test improved the ability to detect restenosis, 20% of patients with restenosis had neither recurrent angina nor a positive stress test. Laarman et al. also addressed whether exercise stress testing can identify patients with silent restenosis (76). They found that exercise stress testing detected silent restenosis with a sensitivity of 24% and with a specificity of 82%. Honan et al. found that exercise stress testing was a particularly poor predictor of restenosis in patients undergoing angioplasty for acute myocardial infarction (77). In 144 patients, exercise stress testing detected restenosis with a sensitivity of only 24% and with a specificity of 88%.

Several investigators have evaluated the utility of thallium stress testing following angioplasty (73,78–83). Wijns et al. studied 91 asymptomatic patients an average of 5 weeks after successful angioplasty (79). Thallium stress testing was able to detect silent restenosis with a positive predictive value of 82%, as compared with a positive predictive value of only 60% for electrocardiographic stress testing alone. Manyari et al. studied 43 patients at average times of 9 days, 3.3 months, and 6.8 months after single-vessel angioplasty (82). They found that early on, thallium scanning could be abnormal, and did not necessarily reflect residual stenosis or recurrence. It appears that thallium stress testing can detect restenosis when properly timed following angioplasty. The predictive value of thallium stress testing to predict restenosis and other cardiac events appears to be better than electrocardiographic stress testing alone, and thallium stress testing may be useful in detecting silent restenosis.

Exercise radionuclide angiography has also been used to detect restenosis or predict patients who will develop restenosis (84–86). This technique appears to be a sensitive method of detecting exercise-induced myocardial ischemia, which may represent restenosis, but the technique is limited in patients with regional wall motion abnormalities due to prior infarctions, and the positive predictive value is low. Exercise echocardiography has also been reported (87), but would also be expected to show false positive results in patients with prior infarctions.

PATHOPHYSIOLOGY OF RESTENOSIS

The pathophysiology of restenosis is a complex subject that has been covered more extensively in other

TABLE 6. *Factors contributing to restenosis*

Elastic vessel recoil
Arterial spasm
Platelet adhesion and aggregation
Thrombus formation
Inflammatory cell infiltration
Smooth muscle cell migration and proliferation
Organization of connective tissue matrix

chapters of this book. From epidemiologic studies and experimental animal studies, it appears that several factors contribute to the occurrence of restenosis, and no one factor is solely responsible. The factors that have been postulated as contributing to restenosis are listed in Tables 6 and 7. Studies evaluating these mechanisms have led investigators to test a number of pharmacologic and mechanical approaches to prevent restenosis. These efforts have been hampered by the lack of an ideal animal model for simulating restenosis. Several agents have been shown to reduce the incidence of restenosis in several animal models, but no pharmacologic agent has yet proved effective in patients.

DRUG THERAPY FOR RESTENOSIS

Because of the early recognition of platelet aggregation following angioplasty, antiplatelet drugs have been extensively studied. Studies have indicated that aspirin reduces the incidence of abrupt vessel closure during angioplasty (88), but aspirin has no effect on restenosis (88–94). Other antiplatelet agents, including dipyridamole and ticlopidine, have proved ineffective (90). A prostacyclin analogue, ciprostene, has shown promise but needs further study (91).

Fish oils have antiplatelet effects as well as antiinflammatory effects. In one study, fish oil was given 1 week prior to angioplasty, and for 6 months after angioplasty (92). The restenosis rate was 19% in the treatment group as compared with 46% in the placebo group. Two other randomized controlled trials failed to show benefit, but in these trials, fish oil was begun after angioplasty (93,94). Fish oils are currently being studied in a larger trial. Several other antiplatelet agents, including a monoclonal antibody to the platelet glycoprotein IIb/IIIa, antibodies to von Willebrand factor, ketanserin (an inhibitor of serotonin), thromboxane synthetase inhibitors, and thromboxane receptor antagonists are being tested.

Trapadil, an agent that inhibits platelet derived growth factor (PDGF) has been shown to inhibit restenosis in animals, and one study has indicated that this agent may have benefit in patients (95). Other inhibitors of PDGF are also being studied.

In two small studies, warfarin did not appear to reduce restenosis (89,96) although a combination of aspirin and warfarin was effective in preventing restenosis in an atherosclerotic rabbit model of angioplasty (97). Heparin has antithrombotic effects, but also has effects on smooth muscle cell proliferation (98). Studies using short-term heparin have shown no benefit on restenosis, but long-term therapy may be necessary. In animals, prolonged therapy with a low molecular weight heparin, enoxaparin, can reduce restenosis (99), and several clinical trials are currently studying this agent. Specific antithrombin therapy with recombinant hirudin is also currently being tested.

Angiotensin II has been shown to stimulate smooth muscle hypertrophy and an inhibitor of angiotensin converting enzyme, cilazapril, has been shown to inhibit smooth muscle thickening after balloon denudation in a rat carotid model (100). This agent is currently being tested in two multicenter trials in Europe and North America.

Because vasospasm may contribute to restenosis, calcium channel antagonists have been tested. Diltiazem, nifedipine, and verapamil have all been ineffective in preventing restenosis (101–103).

Glucocorticoids in combination with heparin have been shown to inhibit smooth muscle cell proliferation in a balloon injury model of restenosis (104). Use of bolus steroids at the time of angioplasty, or oral steroid therapy for 7 days, has been ineffective (105,106). Colchicine potentially limits smooth muscle cell migration (107), however, colchicine has not been beneficial in patients (108). Angiopeptin, an analogue of somatostatin, the pituitary growth hormone has shown potential in experimental studies (109), and a clinical trial is being planned.

Despite enormous efforts, there is no known pharmacologic agent that prevents restenosis. It is likely that further research into the biologic mechanisms of restenosis will lead to an agent or combination of agents that will eventually prove effective.

DEVICES TO PREVENT RESTENOSIS

Investigators have hypothesized that restenosis is a healing response to arterial injury and that by reducing the degree of injury, restenosis will be reduced. Several devices have been developed that could potentially reduce the degree of injury. Laser devices have been tested, and trials using the eximer laser device are currently underway. Preliminary results indicate that laser systems do not reduce restenosis rates (110). Laser balloon angioplasty appears to cause thermal fusion of separated tissues during balloon angioplasty; however, laser balloon angioplasty does not reduce restenosis (111).

The Simpson directional athrectomy device has been developed on the theory that excision of plaque rather than stretching results in a smooth luminal surface which will be less prone to restenosis and abrupt closure. The Athrectomy Multicenter Study recently reported an incidence of restenosis of 30% (112). There is some evi-

dence that the restenosis rate of proximal lesions, particularly ostial LAD lesions is less using this device, although this requires further study.

Stents hold potential for reducing restenosis by reducing elastic recoil and spasm and producing a smooth internal arterial surface. A stent is a foreign object, however, and promotes thrombus formation. No randomized trial has evaluated stents, although retrospective subgroup analyses of stent data suggest that single stents placed for first-time angioplasty in larger arteries may result in a lower restenosis rate (113).

CURRENT APPROACHES TO PREVENTION AND TREATMENT OF RESTENOSIS

At present, no drug or device appears to reduce restenosis, although there are preliminary data on several approaches which show promise. Our current practice includes the routine use of aspirin before, and heparin during, the angioplasty procedure to prevent abrupt occlusion, and calcium channel antagonists for approximately 6 weeks following the angioplasty to prevent spasm. At the present time, other therapeutic regimens or devices cannot be recommended for routine use.

TABLE 7. *Potential mechanisms of restenosis and future directors of therapy*

Mechanism	Potential therapy
Recoil	Prolonged balloon inflations, stents
Platelet deposition	Antibody to glycoproteinIIB/IIIA
	Antibody to von Willebrand factor
Thrombus formation	Thrombin inhibitors
	Warfarin/aspirin
	Heparins
Inflammation	Steroids
	Cyclosporin
	Colchicine
Growth factors	Trapidil, suramin
	Ketanserin
	ACE inhibitors
	Angiopeptin
	GR32191B
	Heparins
Smooth muscle cell	
Migration	ACE inhibitors
	Colchicine
Proliferation	ACE inhibitors
	Lovastatin
	Heparins
	Antimetabolites
	Gene transfer
Hypertrophy	ACE inhibitors
	Thrombin inhibitors
Matrix production	Colchicine
	Heparins
	Thrombin inhibitors
Delayed reendothelialization	Endothelial cell seeding, gene transfer

ACE, angiotensin-converting-enzyme.

When restenosis occurs, the standard treatment at most centers is repeat angioplasty. Williams et al. reported from the NHLBI registry that repeat angioplasty had a higher initial success rate than a first-time angioplasty (114). Recent reports indicate that the success rates for second and third angioplasty are approximately 93% (115,116). The restenosis lesion may differ from the original lesion in terms of length of the lesion and involvement of side branches, as shown in Fig. 5. Usually, repeat angioplasty with the same size balloon and to the same inflation pressure achieves an acceptable result. If the cineangiogram of the initial angioplasty shows any degree of underdilation, it is useful to carefully upsize the balloon size slightly to achieve a better angiographic result.

To determine the restenosis rates after multiple angioplasties, Glazier et al. obtained clinical followup on

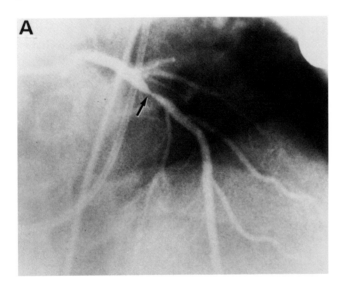

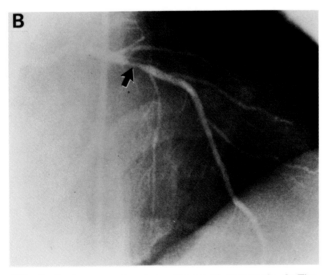

FIG. 5. Angiograms showing patterns of restenosis. **A:** The LAD has a tight discrete stenosis which was successfully dilated. **B:** When the patient returned with recurrent angina, the lesion had restenosed as a longer lesion.

1,162 consecutive patients undergoing angioplasty (117). The clinical restenosis rates were 20%, 26%, 34%, and 50% following the first, second, third, and fourth angioplasties, respectively. In this study, multivariate analysis revealed that patients who develop recurrent symptoms less than 60 days after the initial angioplasty are more likely to have recurrent restenosis (118). Also, as in other studies, a larger number of balloon inflations was associated with a higher restenosis rate. Black et al. found that a second restenosis occurred in 31% of patients undergoing a second angioplasty (119). Multivariate predictors of a second restenosis were a short interval between the first and second angioplasty, male gender, longer lesions, and the need to have an additional site dilated at the time of the second angioplasty. Quigley reported a 32% recurrent restenosis rate in a cohort of 114 patients with 88% angiographic followup (120). Again, the interval between the first and second angioplasty was predictive of recurrent restenosis. Multivariate analysis indicated that unstable angina, diabetes, and hypertension were independent predictors of recurrent restenosis.

When recurrent restenosis occurs, the physician is confronted with a decision whether to continue to perform repeated angioplasties, or to refer the patient for bypass surgery. Brush et al. evaluated the economic consequences of recurrent restenosis and found that repeating the angioplasty for the first restenosis is clearly the less expensive strategy (121). Following the second restenosis, repeat angioplasty or bypass surgery are approximately equal in terms of the charges accrued. Therefore, the decision between repeat angioplasty or bypass surgery for recurrent restenosis is usually made on an individual basis, often based on patient preferences, since neither option is clearly less expensive.

Restenosis has been termed the Achilles heel of angioplasty, and continues to be a major limitation of the procedure. It is the hope of all physicians who care for patients with coronary artery disease that further research will yield an answer to the restenosis question and will thus further improve the efficacy of coronary angioplasty.

REFERENCES

1. Blackshear JL, O'Callaghan WG, Califf RM. Medical approaches to prevention of restenosis after coronary angioplasty. *J Am Coll Cardiol* 1987;9:834–848.
2. McBride W, Lange RA, Hillis LD. Restenosis after successful coronary angioplasty. *N Engl J Med* 1988;318:1734–1737.
3. Kent KM. Restenosis after percutaneous transluminal coronary angioplasty. *Am J Cardiol* 1988;61:67G–70G.
4. Meier B. Restenosis after coronary angioplasty: review of literature. *Eur Heart J* 1988;9[Suppl C]:1–6.
5. Popma JJ, Topol EJ. Factors influencing restenosis after coronary angioplasty. *Am J Med* 1990;88:1N–24N.
6. Roubin GS, King III SB, Douglas JS Jr. Restenosis after percutaneous transluminal coronary angioplasty: the Emory University Hospital experience. *Am J Cardiol* 1987;60:39B–43B.

7. Rosing DR, Cannon RO III, Watson RM, Bonow RO, Mincemoyer R, Ewels C, Leon MB, Lakatos E, Epstein SE, Kent KM. Three year anatomic, functional and clinical follow-up after successful percutaneous transluminal coronary angioplasty. *J Am Coll Cardiol* 1987;9:1–7.

8. Gruentzig AR, King SB III, Schlumpf M, Siegenthaler W. Long-term follow-up after percutaneous transluminal coronary angioplasty. The early Zurich experience. *N Engl J Med* 1987;316:1127–1132.

9. Beatt KJ, Serruys PW, Hugenholtz PG. Restenosis after coronary angioplasty: new standards for clinical studies. *J Am Coll Cardiol* 1990;15:491–498.

9a. Rensing BJ, Hermans WRM, Deckers JW, deFeyter PJ, Tijssen JGP, Serruys PW. Luminal narrowing after percutaneous transluminal coronary balloon angioplasty follows a near Gaussian distribution: a quantitative angiographic study of 1,445 successfully dilated lesions. *J Am Coll Cardiol* (in press).

9b. Beatt KJ, Serruys PW, Hugenholtz PG. Restenosis after coronary angioplasty: new standards for clinical studies [Editorial]. *J Am Coll Cardiol* 1990:15:491–498.

9c. Serruys PW, Foley DP, deFeyter PJ. Angiographic assessment of restenosis after coronary angioplasty and other devices: is it time for a new comparative approach based on quantitative angiography? *J Am Coll Cardiol* (in press).

10. Serruys PW, Luijten HE, Beatt KJ, Geuskens R, DeFeyter PJ, Van DenBrand M, Reiber JHC, Ten Katen HJ, Van Es A, Hugenholtz PG. Incidence of restenosis after successful coronary angioplasty: a time-related phenomenon: a quantitative angiographic study in 342 consecutive patients at 1, 2, 3, and 4 months. *Circulation* 1988;77:361–371.

11. Nobuyoshi M, Kimura T, Nosaka H, Mioka S, Ueno K, Yokoi H, Hamasaki N, Horiuchi H, Ohishi H. Restenosis after successful percutaneous transluminal coronary angioplasty: serial angiographic follow-up of 229 patients. *J Am Coll Cardiol* 1988;12:616–623.

12. Gruentzig A. Results from coronary angioplasty and implications for the future. *Am Heart J* 1982;103:779–783.

13. Bertrand ME, Thieuleux FA, LaBlanche JM, Fourrier JL, Traisnel G. L'angioplastie transluminale coronaire: resultats immediats et à court terme. *Arch Mal Coeur Vaiss* 1986;79:40–46.

14. Kent KM, Bentivoglio LG, Block PC, Cowley MJ, Dorros G, Gosselin AJ, Gruentzig A, Myler RK, Simpson J, Stertzer SH, Williams DO, Fisher L, Gillespie MJ, Detre K, Kelsey S, Mullin SM, Mock MB. Percutaneous transluminal coronary angioplasty: report from the registry of the National Heart, Lung, and Blood Institute. *Am J Cardiol* 1982;49:2011–2019.

15. Kaltenbach M, Kober G, Scherer D, Vallbracht C. Recurrence rate after successful coronary angioplasty. *Eur Heart J* 1985;6:276–281.

16. Leimgruber PP, Roubin GS, Anderson V, Bredlau CE, Whitworth HB, Douglas SJ, King SB, Gruentzig AR. Influence of intimal dissection on restenosis after successful coronary angioplasty. *Circulation* 1985;72:530–535.

17. Mabin TA, Holmes DR, Smith HC, Vlietstra RE, Reeder GS, Bresnahan JF, Bove AA, Hammes LN, Elveback LR, Orszulak TA. Follow-up clinical results in patients undergoing percutaneous transluminal coronary angioplasty. *Circulation* 1985;71:754–760.

18. Holmes DR, Vlietstra RE, Smith HC, Vetrovec GW, Kent KM, Cowley MJ, Faxon DP, Gruentzig AR, Kelsey SF, Detre KM, Van Raden MJ, Mock MB. Restenosis after percutaneous transluminal coronary angioplasty (PTCA): a report from the PTCA Registry of the National Heart, Lung, and Blood Institute. *Am J Cardiol* 1984;53:77C–81C.

19. DiSciascio G, Vetrovec GW, Lewis SA, Nath A, Cole SK, Edwards VL. Clinical and angiographic recurrence following PTCA for nonacute total occlusions: comparison of one-versus-five minute inflations. *Am Heart J* 1990;120:529.

20. Cowley MJ, Mullin SM, Kelsey SF, Kent KM, Gruentzig AR, Detre DM, Passamani ER. Sex differences in early and long-term results of coronary angioplasty in the NHLBI PTCA Registry. *Circulation* 1985;71:90–97.

21. Galan KM, Deligonul U, Kern MJ, Chaitman BR, Vandormael MG. Increased frequency of restenosis in patients continuing to smoke cigarettes after percutaneous transluminal coronary angioplasty. *Am J Cardiol* 1988;61:260–263.

22. Kaltenbach M, Kober G, Scherer D, Vallbracht C. Recurrence rate after successful coronary angioplasty. *Eur Heart J* 1985;6:276–281.

23. Nowak J, Murray JJ, Oates JA, Fitzgerald GA. Biochemical evidence of a chronic abnormality in platelet and vascular function in healthy individuals who smoke cigarettes. *Circulation* 1987;76:6–14.

24. Holmes DR, Vlietstra RE, Smith HC, Vetrovec GW, Kent KM, Cowley MJ, Faxon DP, Gruentzig AR, Kelsey SF, Detre KM, Van Raden MJ, Mock MB. Restenosis after percutaneous transluminal coronary angioplasty (PTCA): a report from the PTCA Registry of the National Heart, Lung, and Blood Institute. *Am J Cardiol* 1984;53:77C–81C.

25. Margolis JR, Krieger R, Glemser E. Coronary angioplasty: increased restenosis rate in insulin dependent diabetics. *Circulation* 1984;70[Suppl II]:175.

26. Banskota NK, Taub R, Zellner K, Olsen P, King GL. Characterization of induction of protooncogene c-myc and cellular growth in human vascular smooth muscle cells by insulin and IGF-I. *Diabetes* 1989;38:123–129.

27. Jacobs AK, Folan DJ, McSweeney SM, Faxon DP, Kellett MA, Sanborn TA, Ryan TJ. Effect of plasma lipids on restenosis following coronary angioplasty. *J Am Coll Cardiol* 1987;9:183A.

28. Bergelson BA, Jacobs AK, Small DM, Tercyak AM, Cupple LA, Garber GR, Erario M, Ruocco NA, Ryan TJ, Faxon DP. Lipoproteins predict restenosis after PTCA. *Circulation* 1989;80[Suppl II]:65.

29. Harlan WR, Fortin DF, Frid DJ, Ramos RF, Lee KL, Rendall D, Califf RM. Are serum lipoproteins important in predicting restenosis after coronary angioplasty? *Circulation* 1989;80[Suppl II]:65.

30. Kahn JK, Rutherford BD, McConahay DR, Johnson WL, Girogi LV, Hartzler GO. Short- and long-term outcome of percutaneous transluminal coronary angioplasty in chronic dialysis patients. *Am Heart J* 1990;119:484.

31. De Feyter PJ, Suryapranata H, Serruys PW, Beatt K, Van Domburg R, Van Den Brand M, Tijssen JJ, Azar AJ, Hugenholtz PG. Coronary angioplasty for unstable angina: immediate and late results in 200 consecutive patients with identification of risk factors for unfavorable early and late outcome. *J Am Coll Cardiol* 1988;12:324–333.

32. Lambert M, Bonan R, Cote G, Crepeau J, De Guise P, Lesperance J, David PR, Waters DD. Multiple coronary angioplasty: a model to discriminate systemic and procedural factors related to restenosis. *J Am Coll Cardiol* 1988;12:310–314.

33. Leimgruber PP, Roubin GS, Hollman J, Cotsonis GA, Meier B, Douglas JS, King SB, Gruentzig AR. Restenosis after successful coronary angioplasty in patients with single-vessel disease. *Circulation* 1986;73:710–717.

34. Simonton CA, Mark DB, Hinohara T, Rendall DS, Phillips HR, Peter RH, Behar VS, Kong Y, O'Callaghan WG, O'Connor C, Califf RM, Stack RS. Late restenosis after emergent coronary angioplasty for acute myocardial infarction: comparison with elective coronary angioplasty. *J Am Coll Cardiol* 1988;11:698–705.

35. Corcos T, David PR, Bourassa MG, Val PG, Robert J, Mata LA, Waters DD. Percutaneous transluminal coronary angioplasty for the treatment of variant angina. *J Am Coll Cardiol* 1985;5:1046–1054.

36. Bertrand ME, LaBlanche JM, Thieuleux FA, Fourrier JL, Traisnel G, Asseman P. Comparative results of percutaneous transluminal coronary angioplasty in patients with dynamic versus fixed coronary stenosis. *J Am Coll Cardiol* 1986;8:504–508.

37. Leish F, Schutzenberger W, Kerschner K, Herbinger. Influence of a variant angina on the results of percutaneous transluminal coronary angioplasty. *Br Heart J* 1986;56:341–345.

38. David PR, Waters DD, Scholl JM, Crepeau J, Szlachcic J, Lesperance J, Hudon G, Bourassa MG. Percutaneous transluminal coronary angioplasty in patients with variant angina. *Circulation* 1982;66:695–702.

39. Bertrand ME, Lablanche JM, Fourrier JL, Gommeaux A, Ruel M. Relation to restenosis after percutaneous transluminal coro-

nary angioplasty to vasomotion of the dilated coronary arterial segment. *Am J Cardiol* 1989;63:277–281.

40. Whitworth HB, Pilcher GS, Roubin GS, Gruentzig AR. Do proximal lesions involving the origin of the left anterior descending artery (LAD) have a higher restenosis rate after coronary angioplasty (PTCA)? *Circulation* 1985;72:III-398.

41. Block PC, Cowley MJ, Kaltenbach M, Kent KM, Simpson J. Percutaneous angioplasty of stenoses of bypass grafts or bypass graft anastomotic sites. *Am J Cardiol* 1984;53:666–668.

42. Platko WP, Hollman J, Whitlow PL, Franco I. Percutaneous transluminal angioplasty of saphenous vein graft stenosis: long-term follow-up. *J Am Coll Cardiol* 1989;14:1645–1650.

43. Dorros G, Johnson WD, Tector AJ, Schmahl TM, Kalush SL, Janke L. Percutaneous transluminal coronary angioplasty in patients with prior coronary artery bypass grafting. *J Thorac Cardiovasc Surg* 1984;87:17–26.

44. Reeder GS, Breshahan JF, Holmes DR, Mock MB, Orszulak TA, Smith HC, Vlietstra RE. Angioplasty for aortocoronary bypass graft stenosis. *Mayo Clin Proc* 1986;61:14–19.

45. Cote G, Myler RK, Stertzer SH, Clark DA, Fishman-Rosen J, Murphy M, Shaw RE. Percutaneous transluminal angioplasty of stenotic coronary artery bypass grafts: 5 years' experience. *J Am Coll Cardiol* 1987;9:8–17.

46. Topol EJ, Ellis SG, Fishman J, Leimgruber P, Myler RK, Stertzer SH, O'Neill WW, Douglas JS, Roubin GS, King SB. Multicenter study of percutaneous transluminal angioplasty for right coronary artery ostial stenosis. *J Am Coll Cardiol* 1987;9:1214–1218.

47. Hall DP, Gruentzig AR. Influence of lesion length on initial success and recurrence rates in coronary angioplasty. *Circulation* 1984;70[Supp II]:176.

48. Hirshfeld JW, Goldberg S, MacDonald R, Vetrovec G, Bass T, Taussig A, Margolis J, Jugo R, Pepine C, for the M-HEART Study Group. Lesion and procedure–related variables predictive of restenosis after PTCA—a report from the M-Heart Study. *Circulation* 1987;76[Suppl IV]:IV-215.

49. Uebis R, von Essen R, vom Dahl J, Schmitz HJ, Seiger K, Effert S. Recurrence rate after PTCA in relationship to the initial length of coronary artery narrowing. *J Am Coll Cardiol* 1986;7:62A.

50. Ellis SG, Roubin GS, King SB, Douglas JS, Cox WR. Importance of stenosis morphology in the estimation of restenosis risk after elective percutaneous transluminal coronary angioplasty. *Am J Cardiol* 1989;63:30–34.

51. Ellis SG, Shaw RE, Gershony G, Thomas R, Roubin GS, Douglas JS, Topol EJ, Stertzer SH, Myler RK, King SB. Risk factors, time course and treatment effect for restenosis after successful percutaneous transluminal coronary angioplasty of chronic total occlusion. *Am J Cardiol* 1989;63:897–901.

52. Finci L, Meier B, Favre J, Righetti A, Rutishauser W. Long-term results of successful and failed angioplasty for chronic total coronary arterial occlusion. *Am J Cardiol* 1990;66:660–662.

53. Tcheng JE, Fortin DF, Frid DJ, Nelson CL, Rendall DS, Lee KL, Stack RS. Conditional probabilities of restenosis following coronary angioplasty. *Circulation* 1990;82[Suppl III]:1.

54. Mata LA, Bosch X, David PR, Rapold HJ, Corcos T, Bourassa MG. Clinical and angiographic assessment 6 months after double vessel percutaneous coronary angioplasty. *J Am Coll Cardiol* 1985;6:1239–1244.

55. Cowley MJ, Vetrovec GW, DiSciascio G, Lewis SA, Hirsh PD, Wolfgand TC. Coronary angioplasty of multiple vessels: short-term outcome and long-term results. *Circulation* 1985;72:1314–1320.

56. Dorros G, Lewin RF, Janke L. Multiple lesion transluminal coronary angioplasty in single and multivessel coronary artery disease: acute outcome and long-term effect. *J Am Coll Cardiol* 1987;10:1007–1013.

57. DiSciascio G, Cowley MJ, Vetrovec GW, Kelly KM, Lewis SA. Triple vessel coronary angioplasty: acute outcome and long-term results. *J Am Coll Cardiol* 1988;12:42–48.

58. O'Keefe JH, Rutherford BD, McConahay DR, Johnson WL, Giorgi LV, Ligon RW, Shimshak TM, Hartzler GO. Multivessel coronary angioplasty from 1980 to 1989: procedural results and long-term outcome. *J Am Coll Cardiol* 1990;16:1097–1102.

59. Lambert M, Bonan R, Cote G, Crepeau J, De Guise P, Lesperance J, David PR, Waters DD. Multiple coronary angioplasty: a model to discriminate systemic and procedural factors related to restenosis. *J Am Coll Cardiol* 1988;12:310–314.

60. Vandormael MG, Deligonul U, Kern MJ, Harper M, Presant 5, Gibson P, Galan K, Chaitman BR. Multilesion coronary angioplasty: clinical and angiographic follow-up. *J Am Coll Cardiol* 1987;10:246–252.

61. Deligonul U, Vandormael MG, Kern MJ, Zelman R, Galan K, Chaitman BR. Coronary angioplasty: a therapeutic option for symptomatic patients with two and three vessel coronary disease. *J Am Coll Cardiol* 1988;11:1173–1179.

62. Finci L, Meier B, De Bruyne B, Steffenino G, Divernois J, Rutishauser W. Angiographic follow-up after multivessel percutaneous transluminal coronary angioplasty. *Am J Cardiol* 1987;60:467–470.

63. DiSciascio G, Cowley MJ, Vetrovec GW. Angiographic patterns of restenosis after angioplasty of multiple coronary arteries. *Am J Cardiol* 1986;58:922–925.

64. Shaw RE, Myler RK, Fishman-Rosen J, Murphy MC, Stertzer SH, Topol EJ. Clinical and morphologic factors in prediction of restenosis after multiple vessel angioplasty. *J Am Coll Cardiol* 1986;7:63A.

65. Lambert M, Bonan R, Cote G, Crepeau J, de Guise P, Lesperance J, David PR, Waters DD. Early results, complications and restenosis rates after multilesion and multivessel percutaneous transluminal coronary angioplasty. *Am J Cardiol* 1987;60:788–791.

66. DiSciascio G, Cowley MJ, Vetrovec GW, Wolfgang TC. Clinical recurrence rates following coronary angioplasty of single lesions, multiple (tandem) lesions, and multiple vessels. *Circulation* 1985;72;[Suppl III]:1590.

67. Roubin GS, Douglas JS, King SB, Hutchison N, Thomas RG, Gruentzig AR. Influence of balloon size on initial success, acute complications, and restenosis after percutaneous transluminal coronary angioplasty. *Circulation* 1988;78:557–565.

68. Nichols AB, Smith R, Berke AD, Shlofmitz RA, Powers ER. Importance of balloon size in coronary angioplasty. *J Am Coll Cardiol* 1989;13:1094–1100.

69. Leimgruber PP, Roubin GS, Anderson V, Bredlau CE, Whitworth HB, Douglas JS, King SB, Gruentzig AR. Influence of intimal dissection on restenosis after successful coronary angioplasty. *Circulation* 1985;72:530–535.

70. Matthews BJ, Ewels CJ, Kent KM. Coronary dissection: a predictor of restenosis? *Am Heart J* 1988;115:547.

71. DiSciascio G, Vetrovec GW, Lewis SA, Nath A, Cole SK, Edwards VL. Clinical and angiographic recurrence following PTCA for nonacute total occlusions: Comparison of one-versus-five minute inflations. *Am Heart J* 1990;120:529.

72. Urban P, Meier B, Finci L, De Bruyne B, Steffenino G, Rutishauser W. Coronary wedge pressure: a predictor of restenosis after coronary balloon angioplasty. *J Am Coll Cardiol* 1987;10:504–509.

73. Wijns W, Serruys PW, Reiber JHC, de Feyter PJ, van den Brand M, Simoons ML, Hugenholtz PG. Early Detection of restenosis after successful percutaneous transluminal coronary angioplasty by exercise-redistribution thallium scintigraphy. *Am J Cardiol* 1985;55:357–361.

74. Deligonul U, Vandormael MG, Shah Y, Galan K, Kern MJ, Chaitman BR. Prognostic value of early exercise stress testing after successful coronary angioplasty: importance of the degree of revascularization. *Am Heart J* 1989;117:509.

75. Bengtson JR, Mark DB, Honan MB, Rendall DS, Hinohara T, Stack RS, Hlatky MA, Califf RM, Lee KL, Pryor DB. Detection of restenosis after elective percutaneous transluminal coronary angioplasty using the exercise treadmill test. *Am J Cardiol* 1990;65:28–34.

76. Laarman G, Luijten HE, van Zeyl LGPM, Beatt KJ, Tijssen JGP, Serruys PW, de Feyter PJ. Assessment of "silent" restenosis and long-term follow-up after successful angioplasty in single vessel coronary artery disease: the value of quantitative exercise electrocardiography and quantitative coronary angiography. *J Am Coll Cardiol* 1990;16:578–585.

77. Honan MB, Bengtson JR, Pryor DB, Rendall DS, Stack RS, Hinohara T, Skelton TN, Califf RM, Hlatky MA, Mark DB. Exercise treadmill testing is a poor predictor of anatomic restenosis after angioplasty for acute myocardial infarction. *Circulation* 1989;80:1585–1594.

78. Scholl JM, Chaitman BR, David PR, Dupras G, Brevers G, Val PG, Crepeau J, Lesperance J, Bourassa MG. Exercise electrocardiography and myocardial scintigraphy in the serial evaluation of the results of percutaneous transluminal coronary angioplasty. *Circulation* 1982;66:380–390.

79. Wijns W, Serruys PW, Simoons ML, van den Brand M, De Feijter PJ, Reiber JHC, Hugenholtz PG. Predictive value of early maximal exercise test and thallium scintigraphy after successful percutaneous transluminal coronary angioplasty. *Br Heart J* 1985;53:194–200.

80. Miller DD, Liu P, Strauss HW, Block PC, Okada RD, Boucher CA. Prognostic value of computer-quantitated exercise thallium imaging early after percutaneous transluminal coronary angioplasty. *J Am Coll Cardiol* 1987;10:275–283.

81. Breisblatt WM, Weiland FL, Spaccavento LJ. Stress thallium-201 imaging after coronary angioplasty predicts restenosis and recurrent symptoms. *J Am Coll Cardiol* 1988;12:1199–1204.

82. Manyari DE, Knudtson M, Kloiber R, Roth D. Sequential thallium-201 myocardial perfusion studies after successful percutaneous transluminal coronary angioplasty: delayed resolution of exercise-induced scintigraphic abnormalities. *Circulation* 1988;77:86–95.

83. Stuckey TD, Burwell LR, Nygaard TW, Gibson RS, Watson DD, Beller GA. Quantitative exercise thallium-201 scintigraphy for predicting angina recurrence after percutaneous transluminal coronary angioplasty. *Am J Cardiol* 1989;63:517–521.

84. O'Keefe JH, Lapeyre AC, Holmes DR, Gibbons RJ. Usefulness of early radionuclide angiography for identifying low-risk patients for late restenosis after percutaneous transluminal coronary angioplasty. *Am J Cardiol* 1988;61:51–54.

85. DePuey EG, Leatherman LL, Leachman RD, Dear WE, Massin EK, Mathur VS, Burdine JA. Restenosis after transluminal coronary angioplasty detected with exercise-gated radionuclide ventriculography. *J Am Coll Cardiol* 1984;4:1103–1113.

86. Rosing DR, Van Raden MJ, Mincemoyer RM, Bonow RO, Bourassa MG, David PR, Ewels CJ, Detre KM, Kent KM. Exercise, electrocardiographic and functional responses after percutaneous transluminal coronary angioplasty. *Am J Cardiol* 1984;53:36C–41C.

87. Kramer PH, Beauchamp GD, Vacek JL, Rowland AJ, Crouse LJ. Exercise echocardiography predicts restenosis after coronary angioplasty. *Circulation* 1990;82[Suppl III]:192.

88. Schwartz L, Bourassa MG, Lesperance J, Aldridge HE, Kazim F, Salvatori VA, Henderson M, Bonan R, David PR. Aspirin and dipyridamole in the prevention of restenosis after percutaneous transluminal coronary angioplasty. *N Engl J Med* 1988;318:1714–1719.

89. Thornton MA, Gruentzig AR, Hollman J, King SB, Douglas Coumadin and aspirin in prevention of recurrence after transluminal coronary angioplasty: a randomized study. *Circulation* 1984;69:721–727.

90. White CW, Knudtson M, Schmidt RJ, Chisholm M, Vandormael M, Morton B, Roy L, Khaja F, Reitman M and the Triclopidine Study Group. Neither Ticlopidine nor aspirin-dipyridamole prevents restenosis post PTCA: results from a randomized placebo-controlled multicenter trial. *Circulation* 1987;76[Suppl IV]:213.

91. Finci L, Meier B, Steffenio G, Rutishauser W. Aspirin versus placebo after coronary angioplasty for prevention of restenosis. *Eur Heart J* 1988;9[Suppl 1]:156(abst).

92. Mufson L, Black A, Roubin G, Wilentz J, Mead S, McFarland K, Weintraub W, Douglas JS, King SB. A randomized trial of aspirin in PTCA: effect of high vs. low dose aspirin on major complications and restenosis. *J Am Coll Cardiol* 1988;[II Suppl A]:236A.

93. Schanzenbacher P, Grillmer M, Maish B, Kochsiek K. Effect of high dose and low dose aspirin on restenosis after primary successful angioplasty. *Circulation* 1988;78[Suppl II]:II-98(abst).

94. Dyckmans J, Thonnes W, Ozbek C, Muller M, Bach R, Schwerdt H, Sen S, Schieffer H, Bette L. High vs low dosage of acetylic salicylic acid for prevention of restenosis after successful PTCA. Preliminary results of a randomized trial. *Eur Heart J* 1988;9[Suppl 1]:5,3(abst).

95. Liu MW, Roubin GS, Robinson KA, et al. Trapidil in preventing restenosis after balloon angioplasty in the atherosclerotic rabbit. *Circulation* 1990;81:1089–1093.

96. Urban P, Buller N, Fo K, Shapiro L, Bayliss J, Rickards A. Lack of effect of warfarin on the restenosis rate or on clinical outcome after balloon coronary angioplasty. *Br Heart J* 1988;60:485–488.

97. Franklin SM, Currier JW, Cannistra A, Leitschuh M, Fiore L, Deykin D, Ryan TJ, Faxon DP. Warfarin/aspirin combination reduces restenosis after angioplasty in atherosclerotic rabbits. *Circulation* 1990;82[Suppl III]:427.

98. Clowes AW, Karnowsky MJ. Supression by heparin of smooth muscle cell proliferation in injured arteries. *Nature* 1977;265:625–626.

99. Currier JW, Pow TK, Haudenshild CC, Minihan AC, Faxon DP. Low molecular weight heparin (Enoxaparin) reduces restenosis after iliac angioplasty in the hypercholesterolemic rabbit. *J Am Coll Cardiol* 1991;17[Suppl B]:118B–125B.

100. Powell JS, Clozel JP, Muller RKM, Kuhn H, Hefti F, Hosang M, Baumgartner HR. Inhibitors of angiotensin-converting enzyme prevent myointimal proliferation after vascular injury. *Science* 1989;249:186–188.

101. Corcos T, David PR, Val PG, et al. Failure of diltiazem to prevent restenosis after percutaneous transluminal coronary angioplasty. *Am Heart J* 1985;109:926–931.

102. Whitworth HB, Roubin GX, Hollman J, et al. Effect of nifedipine on recurrent stenosis after percutaneous transluminal coronary angioplasty. *J Am Coll Cardiol* 1986;8:1271–1276.

103. Hoberg E, Schwarz F, Schomig A, et al. Prevention of restenosis by verapamil. The Verapamil Angioplasty Study (VAS). *Circulation* 1990;82[Suppl III]:428.

104. Gordon JB, Berk BC, Bettmann MA, Selwyn AP, Renke H, Alexander RW. Vascular smooth muscle cell proliferation following balloon injury is synergistically inhibited by low molecular weight heparin and hydrocortisone. *Circulation* 1987;76[Suppl IV]:213.

105. Pepine CJ, Hirshfeld JW, MacDonald RG, et al. M-HEART Group: a controlled trial of corticosteroids to prevent restenosis following coronary angioplasty. *Circulation* 1988;78[Suppl II]:291.

106. Rose TA, Beauchamg BG. Short term, high dose steroid treatment to prevent restenosis in PTCA. *Circulation* 1987;76[Suppl IV]:371.

107. Currier JW, Pow TK, Minihan AC, Haudenschild CC, Faxon DP, Ryan TJ. Colchicine inhibits restenosis after iliac angioplasty in the atherosclerotic rabbit. *Circulation* 1989;80[Suppl II]:66.

108. O'Keefe JG, McCallister BD, Bateman TM, Kuhnlein D, Ligon RW, Hartzler GO. Colchicine for the prevention of restenosis after coronary angioplasty. *J Am Coll Cardiol* 1991;17[Suppl A]:181A.

109. Lundergan CF, Foegh ML, Ramwell PW. Peptide inhibition of myointimal proliferation by angiopeptin: a somatosatin analogue. *J Am Coll Cardiol* 1991;17[Suppl B]:132B–136B.

110. Bresnahan JF, Litvack F, Margolis J, Rothbaum D, Kent K, Untereker W, Cummins F and the ELCA investigators. Eximer laser coronary angioplasty: initial results of a multicenter investigation in 958 patients. *J Am Coll Cardiol* 1991;17[Suppl A]:30A.

111. Spears JR, Reyes VP, Plokker HWT, et al (LBA Study Group). Laser balloon angioplasty: coronary angiographic follow-up of a multicenter trial. *J Am Coll Cardiol* 1990;15:26A.

112. U.S. Directional Coronary Atherectomy Investigator Group. Restenosis following directional coronary atherectomy in a multi-center experience. *Circulation* 1990;82[Suppl III]:679.

113. Schatz RA, Goldberg S, Leon M, Main D, Hirshfeld J, Cleman M, Ellis S, Topol E. Clinical experience with the Palmaz-Schatz coronary stent. *J Am Coll Cardiol* 1991;17[Suppl B]:155B–159B.

114. Williams DO, Gruentzig AR, Kent KM, Detre KM, Kelsey SF, To T. Efficacy of repeat percutaneous transluminal coronary angioplasty for coronary restenosis. *Am J Cardiol* 1984;53:32C–35C.

115. Vallbracht C, Kober G, Klepzig H, Kaltenbach M. Recurrent restenosis after transluminal coronary angioplasty dilatiation or surgery? *Eur Heart J* 1988;9[Suppl C]:7–10.

116. Teirstein PS, Hoover CA, Ligon RW, Giorgi LV, Rutherford BD, McConahay DR, Johnson WL, Hartzler GO. Repeat coronary angioplasty: efficacy of a third angioplasty for a second restenosis. *J Am Coll Cardiol* 1989;13:291–296.

117. Glazier JJ, Varricchione TR, Ryan TJ, Ruocco NA, Jacobs AK, Faxon DP. Outcome in patients with recurrent restenosis after percutaneous transluminal balloon angioplasty. *Br Heart J* 1989;61:485–488.

118. Glazier JJ, Varricchione TR, Ryan TJ, Ruocco NA, Jacobs AK, Faxon DP. Factors predicting recurrent restenosis after percutane-ous transluminal coronary balloon angioplasty. *Am J Cardiol* 1989;63:902–905.

119. Black AJR, Anderson V, Roubin GS, Powelson SW, Douglas JS, King SB. Repeat coronary angioplasty: correlates of a second re-stenosis. *J Am Coll Cardiol* 1988;11:714–718.

120. Quigley PJ, Hlatky MA, Hinohara T, Rendall DS, Perez JA, Phil-lips HR, Califf RM, Stack RS. Repeat percutaneous transluminal coronary angioplasty and predictors of recurrent restenosis. *Am J Cardiol* 1989;63:409–413.

121. Brush JE, Erario M, McGovern W, Jacobs AK, Faxon DP, Ryan TJ. Economic consequences of restenosis: a model to compare relative costs of revascularization strategies. *J Am Coll Cardiol* 1990;15:59A.

Subject Index